2013
YEAR BOOK OF
ENDOCRINOLOGY®

The 2013 Year Book Series

Year Book of Critical Care Medicine®: Drs Dries, Zanotti-Cavazzoni, Latenser, Martinez, Rincon, and Zwank

Year Book of Emergency Medicine®: Drs Hamilton, Bruno, Handly, Minczak, Quintana, and Ramoska

Year Book of Endocrinology®: Drs Schott, Apovian, Clarke, Eugster, Meikle, Oetgen, Ovalle, Schteingart, and Toth

Year Book of Hand and Upper Limb Surgery®: Drs Yao, Adams, Isaacs, and Rizzo

Year Book of Medicine®: Drs Barker, Garrick, Gersh, Khardori, LeRoith, Panush, Talley, and Thigpen

Year Book of Neonatal and Perinatal Medicine®: Drs Fanaroff, Benitz, Donn, Neu, Papile, and Van Marter

Year Book of Neurology and Neurosurgery®: Drs Klimo, Minagar, Gandhi, Liu, Panagariya, Rezania, Riel-Romero, Riesenburger, Robottom, Schwendimann, Shafazand, and Yang

Year Book of Obstetrics, Gynecology, and Women's Health®: Drs Dungan and Shulman

Year Book of Oncology®: Drs Arceci, Bauer, Chiorean, Gordon, Lawton, Murphy, Thigpen, and Tsao

Year Book of Ophthalmology®: Drs Rapuano, Cohen, Flanders, Hammersmith, Milman, Myers, Nagra, Nelson, Penne, Pyfer, Sergott, Shields, Talekar, and Vander

Year Book of Orthopedics®: Drs Morrey, Huddleston, Rose, Swiontkowski, and Trigg

Year Book of Otolaryngology-Head and Neck Surgery®: Drs Sindwani, Balough, Franco, Gapany, and Mitchell

Year Book of Pathology and Laboratory Medicine®: Drs Raab and Bissell

Year Book of Pediatrics®: Dr Stockman

Year Book of Plastic and Aesthetic Surgery™: Drs Miller, Boehmler, Gosman, Gutowski, Ruberg, Salisbury, and Smith

Year Book of Psychiatry and Applied Mental Health®: Drs Talbott, Ballenger, Buckley, Frances, Krupnick, and Mack

Year Book of Pulmonary Disease®: Drs Barker, Jones, Maurer, Spradley, Tanoue, and Willsie

Year Book of Sports Medicine®: Drs Shephard, Cantu, Feldman, Galea, Jankowski, Janssen, Lebrun, and Nieman

Year Book of Surgery®: Drs Behrns, Daly, Fahey, Hines, Howe, Huber, Klodell, Mozingo, and Pruett

Year Book of Urology®: Drs Andriole and Coplen

Year Book of Vascular Surgery®: Drs Gillespie, Bush, Passman, Starnes, and Watkins

2013

The Year Book of ENDOCRINOLOGY®

Editor-in-Chief
Matthias Schott, MD, PhD
Associate Professor, Deputy Director of the Department of Endocrinology, Diabetology and Rheumatology, University Hospital of Düsseldorf, Düsseldorf, Germany

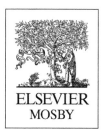

ELSEVIER
MOSBY

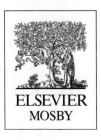

ELSEVIER
MOSBY

Vice President, Continuity: Kimberly Murphy
Developmental Editor: Patrick Manley
Production Supervisor, Electronic Year Books: Donna M. Skelton
Electronic Article Manager: Mike Rainey
Senior Illustrations and Permissions Coordinator: Dawn Vohsen

Composition by TNQ Books and Journals Pvt Ltd, India

Editorial Office:
Elsevier
Suite 1800
1600 John F. Kennedy Blvd
Philadelphia, PA 19103-2899

International Standard Serial Number: 0084-3741
International Standard Book Number: 978-1-4557-7275-9

Printed and bound by CPI Group (UK) Ltd, Croydon, CR0 4YY

Transferred to digital print 2012

Associate Editors

Caroline M. Apovian, MD, FACP, FACN
Associate Professor of Medicine and Pediatrics, Boston University School of Medicine; Director, Center for Nutrition and Weight Management, Boston Medical Center, Boston, Massachusetts

Bart L. Clarke, MD
Associate Professor of Medicine, Mayo Clinic College of Medicine; Consultant, St. Mary's Hospital; Consultant, Rochester Methodist Hospital, Rochester, Minnesota

Erica Eugster, MD
Professor of Pediatrics, Director, Section of Pediatric Endocrinology/ Diabetology, Riley Hospital for Children, Indiana University School of Medicine, Indianapolis, Indiana

A. Wayne Meikle, MD
Professor of Medicine and Pathology, University of Utah School of Medicine; Director of Endocrine Testing, ARUP Laboratories, The University of Utah Hospitals, Salt Lake City, Utah

Elke Oetjen
Professor, Institute of Clinical Pharmacology and Toxicology, University Medical Center Hamburg-Eppendorf, Hamburg, Germany

Peter P. Toth, MD, PhD, FAAFP, FICA, FAHA, FCCP, FACC
Director of Preventive Cardiology, Sterling Rock Falls Clinic, Ltd; Clinical Professor, University of Illinois College of Medicine, Peoria, Illinois

Holger S. Willenberg, MD
Deparment of Endocrinology, Diabetes and Metabolism, University of Duesseldorf, Duesseldorf, Germany

Contributing Editors

Rosane Ness-Abramof, MD
Meir Hospital, Kfar Saba, Israel, and Sackler School of Medicine, Tel Aviv, Israel

Juliana Simonetti, MD
Instructor in Medicine, Division of Endocrinology, Nutrition and Weight Management, Boston University Medical School, Boston, Massachusetts

Table of Contents

JOURNALS REPRESENTED xi

INTRODUCTION xiii

1. Diabetes 1
   Introduction 1
   Complications 1
   Glycemic Control 9
   Pathogenesis 12
   Prevention and Reversal of Diabetes 20
2. Lipoproteins and Atherosclerosis 29
   Introduction 29
   Epidemiology and Diagnosis 30
   Metabolic Syndrome 32
   Nutrition and Nutritional Supplements 34
   Pharmacologic Therapy 36
   Prevention of Atherosclerosis 64
   Stroke and Peripheral Artery Disease 71
3. Obesity 75
   Introduction 75
   Diet and Obesity 76
   Epidemiology and Complications of Obesity 84
   New Developments in Obesity 98
   Surgical Treatment of Obesity 101
4. Thyroid 105
   Introduction 105
   Autoimmunity 106
   Thyroid Cancer 113
   Thyroid Disease in Pregnancy 122
   Thyroid Nodules 125
   Miscellaneous 127

5. Calcium and Bone Metabolism 147

    Introduction 147

    Mineral and Vitamin D Metabolism 152

    Epidemiology and Pathophysiology of Osteoporosis 164

    Current Issues in Osteoporosis Therapy................ 173

    Novel Osteoporosis Therapies 191

    Metabolic Bone Disease 202

    Miscellaneous.................................... 206

6. Adrenal Cortex 209

    Adrenal Hormone Secretion and Pathology 209

    Cushing's Disease: Diagnosis and Treatment 217

    Primary Aldosteronism............................. 218

7. Reproductive Endocrinology......................... 225

    Introduction 225

    Bone Health in Men............................... 227

    Female Reproductive Function....................... 230

    Male Reproductive Function 236

    Polycystic Ovary Syndrome 244

    Metabolic Syndrome 257

    Hypogonadism and Aging 259

8. Neuroendocrinology............................... 263

    ACTH 263

    General 264

    Pituitary—General 265

    Prolactin.. 266

9. Pediatric Endocrinology 269

    Introduction 269

    Growth/Growth Hormone.......................... 270

    Miscellaneous.................................... 276

    ARTICLE INDEX 289

    AUTHOR INDEX 297

Journals Represented

Journals represented in this YEAR BOOK are listed below.
American Journal of Cardiology
American Journal of Clinical Nutrition
American Journal of Clinical Oncology
American Journal of Orthodontics and Dentofacial Orthopedics
Annals of Internal Medicine
Archives of Disease in Childhood
Archives of Internal Medicine
British Journal of Urology International
British Medical Journal
Calcified Tissue International
Cancer Research
Circulation
Clinical Cancer Research
Clinical Endocrinology
Clinical Pharmacology & Therapeutics
Clinical Radiology
Developmental Cell
Diabetes
Diabetes Care
Diabetologia
Endocrinology
European Journal of Endocrinology
European Molecular Biology Organization Journal
Fertility and Sterility
Heart
Human Reproduction
Hypertension
International Journal of Cardiology
International Journal of Obesity
JAMA Internal Medicine
Journal of Bone and Joint Surgery (American)
Journal of Bone Mineral Research
Journal of Clinical Endocrinology & Metabolism
Journal of Clinical Investigation
Journal of Clinical Oncology
Journal of Hypertension
Journal of Neurological Sciences
Journal of Pediatrics
Journal of Pharmacology and Experimental Therapeutics
Journal of the American College of Cardiology
Journal of the American Medical Association
Lancet
Maturitas
Medicine and Science in Sports and Exercise
Metabolism
Nature
Nature Genetics

New England Journal of Medicine
Osteoporosis International
Pediatrics
Proceedings of the National Academy of Sciences of the United States of America

---

STANDARD ABBREVIATIONS

The following terms are abbreviated in this edition: adrenocorticotropin hormone (ACTH); acquired immunodeficiency syndrome (AIDS); cardiopulmonary resuscitation (CPR); central nervous system (CNS); cerebrospinal fluid (CSF); computed tomography (CT); corticotropin-releasing hormone (CRH); deoxyribonucleic acid (DNA); electrocardiography (ECG); follicle-stimulating hormone (FSH); gonadotropin-releasing hormone (GnRH); growth hormone (GH); health maintenance organization (HMO); high-density lipoprotein (HDL); human immunodeficiency virus (HIV); insulin-dependent diabetes mellitus (IDDM); insulin-like growth factor I (IGF-I); intensive care unit (ICU); intermediate-density lipoprotein (IDL); intramuscular (IM); intravenous (IV); low-density lipoprotein (LDL); luteinizing hormone (LH); magnetic resonance (MR) imaging (MRI); multiple endocrine neoplasia (MEN); non-insulin-dependent diabetes mellitus (NIDDM); parathyroid hormone (PTH); prolactin (PRL); releasing hormone (RH); ribonucleic acid (RNA); thyrotropin-releasing hormone (TRH); thyroid-stimulating hormone or thyrotropin (TSH); thyroxine (T_4); triiodothyronine (T_3); ultrasound (US); and very-low-density lipoprotein (VLDL).

NOTE

The YEAR BOOK OF ENDOCRINOLOGY is a literature survey service providing abstracts of articles published in the professional literature. Every effort is made to assure the accuracy of the information presented in these pages. Neither the editor nor the publisher of the YEAR BOOK OF ENDOCRINOLOGY can be responsible for errors in the original materials. The editors' comments are their own opinions. Mention of specific products within this publication does not constitute endorsement.

To facilitate the use of the YEAR BOOK OF ENDOCRINOLOGY as a reference tool, all illustrations and tables included in this publication are now identified as they appear in the original article. This change is meant to help the reader recognize that any illustration or table appearing in the YEAR BOOK OF ENDOCRINOLOGY may be only one of many in the original article. For this reason, figure and table numbers appear to be out of sequence within the YEAR BOOK OF ENDOCRINOLOGY.

Introduction

Within the last year, the world community of endocrinologists and endocrine researchers produced an abundant crop of important publications. Just to give you an idea, by performing a PubMed search for the keyword "thyroid," 6314 articles show up; the keywords "diabetes mellitus" turn up 18 742 articles. As the number and, most importantly, the quality of publications increase each year, the section editors in the YEAR BOOK OF ENDOCRINOLGY have the daunting task of reviewing a large number of articles in each field. Of course, there is a high probability that I and the other coeditors have failed to mention important research that will prove to be of high importance in the future. On the other hand, this probability is minimalized by *Elsevier Science's* preselection process. This helps the editors to evaluate each research article and pick up the most important articles in the field. Out of the selected articles, this year's Editor's Choice is the article by Antonica et al entitled, Generation of Functional Thyroid from Embryonic Stem Cells and published in the journal *Nature*.

The aim of this study was to generate thyroid follicular cells (TFCs) generated from murine embryonic stem cells (ESCs). The authors overexpressed two transcription factors (NKX2-1 and PAX8) which led to the generation of TFCs and subsequently to the self-formation of thyroid follicles. The authors could demonstrate that ESC-derived thyroid cells show full morphological and functional maturation and that these cells are able to form thyroid follicles in mice (under the kidney capsula, where cells were injected). Importantly, the generated thyroid worked under the control of thyroid-stimulating hormone (secreted by the pituitary gland) resulting in an increase of T4 and a rise in body temperature (in comparison to hypothyroid mice without transplantation). In my eyes, this is certainly one of the most important studies published in the thyroid field in the last couple of years. The authors clearly demonstrated the generation of a completely functional thyroid from ESCs. Based on that protocol, functional thyroids might be generated sometimes in the future for patients with dysfunctional or dysplastic thyroids. In addition, similar protocols with other transcription factors might be used in the future to generate other functional organ cells.

Matthias Schott, MD, PhD

1   Diabetes

Introduction

In the aftermath of the ACCORD and the ADVANCE studies, many discussions have arisen as to what targets to choose to ensure a good glycemic control to minimize cardiovascular complications without the danger of hypoglycemia and associated risks. In 2012, the American Diabetes Association and the European Foundation for the Study of Diabetes joined forces and recommended a more patient-centered approach for the management of hyperglycemia in type 2 diabetes. Despite the variety of antidiabetic drugs, the search is still on for new drugs. As such, the agonist of the G protein-coupled receptor 40/Free fatty acid receptor 1 TAK-875 has entered the stage. TAK-875 acts directly on the β cell by increasing glucose-stimulated insulin secretion. Other drug candidates might be the amorfrutins as selective PPARgamma modulators or inhibitors of the vascular endothelial growth factor-B (VEGF-B) action, both having in common the ability to enhance insulin sensitivity. Interfering with glucagon action as a suitable drug target is often neglected. Two studies in mice and a thorough review on glucagon action emphasized that diabetes should be considered a bihormonal disease. Using newer methods like DNA methylation profiling and the study of gut microbiota might help to further our understanding of type 2 diabetes and even reveal new drug targets. Obesity is considered a major risk factor for the development of type 2 diabetes. Two studies seem to contradict this dogma. Further studies are needed to determine whether indeed weight loss in diabetic patients is associated with higher mortality.

Elke Oetjen, MD

Complications

Basal Insulin and Cardiovascular and Other Outcomes in Dysglycemia

The ORIGIN Trial Investigators (McMaster Univ and Hamilton Health Sciences, Ontario, Canada; Institut Universitaire de Cardiologie et de Pneumologie de Québec, Canada; et al)
N Engl J Med 367:319-328, 2012

Background.—The provision of sufficient basal insulin to normalize fasting plasma glucose levels may reduce cardiovascular events, but such a possibility has not been formally tested.

Methods.—We randomly assigned 12,537 people (mean age, 63.5 years) with cardiovascular risk factors plus impaired fasting glucose, impaired glucose tolerance, or type 2 diabetes to receive insulin glargine (with a target fasting blood glucose level of ≤ 95 mg per deciliter [5.3 mmol per liter]) or standard care and to receive n−3 fatty acids or placebo with the use of a 2-by-2 factorial design. The results of the comparison between insulin glargine and standard care are reported here. The coprimary outcomes were nonfatal myocardial infarction, nonfatal stroke, or death from cardiovascular causes and these events plus revascularization or hospitalization for heart failure. Microvascular outcomes, incident diabetes, hypoglycemia, weight, and cancers were also compared between groups.

Results.—The median follow-up was 6.2 years (interquartile range, 5.8 to 6.7). Rates of incident cardiovascular outcomes were similar in the insulin-glargine and standard-care groups: 2.94 and 2.85 per 100 person-years, respectively, for the first coprimary outcome (hazard ratio, 1.02; 95% confidence interval [CI], 0.94 to 1.11; $P = 0.63$) and 5.52 and 5.28 per 100 person-years, respectively, for the second coprimary outcome (hazard ratio, 1.04; 95% CI, 0.97 to 1.11; $P = 0.27$). New diabetes was diagnosed approximately 3 months after therapy was stopped among 30% versus 35% of 1456 participants without baseline diabetes (odds ratio, 0.80; 95% CI, 0.64 to 1.00; $P = 0.05$). Rates of severe hypoglycemia were 1.00 versus 0.31 per 100 person-years. Median weight increased by 1.6 kg in the insulin-glargine group and fell by 0.5 kg in the standard-care group. There was no significant difference in cancers (hazard ratio, 1.00; 95% CI, 0.88 to 1.13; $P = 0.97$).

Conclusions.—When used to target normal fasting plasma glucose levels for more than 6 years, insulin glargine had a neutral effect on cardiovascular outcomes and cancers. Although it reduced new-onset diabetes, insulin glargine also increased hypoglycemia and modestly increased weight. (Funded by Sanofi; ORIGIN ClinicalTrials.gov number, NCT00069784.)

▶ Besides lowering blood glucose levels, insulin has many effects. Evidence suggests that insulin, and especially the long-acting insulin glargine, might induce cancer. In addition, insulin in a dose to normalize fasting plasma glucose levels might reduce cardiovascular events. However, hypoglycemia as an adverse effect of too intensive glucose-lowering therapy negatively influences cardiovascular events. In this study, insulin glargine had no effect on cardiovascular outcome and on cancer induction. As could be expected, insulin glargine induced moderate weight gain. In addition, new-onset diabetes was reduced. This might be explained by insulin's beta-cell protective effect. Thus, the anxiety of insulin glargine—induced cancer is relieved, but this study does not warrant the preventive administration of insulin glargine to impede cardiovascular events. It should be noted that 47% of the participants receiving insulin glargine received metformin as well. Considering the protective effect metformin has on the macrovascular system, any insulin-induced effect might have been mitigated.

E. Oetjen, MD

Association of Weight Status With Mortality in Adults With Incident Diabetes

Carnethon MR, De Chavez PJD, Biggs ML, et al (Northwestern Univ, Chicago, IL; Univ of Washington, Seattle; et al)
JAMA 308:581-590, 2012

Context.—Type 2 diabetes in normal-weight adults (body mass index [BMI] <25) is a representation of the metabolically obese normal-weight phenotype with unknown mortality consequences.

Objective.—To test the association of weight status with mortality in adults with new onset diabetes in order to minimize the influence of diabetes duration and voluntary weight loss on mortality.

Design, Setting, and Participants.—Pooled analysis of 5 longitudinal cohort studies: Atherosclerosis Risk in Communities study, 1990-2006; Cardiovascular Health Study, 1992-2008; Coronary Artery Risk Development in Young Adults, 1987-2011; Framingham Offspring Study, 1979-2007; and Multi-Ethnic Study of Atherosclerosis, 2002-2011. A total of 2625 participants with incident diabetes contributed 27 125 person-years of follow-up. Included were men and women (age > 40 years) who developed incident diabetes based on fasting glucose 126 mg/dL or greater or newly initiated diabetes medication and who had concurrent measurements of BMI. Participants were classified as normal weight if their BMI was 18.5 to 24.99 or overweight/obese if BMI was 25 or greater.

Main Outcome Measures.—Total, cardiovascular, and noncardiovascular mortality.

Results.—The proportion of adults who were normal weight at the time of incident diabetes ranged from 9% to 21% (overall 12%). During follow-up, 449 participants died: 178 from cardiovascular causes and 253 from noncardiovascular causes (18 were not classified). The rates of total, cardiovascular, and noncardiovascular mortality were higher in normal-weight participants (284.8, 99.8, and 198.1 per 10 000 person-years, respectively) than in overweight/obese participants (152.1, 67.8, and 87.9 per 10 000 person-years, respectively). After adjustment for demographic characteristics and blood pressure, lipid levels, waist circumference, and smoking status, hazard ratios comparing normal-weight participants with overweight/obese participants for total, cardiovascular, and noncardiovascular mortality were 2.08 (95% CI, 1.52-2.85), 1.52 (95% CI, 0.89-2.58), and 2.32 (95% CI, 1.55-3.48), respectively.

Conclusion.—Adults who were normal weight at the time of incident diabetes had higher mortality than adults who are overweight or obese.

▶ Obesity is considered a major risk factor for the development of type 2 diabetes. An obesity paradox has been observed for many chronic diseases, implying that weight loss might result in higher mortality. In this meta-analysis of 5 longitudinal cohort studies, total cardiovascular and noncardiovascular mortality of normal-weight and overweight/obese participants with incident diabetes (defined as fasting glucose ≥126 mg/dL) were compared. Weight was defined by body mass index. Participants who were normal weight at the time of incident diabetes had a higher total and noncardiovascular mortality than over-weight or obese patients. There was no difference in cardiovascular mortality. Although this is an interesting analysis, information about insulin sensitivity and fat mass distribution are lacking. In addition, the type of diabetes was not further investigated (ie, latent autoimmune diabetes in adults). Hence, the obesity paradox might hold true for diabetes, but this analysis cannot provide sufficient evidence.

E. Oetjen, MD

Altered MAPK Signaling in Progressive Deterioration of Endothelial Function in Diabetic Mice

Huang A, Yang Y-M, Yan C, et al (New York Med College, Valhalla; Xuzhou Med College, China)
Diabetes 61:3181-3188, 2012

We aimed to investigate specific roles of mitogen-activated protein kinases (MAPK) in the deterioration of endothelial function during the progression of diabetes and the potential therapeutic effects of MAPK inhibitors and agonists in the amelioration of endothelial function. Protein expression and phosphorylation of p38, c-Jun NH_2-terminal kinase (JNK), and extra-cellular signal—regulated kinase (Erk) were assessed in mesenteric arteries of 3- (3M) and 9-month-old (9M) male diabetic and control mice. The expression of p38, JNK, and Erk was comparable in all groups of mice, but the phosphorylation of p38 and JNK was increased in 3M and further increased in 9M diabetic mice, whereas the phosphorylation of Erk was substantially reduced in 9M diabetic mice. NADPH oxidase—dependent superoxide production was significantly increased in vessels of two ages of diabetic mice. Inhibition of either p38 with SB203580 or JNK with SP600125 reduced superoxide production and improved shear stress—induced dilation (SSID) in 3M, but not in 9M, diabetic mice. Treating the vessels of 9M diabetic mice with resveratrol increased Erk phosphorylation and shear stress—induced endothelial nitric oxide synthase (eNOS) phos-phorylation and activity, but resveratrol alone did not improve SSID. Administration of resveratrol and SB203580 or resveratrol and SP600125 together significantly improved SSID in vessels of 9M diabetic mice. The improved response was prevented by U0126, an Erk inhibitor. Thus, p38/JNK-dependent increase in oxidative stress diminished nitric oxide—mediated dilation in vessels of 3M diabetic mice. Oxidative stress and impaired Erk-dependent activation of eNOS exacerbates endothelial dysfunction in the advanced stage of diabetes.

▶ Endothelial dysfunction caused by increased oxidative stress with impaired endothelial nitric oxide synthase (eNOS) activation is associated with diabetes and contributes to cardiovascular diseases. In this study, the role of 3 mitogen-activated protein kinases (extracellular signal—regulated kinase [Erk], c-Jun

NH$_2$-terminal kinase [JNK], and p38) in the development of endothelial dysfunction was investigated in diabetic mice (*db/db* mice). In mesenteric arteries of 3- and 9-month-old *db/db* mice, JNK and p38 activation were increased as well as NADPH oxidase-dependent superoxide production, whereas Erk activity was reduced in 9-month-old mice. Inhibition of either JNK or p38 reduced superoxide production and improved sheer stress—induced dilation in 3-month-old mice. A combination of resveratrol to enhance Erk activation with either a JNK or p38 inhibitor was required to improve eNOS activity and sheer stress—induced dilation in 9-month-old diabetic mice. In this study, diabetes interferes with endothelial function by distinct mechanisms depending on its duration. Because this study was performed in *db/db* mice, the effect of hyperleptinemia cannot be excluded.

E. Oetjen, MD

Association Between Coronary Vascular Dysfunction and Cardiac Mortality in Patients With and Without Diabetes Mellitus
Murthy VL, Naya M, Foster CR, et al (Brigham and Women's Hosp, Boston, MA)
Circulation 126:1858-1868, 2012

Background.—Diabetes mellitus increases the risk of adverse cardiac outcomes and is considered a coronary artery disease (CAD) equivalent. We examined whether coronary vascular dysfunction, an early manifestation of CAD, accounts for increased risk among diabetics compared with nondiabetics.

Methods and Results.—A total of 2783 consecutive patients (1172 diabetics and 1611 nondiabetics) underwent quantification of coronary flow reserve (CFR; CFR = stress divided by rest myocardial blood flow) by positron emission tomography and were followed up for a median of 1.4 years (quartile 1—3, 0.7—3.2 years). The primary end point was cardiac death. Impaired CFR (below the median) was associated with an adjusted 3.2- and 4.9-fold increase in the rate of cardiac death for diabetics and nondiabetics, respectively ($P = 0.0004$). Addition of CFR to clinical and imaging risk models improved risk discrimination for both diabetics and nondiabetics (c index, 0.77—0.79, $P = 0.04$; 0.82—0.85, $P = 0.03$, respectively). Diabetic patients without known CAD with impaired CFR experienced a rate of cardiac death comparable to that for nondiabetic patients with known CAD (2.8%/y versus 2.0%/y; $P = 0.33$). Conversely, diabetics without known CAD and preserved CFR had very low annualized cardiac mortality, which was similar to patients without known CAD or diabetes mellitus and normal stress perfusion and systolic function (0.3%/y versus 0.5%/y; $P = 0.65$).

Conclusions.—Coronary vasodilator dysfunction is a powerful, independent correlate of cardiac mortality among both diabetics and nondiabetics and provides meaningful incremental risk stratification. Among diabetic patients without CAD, those with impaired CFR have event rates comparable to those of patients with prior CAD, whereas those with preserved CFR have event rates comparable to those of nondiabetics.

▶ Diabetes increases cardiovascular risk and is itself considered a coronary artery disease (CAD) equivalent. An early manifestation of CAD is coronary vascular dysfunction. In this single-center, nonrandomized, observational study, coronary flow reserve (CFR) as a measure of coronary vascular dysfunction was quantified by positron emission tomography and correlated with the primary endpoint (cardiac death). The follow-up was a median of 1.4 years. Diabetic patients without known CAD with impaired CFR experienced a rate of cardiac death comparable to that of nondiabetic patients with known CAD. The annualized cardiac mortality of diabetics without known CAD and preserved CFR was similar to that of patients without known CAD or diabetes and normal stress perfusion and systolic function. This analysis suggests that measurement of CFR, especially in diabetics, provides a good estimation for cardiovascular risk assessment. In addition, it emphasizes the importance of preventing vascular dysfunction in diabetic patients.

E. Oetjen, MD

Inverse relation of body weight and weight change with mortality and morbidity in patients with type 2 diabetes and cardiovascular co-morbidity: An analysis of the PROactive study population
Doehner W, Erdmann E, Cairns R, et al (Ctr for Stroke Res Berlin, Charité, Germany; Univ Cologne, Germany; Clinical Trials Centre, Nottingham, UK; et al)
Int J Cardiol 162:20-26, 2012

Context.—Although weight reduction is a recommended goal in type 2 diabetes mellitus (T2DM), weight loss is linked to impaired survival in patients with some chronic cardiovascular diseases.

Objective.—To assess the association of weight and weight change with mortality and non-fatal cardiovascular outcomes (hospitalisation, myocardial infarction and stroke) in T2DM patients with cardiovascular co-morbidity and the effect of pioglitazone-induced weight change on mortality.

Setting and Participants.—We assessed in a post hoc analysis body weight and weight change in relation to outcome in 5202 patients from the PROactive trial population who had T2DM and evidence of pre-existing cardiovascular disease. Patients were randomized to treatment with pioglitazone or placebo in addition to their concomitant glucose-lowering and cardiovascular medication. Mean follow up was 34.5 months.

Main Outcome Measure.—The impact of body weight and body weight change on all-cause mortality, cardiovascular mortality, on non-fatal cardiovascular events and on hospitalisation.

Results.—The lowest mortality was seen in patients with BMI 30–35 kg/m^2 at baseline. In comparison to this (reference group), patients in the placebo group with BMI <22 kg/m^2 (Hazard Ratio (95% confidence intervals) 2.96 [1.27 to 6.86]; $P = 0.012$) and BMI 22 to 25 kg/m^2 (HR

1.88 [1.11 to 3.21]; $P = 0.019$) had a higher all-cause mortality. Weight loss was associated with increased total mortality (HR per 1% body weight: 1.13 [1.11 to 1.16]; $P < 0.0001$), with increased cardiovascular mortality, all-cause hospitalisation and the composite of death, myocardial infarction and stroke. Weight loss of ≥7.5% body weight (seen in 18.3% of patients) was the strongest cut-point to predict impaired survival (multivariable adjusted HR 4.42 [3.30 to 5.94]. Weight gain was not associated with increased mortality. Weight gain in patients treated with pioglitazone (mean + 4.0 ± 6.1 kg) predicted a better prognosis (HR per 1% weight gain: 0.96 [0.92 to 1.00] $P = 0.037$) compared to patients without weight gain.

Conclusion.—Among patients with T2DM and cardiovascular comorbidity, overweight and obese patients had a lower mortality compared to patients with normal weight. Weight loss but not weight gain was associated with increased mortality and morbidity. There may be an "obesity paradox" in patients with type 2 diabetes and cardiovascular risk.

The original PROactive trial is registered as an International Standard Randomized Controlled Trial (Number ISRCTN NCT00174993).

▶ One goal in the treatment of type 2 diabetes is weight reduction, but weight loss has been linked to impaired survival in patients with certain cardiovascular diseases. In this post hoc analysis, the association of body weight and weight change with mortality and nonfatal cardiovascular events (hospitalization, myocardial infarction, stroke) was studied in type 2 diabetic patients with cardiovascular comorbidity from the PROactive trial population. The mean follow-up was 34.5 months. Overweight and obese patients with type 2 diabetes and cardiovascular comorbidity had lower mortality rates compared with normal-weight patients. Weight loss was associated with increased mortality and morbidity. The identification of obesity as an independent risk factor for the development of cardiovascular diseases points to a beneficial effect of weight reduction in primary prevention, which might become overridden once diabetes and cardiovascular diseases are established.

E. Oetjen, MD

Relationship between HbA$_{1c}$ levels and risk of cardiovascular adverse outcomes and all-cause mortality in overweight and obese cardiovascular high-risk women and men with type 2 diabetes

Andersson C, van Gaal L, Caterson ID, et al (Gentofte Univ Hosp of Copenhagen, Hellerup, Denmark; Antwerp Univ Hosp, Belgium; Univ of Sydney, Victoria, Australia; et al)
Diabetologia 55:2348-2355, 2012

Aims/Hypothesis.—The optimal HbA$_{1c}$ concentration for prevention of macrovascular complications and deaths in obese cardiovascular high-risk patients with type 2 diabetes remains to be established and was therefore studied in this post hoc analysis of the Sibutramine Cardiovascular

OUTcomes (SCOUT) trial, which enrolled overweight and obese patients with type 2 diabetes and/or cardiovascular disease.

Methods.—HRs for meeting the primary endpoint (nonfatal myocardial infarction, nonfatal stroke, resuscitated cardiac arrest or cardiovascular death) and all-cause mortality were analysed using Cox regression models.

Results.—Of 8,252 patients with type 2 diabetes included in SCOUT, 7,479 had measurements of HbA_{1c} available at baseline (i.e. study random-isation). Median age was 62 years (range 51–86 years), median BMI was 34.0 kg/m^2 (24.8–65.1 kg/m^2) and 44% were women. The median HbA_{1c} concentration was 7.2% (3.8–15.9%) (55 mmol/l [18–150 mmol/l]) and median diabetes duration was 7 years (0–57 years). For each 1 percentage point HbA_{1c} increase, the adjusted HR for the primary endpoint was 1.17 (95% CI 1.11, 1.23); no differential sex effect was observed ($p = 0.12$ for interaction). In contrast, the risk of all-cause mortality was found to be greater in women than in men: HR 1.22 (1.10, 1.34) vs 1.12 (1.04, 1.20) for each 1 percentage point HbA_{1c} increase ($p = 0.02$ for interaction). There was no evidence of increased risk associated with $HbA_{1c} \leq 6.4\%$ (≤ 46 mmol/l). Glucose-lowering treatment regimens, diabetes duration or a history of cardiovascular disease did not modify the associations.

Conclusions/Interpretation.—In overweight, cardiovascular high-risk patients with type 2 diabetes, increasing HbA_{1c} concentrations were associated with increasing risks of cardiovascular adverse outcomes and all-cause mortality.

▶ Macrovascular complications are the main, potentially lethal consequences of diabetes. In a post-hoc analysis of the Sibutramine Cardiovascular OUTcomes trial (a weight-loss trial), the optimal HbA_{1c} concentration to prevent macrovascular complications and deaths in obese patients with type 2 diabetes and high cardiovascular risk was evaluated. Median age was 62 years, with a median body mass index of 34 kg/m^2, median HbA_{1c} of 7.2%, and median diabetes duration of 7 years. The adjusted hazard ratio of the primary endpoint (nonfatal myocardial infarction, nonfatal stroke, resuscitated cardiac arrest, cardiovascular death) was 1.17 for each 1 percentage point increase in HbA_{1c}, independent of sex. Risk of all-cause mortality was higher in women than in men. Importantly, no increased risk was associated with $HbA_{1c} \leq 6.4\%$. In this analysis, glucose-lowering treatments, diabetes duration, or a history of cardiovascular events did not modify the associations. Limitations are the lack of data on hypoglycemic events.

E. Oetjen, MD

Glycemic Control

Management of hyperglycaemia in type 2 diabetes: a patient-centered approach. Position statement of the American Diabetes Association (ADA) and the European Association for the Study of Diabetes (EASD)
Inzucchi SE, Bergenstal RM, Buse JB, et al (Yale Univ School of Medicine and Yale-New Haven Hosp, CT; International Diabetes Ctr at Park Nicollet, Minneapolis, MN; Univ of North Carolina School of Medicine, Chapel Hill; et al)
Diabetologia 55:1577-1596, 2012

Background.—Glycemic management in patients with type 2 diabetes mellitus is growing more complex and somewhat more controversial. More pharmacologic approaches are available, but come with concern about potential adverse effects and a lack of information about the benefits of intensive control methods on macrovascular complications. The American Diabetes Association (ADA) and the European Association for the Study of Diabetes (EASD) produced recommendations for anti-hyperglycemic therapy in non-pregnant adults with type 2 diabetes. An update was developed in light of contemporary information on the benefits and risks associated with glycemic control, the availability of evidence on the efficacy and safety of new drug classes, the removal or restriction of older agents, and the increased focus on patient-centered care.

Patient-Centered Considerations.—Patient-centered care is an approach focused on providing care that respects the patient's preferences, needs, and values; responds accordingly; and ensures that clinical decisions are guided by patient values. During clinical encounters, clinicians gauge the patient's preferred level of involvement, explore treatment choices, and engage the patient in health care decisions to increase adherence to therapy. Goals include lowering the HbA_{1c} to less than 7.0% in most patients to reduce the incidence of microvascular disease. Mean plasma glucose level should be between about 8.3 and 8.9 mmol/L, fasting and pre-meal glucose should be maintained at less than 7.2 mmol/L, and postprandial glucose should be less than 10 mmol/L. Select patients may be managed with more stringent targets, but treatment must weigh the possibility of inducing significant hypoglycemia or other adverse effects. Other considerations when making treatment decisions include the patient's age, weight, sex/racial/ethnic/genetic status, comorbidities such as heart failure or chronic kidney disease, and hypoglycemic status.

Treatments.—Therapeutic approaches target lifestyle changes, specifically, the patient's physical activity levels and food intake. Weight reduction improves glycemic control and other cardiovascular risk factors. Patients should receive dietary advice tailored to their specific needs and situation. The approach is reevaluated regularly and adjusted as needed.

Oral agents and non-insulin injectable agents are used first to control glycemia, avoid acute osmotic symptoms of hyperglycemia, avoid instability of blood glucose levels over time, and prevent or delay the development of diabetic complications without adversely affecting quality of life. Metformin is the most widely used first-line agent. Others include sulfonylurea insulin secretagogues, thiazolidinediones (TZDs), and new agents focused on the incretin system. Agent- and patient-specific factors are considered to guide the selection of agent. Insulin replacement therapy is often required with progressive beta cell dysfunction. The strategy for insulin delivery is designed specifically for individual patients. It is tailored to fit the patient's dietary and exercise habits and prevailing glucose trends.

Initial therapy is metformin, which is begun at or soon after diagnosis. Because it has gastrointestinal side effects, it should be started at a low dose with gradual titration. For patients with a high baseline $HBbA_{1c}$ and a low probability of achieving a near-normal target with monotherapy, a combination of two non-insulin agents or metformin plus insulin may be justified. Depending on the patient's condition, the patient may be advanced to dual combination therapy, triple combination therapy, and insulin, delivered according to various protocols.

Conclusions.—High-quality research is needed to determine the comparative effectiveness of the various approaches and agents and to measure effects on the patient's quality of life. We also lack information on the durability of effectiveness and how phenotype and other patient/disease characteristics interact with the available drugs.

▶ Because of the increasing complexity in management of glycemic control in type 2 diabetic patients caused by an increase in drugs with their potential adverse effects and the controversies concerning the benefits of intensive control elicited by the ACCORD (Action to Control Cardiovascular Risk in Diabetes) and the ADVANCE (Action in Diabetes and Vascular Disease: Preterax and Diamicron MR Controlled Evaluation) studies, the American Diabetes Association and the European Association for the Study of Diabetes developed recommendations for the antiglycemic treatment in nonpregnant adults suffering from type 2 diabetes. The key points, among others, are: (1) glucose-lowering therapy should be individualized according to the patient's needs, with diet, exercise, and education as foundation; (2) metformin is the optimal first-line drug unless there are prevalent contradictions; (3) many patients will ultimately require insulin therapy alone or in combination with other drugs; and (4) a comprehensive reduction of cardiovascular risk (ie, lowering of blood pressure) must be a major therapeutic focus. This recommendation opens the way to a more individualized antidiabetic therapy by attenuating the previously strict limits of HbA_{1c} concentrations.

E. Oetjen, MD

A Clinical Trial to Maintain Glycemic Control in Youth with Type 2 Diabetes
TODAY Study Group (Univ of Colorado Denver, Aurora; George Washington Univ, DC; et al)
N Engl J Med 366:2247-2256, 2012

Background.—Despite the increasing prevalence of type 2 diabetes in youth, there are few data to guide treatment. We compared the efficacy of three treatment regimens to achieve durable glycemic control in children and adolescents with recent-onset type 2 diabetes.

Methods.—Eligible patients 10 to 17 years of age were treated with metformin (at a dose of 1000 mg twice daily) to attain a glycated hemoglobin level of less than 8% and were randomly assigned to continued treatment with metformin alone or to metformin combined with rosiglitazone (4 mg twice a day) or a lifestyle-intervention program focusing on weight loss through eating and activity behaviors. The primary outcome was loss of glycemic control, defined as a glycated hemoglobin level of at least 8% for 6 months or sustained metabolic decompensation requiring insulin.

Results.—Of the 699 randomly assigned participants (mean duration of diagnosed type 2 diabetes, 7.8 months), 319 (45.6%) reached the primary outcome over an average follow-up of 3.86 years. Rates of failure were 51.7% (120 of 232 participants), 38.6% (90 of 233), and 46.6% (109 of 234) for metformin alone, metformin plus rosiglitazone, and metformin plus lifestyle intervention, respectively. Metformin plus rosiglitazone was superior to metformin alone ($P = 0.006$); metformin plus lifestyle intervention was intermediate but not significantly different from metformin alone or metformin plus rosiglitazone. Prespecified analyses according to sex and race or ethnic group showed differences in sustained effectiveness, with metformin alone least effective in non-Hispanic black participants and metformin plus rosiglitazone most effective in girls. Serious adverse events were reported in 19.2% of participants.

Conclusions.—Monotherapy with metformin was associated with durable glycemic control in approximately half of children and adolescents with type 2 diabetes. The addition of rosiglitazone, but not an intensive lifestyle intervention, was superior to metformin alone. (Funded by the National Institute of Diabetes and Digestive and Kidney Diseases and others; TODAY ClinicalTrials.gov number, NCT00081328.)

▶ An increasing number of children and adolescents have type 2 diabetes. However, few trials guide appropriate therapy. The study of the TODAY study group compared the effectiveness of treatment with metformin alone, metformin plus rosiglitazone, or metformin plus lifestyle intervention in maintaining glycemic control in patients 10 to 17 years of age with recently diagnosed diabetes. Loss of glycemic control, defined as HbA$_{1c}$ greater than 8% for 6 months, or sustained metabolic decompensation requiring insulin were the primary endpoints. Approximately 50% of the patients reached a primary endpoint over an average follow-up of 3.86 years. Comparison of the treatments found that metformin plus rosiglitazone, but not metformin plus lifestyle intervention, was superior to metformin monotherapy in maintaining glycemic control. However, considering the adverse effects of rosiglitazone, including cardiovascular events, bladder cancer, and bone resorption, this drug seems to be unsuitable for adolescents. In addition, this study supports the pivotal role of metformin in the treatment of type 2 diabetes.

E. Oetjen, MD

Pathogenesis

Large-scale association analysis provides insights into the genetic architecture and pathophysiology of type 2 diabetes
Morris AP, DIAbetes Genetics Replication And Meta-analysis (DIAGRAM) Consortium (Univ of Oxford, UK; et al)
Nat Genet 44:981-990, 2012

To extend understanding of the genetic architecture and molecular basis of type 2 diabetes (T2D), we conducted a meta-analysis of genetic variants on the Metabochip, including 34,840 cases and 114,981 controls, overwhelmingly of European descent. We identified ten previously unreported T2D susceptibility loci, including two showing sex-differentiated association. Genome-wide analyses of these data are consistent with a long tail of additional common variant loci explaining much of the variation in susceptibility to T2D. Exploration of the enlarged set of susceptibility loci implicates several processes, including CREBBP-related transcription, adipocytokine signaling and cell cycle regulation, in diabetes pathogenesis.

▶ Many genome-wide association studies (GWAS) have been undertaken to identify mutations or single nucleotide polymorphism (SNP) related to type 2 diabetes. In this study, a GWAS meta-analysis was undertaken with almost 150 000 individuals. In addition to identifying 10 new loci associated with diabetes, the authors tried to connect the multitude of SNPs in different genes into a network by analyzing protein-protein interactions. It turned out the cell cycle regulation, adipocyte signaling, and the transcriptional coactivator, CBP or CREBBP (CREB binding protein), are key processes involved in the pathogenesis of type 2 diabetes. Despite its namesake, CBP interacts with many transcription factors. CBP is regulated by diverse signals, among them insulin. It contains a histone acetyl transferase domain, thereby implicating CBP in the coupling of chromatin remodeling to transcription factor recognition. This meta-GWAS goes a step beyond common GWAS trying, albeit tentatively, to show mechanisms involved in the pathogenesis of type 2 diabetes.

E. Oetjen, MD

DNA methylation profiling identifies epigenetic dysregulation in pancreatic islets from type 2 diabetic patients

Volkmar M, Dedeurwaerder S, Cunha DA, et al (Université Libre de Bruxelles, Brussels, Belgium; et al)
EMBO J 31:1405-1426, 2012

In addition to genetic predisposition, environmental and lifestyle factors contribute to the pathogenesis of type 2 diabetes (T2D). Epigenetic changes may provide the link for translating environmental exposures into pathological mechanisms. In this study, we performed the first comprehensive DNA methylation profiling in pancreatic islets from T2D and non-diabetic donors. We uncovered 276 CpG loci affiliated to promoters of 254 genes displaying significant differential DNA methylation in diabetic islets. These methylation changes were not present in blood cells from T2D individuals nor were they experimentally induced in non-diabetic islets by exposure to high glucose. For a subgroup of the differentially methylated genes, concordant transcriptional changes were present. Functional annotation of the aberrantly methylated genes and RNAi experiments highlighted pathways implicated in β-cell survival and function; some are implicated in cellular dysfunction while others facilitate adaptation to stressors. Together, our findings offer new insights into the intricate mechanisms of T2D pathogenesis, underscore the important involvement of epigenetic dysregulation in diabetic islets and may advance our understanding of T2D aetiology.

▶ To investigate the role of environmental and lifestyle factors in the pathogenesis of type 2 diabetes, DNA methylation profiling was performed in islets of type 2 diabetic and nondiabetic donors. A total of 276 CpG loci with differentially methylated DNA were identified in diabetic islets. These epigenetic changes were not present in the blood cells from type 2 diabetics nor was it possible to induce these changes in the islets of nondiabetic donors exposed to high glucose. Functional annotation of these distinctly methylated genes found pathways implicated in β cell survival and function, in cellular dysfunction, and in the adaptation to stressors. Although this study does not provide a simple method to assess diabetes, it opens the door to the relatively new field: how environmental and lifestyle factors by causing epigenetic changes influence the pathogenesis of diabetes.

E. Oetjen, MD

A metagenome-wide association study of gut microbiota in type 2 diabetes

Qin J, Li Y, Cai Z, et al (BGI-Shenzhen, China; The First Affiliated Hosp of Shenzhen Univ, China; et al)
Nature 490:55-60, 2012

Assessment and characterization of gut microbiota has become a major research area in human disease, including type 2 diabetes, the most prevalent endocrine disease worldwide. To carry out analysis on gut microbial content in patients with type 2 diabetes, we developed a protocol for a metagenome-wide association study (MGWAS) and undertook a two-stage MGWAS based on deep shotgun sequencing of the gut microbial DNA from 345 Chinese individuals. We identified and validated approximately 60,000 type-2-diabetes-associated markers and established the concept of a metagenomic linkage group, enabling taxonomic species-level analyses. MGWAS analysis showed that patients with type 2 diabetes were characterized by a moderate degree of gut microbial dysbiosis, a decrease in the abundance of some universal butyrate-producing bacteria and an increase in various opportunistic pathogens, as well as an enrichment of other microbial functions conferring sulphate reduction and oxidative stress resistance. An analysis of 23 additional individuals demonstrated that these gut microbial markers might be useful for classifying type 2 diabetes.

▶ The intestinal microbiome or the gut metagenome and their changes in disease have increasingly gained attention. To investigate gut microbial compositional changes and their impact on type 2 diabetes, a 2-stage, case-control metagenome-wide association study based on deep next-generation shogun sequencing of DNA extracted from the stool samples of 345 Chinese type 2 diabetic and nondiabetic participants was carried out. This study found moderate dysbiosis in the gut microbiota of diabetic patients. In particular, enrichment of membrane transport of sugars and branched-chain amino acids, methane metabolism, xenobiotics degradation and metabolism, and sulfate reduction as well as decreased bacterial chemotaxis, butyrate synthesis, and metabolism of cofactors and vitamins were observed. Furthermore, the identified gut metagenomic markers differentiated between diabetic and nondiabetic participants with a higher level of specificity than similar analyses based on human genome variations. Thus, evaluating gut metagenome might be an approach for risk assessment of diabetes.

E. Oetjen, MD

Early Loss of the Glucagon Response to Hypoglycemia in Adolescents With Type 1 Diabetes
Siafarikas A, Johnston RJ, Bulsara MK, et al (Princess Margaret Hosp for Children, Perth, Western Australia, Australia; Univ of Notre Dame Fremantle, Western Australia, Australia)
Diabetes Care 35:1757-1762, 2012

Objective.—To assess the glucagon response to hypoglycemia and identify influencing factors in patients with type 1 diabetes compared with nondiabetic control subjects.

Research Design and Methods.—Hyperinsulinemic hypoglycemic clamp studies were performed in all participants. The glucagon response to both hypoglycemia and arginine was measured, as well as epinephrine, cortisol, and growth hormone responses to hypoglycemia. Residual β-cell function was assessed using fasting and stimulated C-peptide.

Results.—Twenty-eight nonobese adolescents with type 1 diabetes (14 female, mean age 14.9 years [range 11.2—19.8]) and 12 healthy control subjects (6 female, 15.3 years [12.8—18.7]) participated in the study. Median duration of type 1 diabetes was 0.66 years (range 0.01—9.9). The glucagon peak to arginine stimulation was similar between groups ($P = 0.27$). In contrast, the glucagon peak to hypoglycemia was reduced in the group with diabetes (95% CI): 68 (62—74) vs. 96 (87—115) pg/mL ($P < 0.001$). This response was greater than 3 SDs from baseline for only 7% of subjects with type 1 diabetes in comparison with 83% of control subjects and was lost at a median duration of diabetes of 8 months and as early as 1 month after diagnosis ($R = -0.41$, $P < 0.01$). There was no correlation in response with height, weight, BMI, and HbA_{1c}. Epinephrine, cortisol, and growth hormone responses to hypoglycemia were present in both groups.

Conclusions.—The glucagon response to hypoglycemia in adolescents with type 1 diabetes is influenced by the duration of diabetes and can be lost early in the course of the disease.

▶ The often unphysiologic nature of insulin substitution in type 1 diabetic patients often results in hypoglycemic events. Under physiologic conditions, glucagon secretion is triggered by hypoglycemia, resulting in hepatic glucose production and an increase in the blood glucose levels. Siafarikas et al investigated whether glucagon secretion in adolescents was impaired, thus aggravating hypoglycemia. Using hyperinsulinemic hypoglycemic clamp studies in 28 adolescent type 1 diabetic patients and 14 age-matched healthy volunteers, the authors measured glucagon response to hypoglycemia and arginine. In both groups, glucagon plasma concentrations in response to arginine were similar, whereas the diabetic group showed a reduced glucagon response to hypoglycemia. The hypoglycemia-induced glucagon response correlated with the duration of diabetes. These data suggest that besides the loss of β cells, an α-cell dysfunction might develop in diabetes mellitus type 1, resulting in the aggravation of hypoglycemic events.

E. Oetjen, MD

Glucagon regulates its own synthesis by autocrine signaling
Leibiger B, Moede T, Muhandiramlage TP, et al (Karolinska Institutet, Stockholm, Sweden)
Proc Natl Acad Sci U S A 109:20925-20930, 2012

Peptide hormones are powerful regulators of various biological processes. To guarantee continuous availability and function, peptide hormone secretion must be tightly coupled to its biosynthesis. A simple but efficient way to provide such regulation is through an autocrine feedback mechanism in which the secreted hormone is "sensed" by its respective receptor and initiates synthesis at the level of transcription and/or translation. Such a secretion—biosynthesis coupling has been demonstrated for insulin; however, because of insulin's unique role as the sole blood glucose-decreasing peptide hormone, this coupling is considered an exception rather than a more generally used mechanism. Here we provide evidence of a secretion—biosynthesis coupling for glucagon, one of several peptide hormones that increase blood glucose levels. We show that glucagon, secreted by the pancreatic α cell, up-regulates the expression of its own gene by signaling through the glucagon receptor, PKC, and PKA, supporting the more general applicability of an autocrine feedback mechanism in regulation of peptide hormone synthesis.

▶ "Alpha-cells of the endocrine pancreas: 35 years of research but the enigma remains." This sigh was uttered in 2007 by Gromada et al, the authors of that review.[1] Leibiger et al try to elucidate a bit more the still enigmatic α cell and the regulation of glucagon synthesis. They show mainly in the glucagon-producing α-cell line, αTC1-9, that glucagon by binding to the glucagon receptor initiates a signaling cascade that results in the phosphorylation of the transcription factor CREB and enhances glucagon gene transcription. The expression of the glucagon receptor was demonstrated on αTC1-9 cells and on murine and human islets. Thus, like insulin, glucagon biosynthesis is regulated by an autocrine feedback mechanism resulting in a secretion-biosynthesis coupling that ensures the replenishment of glucagon stores. The question remains whether the regulation of glucagon secretion is distinct in diabetes.

E. Oetjen, MD

Reference

1. Gromada J, Franklin I, Wollheim CB. Alpha-cells of the endocrine pancreas: 35 years of research but the enigma remains. *Endocr Rev.* 2007 Feb;28(1):84-116.

Glucose activates free fatty acid receptor 1 gene transcription via phosphatidylinositol-3-kinase-dependent *O*-GlcNAcylation of pancreas-duodenum homeobox-1

Kebede M, Ferdaoussi M, Mancini A, et al (Univ of Montreal, Quebec, Canada; et al)
Proc Natl Acad Sci U S A 109:2376-2381, 2012

The G protein-coupled free fatty acid receptor-1 (FFA1/GPR40) plays a major role in the regulation of insulin secretion by fatty acids. GPR40 is considered a potential therapeutic target to enhance insulin secretion in type 2 diabetes; however, its mode of regulation is essentially unknown. The aims of this study were to test the hypothesis that glucose regulates GPR40 gene expression in pancreatic β-cells and to determine the mechanisms of this regulation. We observed that glucose stimulates GPR40 gene transcription in pancreatic β-cells via increased binding of pancreas-duodenum homeobox-1 (Pdx-1) to the A-box in the HR2 region of the GPR40 promoter. Mutation of the Pdx-1 binding site within the HR2 abolishes glucose activation of GPR40 promoter activity. The stimulation of

GPR40 expression and Pdx-1 binding to the HR2 in response to glucose are mimicked by N-acetyl glucosamine, an intermediate of the hexosamine biosynthesis pathway, and involve PI3K-dependent O-GlcNAcylation of Pdx-1 in the nucleus. We demonstrate that O-GlcNAc transferase (OGT) interacts with the product of the PI3K reaction, phosphatidylinositol 3,4,5-trisphosphate (PIP$_3$), in the nucleus. This interaction enables OGT to catalyze O-GlcNAcylation of nuclear proteins, including Pdx-1. We conclude that glucose stimulates GPR40 gene expression at the transcriptional level through Pdx-1 binding to the HR2 region and via a signaling cascade that involves an interaction between OGT and PIP$_3$ at the nuclear membrane. These observations reveal a unique mechanism by which glucose metabolism regulates the function of transcription factors in the nucleus to induce gene expression.

▶ Given that G protein—coupled free fatty acid receptor-1 (GPR40/FFAR1) provides a novel target for the antidiabetic therapy, the regulation of this receptor by glucose was investigated by Kebede et al. In isolated murine and human islets, glucose enhanced the expression of GPR40 mRNA and protein levels. This increase was associated with a greater ability of oleic acid to potentiate glucose-induced insulin secretion. Using the β-cell line MIN6 it was shown that glucose feeding into the hexosamine biosynthesis pathway leads to O-linked GlcNAcylation of the transcription factor pancreas-duodenum homeobox-1 and consecutively to the activation of GPR40 gene transcription. Thus, via increased expression of GPR40 and subsequent augmentation of glucose-induced insulin secretion, glucose potentiates its own effect on insulin secretion. It remains to be investigated whether this mechanism holds true in animal models of diabetes or whether in the diabetic state the sensitivity or the expression of GPR40 is reduced, thereby attenuating GPR40-mediated insulin secretion.

E. Oetjen, MD

Neonatal β Cell Development in Mice and Humans Is Regulated by Calcineurin/NFAT

Goodyer WR, Gu X, Liu Y, et al (Stanford Univ School of Medicine, CA; et al)
Dev Cell 23:21-34, 2012

Little is known about the mechanisms governing neonatal growth and maturation of organs. Here we demonstrate that calcineurin/Nuclear Factor of Activated T cells (Cn/NFAT) signaling regulates neonatal pancreatic development in mouse and human islets. Inactivation of *calcineurin b1* (*Cnb1*) in mouse islets impaired dense core granule biogenesis, decreased insulin secretion, and reduced cell proliferation and mass, culminating in lethal diabetes. Pancreatic β cells lacking *Cnb1* failed to express genes revealed to be direct NFAT targets required for replication, insulin storage, and secretion. In contrast, glucokinase activation stimulated Cn-dependent expression of these genes. Calcineurin inhibitors, such as tacrolimus, used for human immunosuppression, induce diabetes. Tacrolimus exposure reduced Cn/NFAT-dependent expression of factors essential for insulin dense core granule formation and secretion and neonatal β cell proliferation, consistent with our genetic studies. Discovery of conserved pathways regulating β cell maturation and proliferation suggests new strategies for controlling β cell growth or replacement in human islet diseases.

▶ Islet transplantation is considered the ultimate treatment for type 1 diabetic patients with a volatile glucose homeostasis. However, organs are scarce. Differentiation of progenitor cells into mature β cells or propagation of β cells might be a source for β cells. Therefore, the elucidation of mechanism governing the development and the proliferation of β cells might be a first step toward an unlimited supply of β cells. Using conditional knock-out mice and human islets, Goodyer et al show that the phosphatase calcineurin is indispensable for postnatal maturation (synthesis of proteins building the dense core granules) and proliferation of β cells. They demonstrate that glucose-induced membrane depolarization results in the activation of calcineurin and that the inhibition of the transcription factor nuclear factor of activated T cells mediates the effects of calcineurin deficiency. It should be noted that there are more calcineurin-responsive transcription factor in β cells. As such, CRTC2 (cAMP-regulated transcriptional coactivator 2) was stimulated in a calcineurin-dependent way by glucose-induced membrane depolarization in β cells (Jansson et al).[1] This study provides additional evidence that calcineurin is important for β-cells' function and proliferation and inhibition of calcineurin for immunosuppressive therapy after transplantation contributes to posttransplant diabetes.

E. Oetjen, MD

Reference

1. Jansson D, Ng AC, Fu A, et al. Glucose controls CREB activity in islet cells via regulated phosphorylation of TORC2. *Proc Natl Acad Sci USA*. 2008;105: 10161-10166.

Metabolic manifestations of insulin deficiency do not occur without glucagon action

Lee Y, Berglund ED, Wang M-Y, et al (Univ of Texas Southwestern Med Ctr, Dallas; et al)
Proc Natl Acad Sci U S A 109:14972-14976, 2012

To determine unambiguously if suppression of glucagon action will eliminate manifestations of diabetes, we expressed glucagon receptors in livers of glucagon receptor-null ($GcgR^{-/-}$) mice before and after β-cell destruction by high-dose streptozotocin. Wild type (WT) mice developed fatal diabetic ketoacidosis after streptozotocin, whereas $GcgR^{-/-}$ mice with similar β-cell destruction remained clinically normal without hyperglycemia, impaired glucose tolerance, or hepatic glycogen depletion. Restoration of receptor expression using adenovirus containing the GcgR cDNA restored hepatic GcgR, phospho-cAMP response element binding protein (P-CREB), and phosphoenol pyruvate carboxykinase, markers of glucagon action, rose dramatically and severe hyperglycemia appeared. When GcgR mRNA spontaneously disappeared 7 d later, P-CREB declined and hyperglycemia disappeared. In conclusion, the metabolic manifestations of diabetes cannot occur without glucagon action and, once present, disappear promptly when glucagon action is abolished. Glucagon suppression should be a major therapeutic goal in diabetes.

▶ To investigate whether suppression of glucagon action affects the manifestations of diabetes, an elegant model was employed by Lee et al. In mice lacking the glucagon receptor and made diabetic by multiple injections of streptozotocin, the glucagon receptor was adenovirally overexpressed. This approach results in mainly hepatic expression of the glucagon receptor. In contrast to streptozotocin-treated glucagon receptor—deficient mice, these mice showed severe hyperglycemia and markers of glucagon action reappeared in their livers. Spontaneous disappearance of glucagon receptor messenger RNA 7 days after injection abolished hyperglycemia. These data suggest that glucagon in the face of insulin deficiency results in the metabolic manifestations of diabetes. The authors conclude that it is not sufficient to supplement insulin, but that hyperglucagonemia needs to be treated in type 1 diabetes as well. Thus, this study might change the prevailing view of antidiabetic therapy.

E. Oetjen, MD

Glucagonocentric restructuring of diabetes: a pathophysiologic and therapeutic makeover
Unger RH, Cherrington AD (Univ of Texas Southwestern Med Ctr, Dallas; Vanderbilt Univ School of Medicine, Nashville, TN)
J Clin Invest 122:4-12, 2012

The hormone glucagon has long been dismissed as a minor contributor to metabolic disease. Here we propose that glucagon excess, rather than insulin deficiency, is the sine qua non of diabetes. We base this on the following evidence: (a) glucagon increases hepatic glucose and ketone production, catabolic features present in insulin deficiency; (b) hyperglucagonemia is present in every form of poorly controlled diabetes; (c) the glucagon suppressors leptin and somatostatin suppress all catabolic manifestations of diabetes during total insulin deficiency; (d) total β cell destruction in glucagon receptor—null mice does not cause diabetes; and (e) perfusion of normal pancreas with anti-insulin serum causes marked hyperglucagonemia. From this and other evidence, we conclude that glucose-responsive β cells normally regulate juxtaposed α cells and that without intraislet insulin, unregulated α cells hypersecrete glucagon, which directly causes the symptoms of diabetes. This indicates that glucagon suppression or inactivation may provide therapeutic advantages over insulin monotherapy.

▶ In this comprehensive review, Unger and Cherrington describe the role of glucagon in the regulation of glucose homeostasis and in the pathophysiology of diabetes mellitus. The intricate relationship between insulin and glucagon within the islets and the regulation of glucagon secretion (and biosynthesis) by insulin are depicted. Being slightly provocative, the authors postulate that it is not the insulin deficiency but the hyperglucagonemia that elicits the metabolic defects seen in diabetes. They propose that insulin substitution and the inhibition of glucagon secretion, or at least glucagon action, constitutes an appropriate treatment of type 1 diabetes. This well-written review will give the reader a thorough insight into the role of glucagon and convince him or her that diabetes is indeed a bihormonal disease.

E. Oetjen, MD

Prevention and Reversal of Diabetes

TAK-875 versus placebo or glimepiride in type 2 diabetes mellitus: a phase 2, randomised, double-blind, placebo-controlled trial
Burant CF, Viswanathan P, Marcinak J, et al (Univ of Michigan, Ann Arbor; Takeda Global Res and Development Ctr, Deerfield, IL)
Lancet 379:1403-1411, 2012

Background.—Activation of free fatty acid receptor 1 (FFAR1; also known as G-protein-coupled receptor 40) by fatty acids stimulated glucose-dependent β-cell insulin secretion in preclinical models. We aimed to assess whether selective pharmacological activation of this receptor by TAK-875 in patients with type 2 diabetes mellitus improved glycaemic control without hypoglycaemia risk.

Methods.—We undertook a phase 2, randomised, double-blind, and placebo-controlled and active-comparator-controlled trial in outpatients with type 2 diabetes who had not responded to diet or metformin treatment. Patients were randomly assigned equally to receive placebo, TAK-875 (6·25, 25, 50, 100, or 200 mg), or glimepiride (4 mg) once daily for 12 weeks. Patients and investigators were masked to treatment assignment. The primary outcome was change in haemoglobin A_{1c} (HbA_{1c}) from baseline. Analysis included all patients randomly assigned to treatment groups who received at least one dose of double-blind study drug. The trial is registered at ClinicalTrials.gov, NCT01007097.

Findings.—426 patients were randomly assigned to TAK-875 (n = 303), placebo (n = 61), and glimepiride (n = 62). At week 12, significant least-squares mean reductions in HbA_{1c} from baseline occurred in all TAK-875 (ranging from −1·12% [SE 0·113] with 50 mg to −0·65% [0·114] with 6·25 mg) and glimepiride (−1·05% [SE 0·111]) groups versus placebo (−0·13% [SE 0·115]; p value range 0·001 to <0·0001). Treatment-emergent hypoglycaemic events were similar in the TAK-875 and placebo groups (2% [n = 7, all TAK-875 groups] *vs* 3% [n = 2]); significantly higher rates were reported in the glimepiride group (19% [n = 12]; *p* value range 0·010–0·002 *vs* all TAK-875 groups). Incidence of treatment-emergent adverse events was similar in the TAK-875 overall (49%; n = 147, all TAK-875 groups) and placebo groups (48%, n = 29) and was lower than in the glimepiride group (61%, n = 38).

Interpretation.—TAK-875 significantly improved glycaemic control in patients with type 2 diabetes with minimum risk of hypoglycaemia. The results show that activation of FFAR1 is a viable therapeutic target for treatment of type 2 diabetes.

▶ In this trial, the glucose-lowering effect of TAK-875 was compared with that of the insulin secretagogue, glimepiride, in type 2 diabetic patients. Patients received either TAK-875 in ascending doses, glimepiride, or placebo. The reduction of hemoglobin A1c (HbA_{1c}) after a 12-week treatment was the primary endpoint. In all patients receiving TAK-875 or glimepiride, HbA_{1c} was decreased. Hypoglycemic events and other treatment-emergent adverse effects were similar in the TAK-875 and placebo groups and higher in the glimepiride group. A gain in body weight was observed after 12 weeks of treatment with glimepiride and with TAK-875, an outcome that was not dose-dependent in the TAK-875 groups. This trial suggests that activation of G-protein-coupled receptor 40 by TAK-875 represents a novel therapeutic target for treating type 2 diabetes with few glycemic events. It should be noted, however, that patients are treated for much longer periods of time with drugs. The long-term effects of TAK-875 remain to be evaluated.

E. Oetjen, MD

Targeting VEGF-B as a novel treatment for insulin resistance and type 2 diabetes

Hagberg CE, Mehlem A, Falkevall A, et al (Karolinska Institutet, Stockholm, Sweden; et al)
Nature 490:426-430, 2012

The prevalence of type 2 diabetes is rapidly increasing, with severe socio-economic impacts. Excess lipid deposition in peripheral tissues impairs insulin sensitivity and glucose uptake, and has been proposed to contribute to the pathology of type 2 diabetes. However, few treatment options exist that directly target ectopic lipid accumulation. Recently it was found that vascular endothelial growth factor B (VEGF-B) controls endothelial uptake and transport of fatty acids in heart and skeletal muscle. Here we show that decreased VEGF-B signalling in rodent models of type 2 diabetes restores insulin sensitivity and improves glucose tolerance. Genetic deletion of *Vegfb* in diabetic *db/db* mice prevented ectopic lipid deposition, increased muscle glucose uptake and maintained normoglycaemia. Pharmacological inhibition of VEGF-B signalling by antibody administration to *db/db* mice enhanced glucose tolerance, preserved pancreatic islet architecture, improved β-cell function and ameliorated dyslipidaemia, key elements of type 2 diabetes and the metabolic syndrome. The potential use of VEGF-B neutralization in type 2 diabetes was further elucidated in rats fed a high-fat diet, in which it normalized insulin sensitivity and increased glucose uptake in skeletal muscle and heart. Our results demonstrate that the vascular endothelium can function as an efficient barrier to excess muscle lipid uptake even under conditions of severe obesity and type 2 diabetes, and that this barrier can be maintained by inhibition of VEGF-B signalling. We propose VEGF-B antagonism as a novel pharmacological approach for type 2 diabetes, targeting the lipid-transport properties of the endothelium to improve muscle insulin sensitivity and glucose disposal.

▶ Many antidiabetic drugs are available, but the search for novel targets is ongoing. One of these novel targets might be vascular endothelial growth factor B (VEGF-B). VEGF-B is expressed in cardiac and skeletal myocytes, in brown adipocytes, and in β cells, from where it signals to the endothelial VEGF receptor 1 and induces upregulation of fatty acid transport proteins 3 and 4. VEGF-B—deficient mice show decreased fatty acid uptake and lipid deposition in muscles, with lipids shunted into white adipocytes, resulting in weight gain. Thus, VEGF-B interferes with impaired lipid deposition in peripheral tissues. Genetic deletion of VEGF-B in diabetic (*db/db*) mice prevents ectopic lipid deposition and maintains normoglycemia. Pharmacologic inhibition of VEGF-B signaling by an antibody in *db/db* mice enhanced glucose tolerance, preserved β-cell function and islet architecture, and ameliorated dyslipidemia. Thus, inhibiting VEGF-B and, thereby, endothelial lipid transport, improves muscle insulin sensitivity and glucose disposal, which delays the loss of β-cell function and mass. By enhancing muscle insulin sensitivity, inhibitors of VEGF-B target an important pathomechanism in diabetes and might become useful antidiabetic drugs.

E. Oetjen, MD

The Effects of TAK-875, a Selective G Protein-Coupled Receptor 40/Free Fatty Acid 1 Agonist, on Insulin and Glucagon Secretion in Isolated Rat and Human Islets

Yashiro H, Tsujihata Y, Takeuchi K, et al (Takeda Pharmaceutical Company Limited, Osaka, Japan; et al)
J Pharmacol Exp Ther 340:483-489, 2012

G protein-coupled receptor 40 (GPR40)/free fatty acid 1 (FFA1) is a G protein-coupled receptor involved in free fatty acid-induced insulin secretion. To analyze the effect of our novel GPR40/FFA1-selective agonist, [(3S)-6-({2′,6′-dimethyl-4′-[3-(methylsulfonyl) propoxy]biphenyl-3-yl} methoxy)-2,3-dihydro-1-benzofuran-3-yl] acetic acid hemi-hydrate (TAK-875), on insulin and glucagon secretion, we performed hormone secretion assays and measured intracellular Ca^{2+} concentration ($[Ca^{2+}]_i$) in both human and rat islets. Insulin and glucagon secretion were measured in static and dynamic conditions by using groups of isolated rat and human pancreatic islets. $[Ca^{2+}]_i$ was recorded by using confocal microscopy. GPR40/FFA1 expression was measured by quantitative polymerase chain reaction. In both human and rat islets, TAK-875 enhanced glucose-induced insulin secretion in a glucose-dependent manner. The stimulatory effect of TAK-875 was similar to that produced by glucagon-like peptide-1 and correlated with the elevation of β-cell $[Ca^{2+}]_i$. TAK-875 was without effect on glucagon secretion at both 1 and 16 mM glucose in human islets. These data indicate that GPR40/FFA1 influences mainly insulin secretion in a glucose-dependent manner. The β-cell-specific action of TAK-875 in human islets may represent a therapeutically useful feature that allows plasma glucose control without compromising counter-regulation of glucagon secretion, thus minimizing the risk of hypoglycemia.

▶ Although glucose is the main stimulus for insulin secretion, other agents binding to distinct receptors in the β cell augment glucose-induced insulin secretion. Besides the well-known glucagon-like peptide 1 (GLP-1) binding to its G protein–coupled receptor, free fatty acids (FFA) stimulate insulin secretion. The previous orphan receptor G protein–coupled receptor 40 (GPR40) has been identified as the receptor bound and activated by FFA. Activation of this receptor results in increased intracellular calcium concentrations and the activation of the protein kinase C, thereby potentiating glucose-induced insulin secretion. The synthetic ligand TAK-875 binds with high affinity specifically to GPR40/FFAR1 (free fatty acid receptor 1). The study by Yashiro et al provides evidence that TAK-875 enhances glucose-stimulated insulin secretion in a manner similar to GLP-1 in isolated rat and in human islets. In addition, TAK-875 had no effect on glucagon secretion in human islets. Their data suggest that TAK-875 might lower blood glucose levels without the danger of hypoglycemia.

E. Oetjen, MD

Cardiovascular benefits and diabetes risks of statin therapy in primary prevention: an analysis from the JUPITER trial
Ridker PM, Pradhan A, MacFadyen JG, et al (Brigham and Women's Hosp, Boston, MA)
Lancet 380:565-571, 2012

Background.—In view of evidence that statin therapy increases risk of diabetes, the balance of benefit and risk of these drugs in primary prevention has become controversial. We undertook an analysis of participants from the JUPITER trial to address the balance of vascular benefits and diabetes hazard of statin use.

Methods.—In the randomised, double-blind JUPITER trial, 17 603 men and women without previous cardiovascular disease or diabetes were randomly assigned to rosuvastatin 20 mg or placebo and followed up for up to 5 years for the primary endpoint (myocardial infarction, stroke, admission to hospital for unstable angina, arterial revascularisation, or cardiovascular death) and the protocol-prespecified secondary endpoints of venous thromboembolism, all-cause mortality, and incident physician-reported diabetes. In this analysis, participants were stratified on the basis of having none or at least one of four major risk factors for developing diabetes: metabolic syndrome, impaired fasting glucose, body-mass index 30 kg/m^2 or higher, or glycated haemoglobin A_{1c} greater than 6%. The trial is registered at ClinicalTrials.gov, NCT00239681.

Findings.—Trial participants with one or more major diabetes risk factor (n=11 508) were at higher risk of developing diabetes than were those without a major risk factor (n=6095). In individuals with one or more risk factors, statin allocation was associated with a 39% reduction in the primary endpoint (hazard ratio [HR] 0·61, 95% CI 0·47−0·79, p=0·0001), a 36% reduction in venous thromboembolism (0·64, 0·39−1·06, p=0·08), a 17% reduction in total mortality (0·83, 0·64−1·07, p=0·15), and a 28% increase in diabetes (1·28, 1·07−1·54, p=0·01). Thus, for those with diabetes risk factors, a total of 134 vascular events or deaths were avoided for every 54 new cases of diabetes diagnosed. For trial participants with no major diabetes risk factors, statin allocation was associated with a 52% reduction in the primary endpoint (HR 0·48, 95% CI 0·33−0·68, p=0·0001), a 53% reduction in venous thromboembolism (0·47, 0·21−1·03, p=0·05), a 22% reduction in total mortality (0·78, 0·59−1·03, p=0·08), and no increase in diabetes (0·99, 0·45−2·21, p=0·99). For such individuals, a total of 86 vascular events or deaths were avoided with no new cases of diabetes diagnosed. In analysis limited to the 486 participants who developed diabetes during follow-up (270 on rosuvastatin vs 216 on placebo; HR 1·25, 95% CI 1·05−1·49, p=0·01), the point estimate of cardiovascular risk reduction associated with statin therapy (HR 0·63, 95% CI 0·25−1·60) was consistent with that for the trial as a whole (0·56, 0·46−0·69). By comparison with placebo, statins accelerated the average time to diagnosis of diabetes by 5·4 weeks (84·3 [SD 47·8] weeks on rosuvastatin vs 89·7 [50·4] weeks on placebo).

Interpretation.—In the JUPITER primary prevention trial, the cardiovascular and mortality benefits of statin therapy exceed the diabetes hazard, including in participants at high risk of developing diabetes.

▶ The lipid-lowering statins may increase risk of diabetes. To study whether the benefit of statins in preventing cardiovascular events overcomes the risk of diabetes, a subanalysis of participants from the JUPITER (Justification of Use of Statins in Prevention: an Intervention Trial Evaluating Rosuvastatin) trial was undertaken. For participants with at least 1 major diabetes risk factor (ie, metabolic syndrome, impaired fasting glucose, body mass index > 30 kg/m^2, HbA$_{1c}$ > 6%), a total of 134 vascular events or deaths was avoided for every 54 newly diagnosed cases of diabetes. For participants without major diabetes risk factors, a total of 86 vascular events or deaths were avoided with no newly diagnosed cases of diabetes. Hence, in the JUPITER trial, cardiovascular and mortality benefits of rosuvastatin therapy exceeds the risks of developing diabetes, including patients with major diabetes risk factors. The benefit of other statins comparing cardiovascular endpoints and diabetes risk is still unknown.

E. Oetjen, MD

Amorfrutins are potent antidiabetic dietary natural products

Weidner C, de Groot JC, Prasad A, et al (Max Planck Inst for Molecular Genetics, Berlin, Germany; Helmholtz Centre for Infection Res, Braunschweig, Germany; Cornell Univ, Ithaca, NY; et al)
Proc Natl Acad Sci U S A 109:7257-7262, 2012

Given worldwide increases in the incidence of obesity and type 2 diabetes, new strategies for preventing and treating metabolic diseases are needed. The nuclear receptor PPARγ (peroxisome proliferator-activated receptor gamma) plays a central role in lipid and glucose metabolism; however, current PPARγ-targeting drugs are characterized by undesirable side effects. Natural products from edible biomaterial provide a structurally diverse resource to alleviate complex disorders via tailored nutritional intervention. We identified a family of natural products, the amorfrutins, from edible parts of two legumes, *Glycyrrhiza foetida* and *Amorpha fruticosa*, as structurally new and powerful antidiabetics with unprecedented effects for a dietary molecule. Amorfrutins bind to and activate PPARγ, which results in selective gene expression and physiological profiles markedly different from activation by current synthetic PPARγ drugs. In diet-induced obese and db/db mice, amorfrutin treatment strongly improves insulin resistance and other metabolic and inflammatory parameters without concomitant increase of fat storage or other unwanted side effects such as hepatoxicity. These results show that selective PPARγ-activation by diet-derived ligands may constitute a promising approach to combat metabolic disease.

▶ Despite the multiple adverse effects of the thiazolidinediones such as rosiglitazone and pioglitazone, activation of their receptor peroxisome proliferator-activated receptor gamma (PPARγ) still remains an eligible drug target in the treatment of diabetes mellitus. The perfect PPARγ agonist would enhance insulin sensitivity and decrease fatty acid oxidation without fluid retention, cardiovascular events, weight gain, danger of bladder cancer, or increased bone resorption. Weidner et al identified the amorfrutins from edible parts of 2 legumes as selective PPARγ agonists. Amorfrutin 1 improved insulin sensitivity in mice fed a high-fat diet and in diabetic mice without an increase in fat storage or hepatotoxicity. In addition, no genotoxicity was observed. Other adverse effects of PPARγ activation, such as bone resorption or heart failure, were not studied. Nonetheless, amorfrutins expand the group of selective PPARγ modulators, which increase insulin sensitivity without the adverse effect inherent to full PPARγ activation in all tissues.

E. Oetjen, MD

A Multiple-Ascending-Dose Study to Evaluate Safety, Pharmacokinetics, and Pharmacodynamics of a Novel GPR40 Agonist, TAK-875, in Subjects With Type 2 Diabetes

Leifke E, Naik H, Wu J, et al (Takeda Global Res & Development Ctr, Inc, Deerfield, IL; et al)
Clin Pharmacol Ther 92:29-39, 2012

G-protein-coupled receptor 40 (GPR40), highly expressed in pancreatic β-cells, mediates free fatty acid (FFA)-induced insulin secretion. This phase I, double-blind, randomized study investigated the safety, tolerability, pharmacokinetics (PK), and pharmacodynamics (PD) of a novel, glucose-lowering GPR40 agonist, TAK-875 (q.d., orally × 14 days), in type 2 diabetics (placebo, $n = 14$; at 25, 50, 100, 200, or 400 mg, $n = 45$). Approximately dose-proportional increases in AU C_{0-24} and C_{max} occurred. TAK-875 showed good tolerability with no dose-limiting side effects. Two subjects (on TAK-875) had mild hypoglycemia, probably related to prolonged fasting after oral glucose tolerance tests (OGTTs). TAK-875 showed reductions from baseline in fasting (2 to −93 mg/dl) and post-OG TT glucose (26 to −172 mg/dl), with an apparent dose-dependent increase in post-OGTT C-peptide over 14 days. Consistent with preclinical data, TAK-875 apparently acts as a glucose-dependent insulinotropic agent with low hypoglycemic risk. Its PK is suitable for once-daily oral administration.

▶ Activation of GPR40, highly expressed in β cells, potentiates glucose-induced insulin secretion without the danger of hypoglycemia. Hence, the GPR40 agonist TAK-875 might represent a novel antidiabetic drug. In this phase I, double-blind, randomized study, Leifke et al investigated essential pharmacological parameters of TAK-875 in diabetic subjects. Ascending doses of TAK-875 were given once daily orally for 14 days. The drug was well tolerated with no dose-limiting side effects; mild hypoglycemia was observed in a few patients. Pharmacokinetic studies suggest that TAK-875 is eliminated by the liver with a half-life of 31 to 51 h. Consistent with this, steady-state levels were reached after 12 days of treatment. This study shows that TAK-875 decreases blood glucose levels and improves β-cell function in diabetic subjects without inducing severe hypoglycemia. However, given that antidiabetics have been taken for years, this study is hampered by the short duration of treatment and the small number of participants per group.

E. Oetjen, MD

Ectopic expression of glucagon receptor in skeletal muscles improves glucose homeostasis in a mouse model of diabetes

Maharaj A, Zhu L, Huang F, et al (St Michael's Hosp, Toronto, Ontario, Canada; et al)
Diabetologia 55:1458-1468, 2012

Aims/Hypothesis.—Excessive secretion of glucagon partially contributes to the development of diabetic hyperglycaemia. However, complete blocking of glucagon action will lead to adverse effects, since glucagon exerts certain beneficial effects via its receptor in many organs. We aimed to study the effects of a 'decoy receptor' for circulating glucagon on modulating beta cell function and glucose homeostasis in mice by overproducing the glucagon receptor (GCGR) in skeletal muscles.

Methods.—We generated transgenic mice in which the expression of Gcgr is driven by the muscle specific creatine kinase (*Mck*) promoter, and assessed the effects of glucagon on the modulation of glucose homeostasis under conditions of extremes of glucose influx or efflux.

Results.—*Mck/Gcgr* mice showed increased circulating levels of glucagon and insulin, resulting in an unchanged ratio of glucagon-to-insulin. The levels of hepatic glucose-6-phosphatase (G6PC) and fructose-1,6-bisphosphatase (F1,6P2ase) were significantly decreased, whereas the phosphorylation level of pancreatic cAMP-response-element-binding-protein (CREB) was significantly increased in these transgenic mice. Under basal conditions, the mice displayed normal blood glucose levels and unchanged glucose tolerance and insulin sensitivity when compared with their age-matched wild-type (WT) littermates. However, following multiple low-dose streptozotocin injections, *Mck/Gcgr* mice exhibited a delay in the onset of hyperglycaemia compared with the WT controls. This was associated with preserved beta cell mass and beta cell secretory capacity in response to glucose challenge.

Conclusions/Interpretation.—We suggest that mild and chronic hyperglucagonaemia, through a strategy involving neutralising peripheral glucagon action, provides beneficial effects on beta cell function and glucose homeostasis. *Mck/Gcgr* mice thus represent a novel mouse model for studying the physiological effects of glucagon.

▶ The role of glucagon in the pathogenesis of diabetes and the best way to alleviate glucagon action is still a matter of debate. Maharaj employs a decoy strategy whereby in mice the glucagon receptor is expressed in skeletal muscles. These mice exhibit increased circulating glucagon and insulin levels, keeping the glucagon-to-insulin ration intact. The levels of hepatic glucagon-regulated genes were reduced but increased phosphorylation of the β-cell protective transcription factor cAMP-response-element-binding protein was observed in β cells. Treatment with the β-cell toxic streptozotocin induced hyperglycemia in wild-type but not in the transgenic mice. In addition, in transgenic mice the β cell mass was conserved, suggesting a β-cell-protective effect of glucagon. These data suggest that paracrine and autocrine actions within the islets regulate β-cell function. In addition, glucagon action might even retard diabetes, given that it acts directly on the β cells.

E. Oetjen, MD

2 Lipoproteins and Atherosclerosis

Introduction

Basic scientific and clinical investigation of lipids, lipoproteins, and atherosclerosis continue to yield fascinating insights. There are no new large outcome trials to report this year. Although it is well known that the Heart Protection Study-2 Treatment of high-density lipoprotein (HDL) to Reduce the Incidence of Vascular Events trial is negative, I do not cover it herein because the study is not yet published. If all goes well, it will be a number of years before outcomes trials with dalcetrapib and evacetrapib are available.

On a positive note, great strides have occurred with the development of new drugs to lower serum levels of atherogenic lipoproteins, including very-low-density lipoprotein (VLDL), low-density lipoprotein (LDL), Lp(a), non-HDL, and apoprotein B100. During the last year, two new LDL lowering drugs were approved, including lomitapide and mipomersen. The monoclonal antibodies against proprotein convertase subtilisin/kexin type 9 are moving through phase 3 development trials and also show exciting capacity to lower serum levels of apoB-containing lipoproteins to impressive degrees. Studies with all 3 of these approaches to lipid lowering are reviewed herein. The use of fish oil comprised solely of eicosapentaenoic acid to treat triglycerides in the 200-499 mg/dL range is also addressed in discussion of the ANCHOR trial. The results of an outcomes trial with this ω-3 fatty acid is eagerly awaited now that the REDUCE-IT trial is nearly fully enrolled.

The controversies with HDL continue to abound, though we are beginning to learn that understanding HDL is no small task. Two studies are included which demonstrate that in patients with end-stage renal disease and coronary artery disease, HDL functionality is markedly impaired. Another intriguing study from the ADVANCE investigators suggests that low serum HDL-C is associated with greater risk for diabetic nephropathy. It will be some time before we will be able to establish the place of HDL management in clinical medicine.

The Copenhagen Heart Study investigators convincingly demonstrate that remnant lipoproteins are important players in the overall scheme of atherogenesis and risk for cardiovascular disease. This substantiates what many investigators have believed for years. The Cholesterol Treatment Trialists Collaborators showed in a very large patient-level meta-analysis of 27 prospective randomized studies that patients at low risk for cardiovascular disease experience as much benefit from statin therapy as those at high risk. This provides important new information to help reassure both patients and physicians that statin therapy in primary prevention is efficacious and should be instituted as appropriate.

An interesting analysis of a managed care database suggests that ezetimibe monotherapy impacts risk for cardiovascular events, including all-cause mortality. Okuzumi present fascinating data linking the LDL-/HDL-C ratio to aortic, mobile, ulcerated, atherosclerotic plaque and how it associates with risk for unexplained ischemic stroke. Aronis et al demonstrate in a meta-analysis that *trans* fat does not increase risk for insulin resistance or diabetes mellitus.

Peter P. Toth, MD, PhD

Epidemiology and Diagnosis

Remnant Cholesterol as a Causal Risk Factor for Ischemic Heart Disease
Varbo A, Benn M, Tybjærg-Hansen A, et al (Copenhagen Univ Hosp, Herlev, Denmark)
J Am Coll Cardiol 61:427-436, 2013

Objectives.—The aim of this study was to test the hypothesis that elevated nonfasting remnant cholesterol is a causal risk factor for ischemic heart disease independent of reduced high-density lipoprotein (HDL) cholesterol.

Background.—Elevated remnant cholesterol is associated with elevated levels of triglyceride-rich lipoproteins and with reduced HDL cholesterol, and all are associated with ischemic heart disease.

Methods.—A total of 73,513 subjects from Copenhagen were genotyped, of whom 11,984 had ischemic heart disease diagnosed between 1976 and 2010. Fifteen genetic variants were selected, affecting: 1) nonfasting remnant cholesterol alone; 2) nonfasting remnant cholesterol and HDL cholesterol combined; 3) HDL cholesterol alone; or 4) low-density lipoprotein (LDL) cholesterol alone as a positive control. The variants were used in a Mendelian randomization design.

Results.—The causal odds ratio for a 1 mmol/l (39 mg/dl) genetic increase of nonfasting remnant cholesterol was 2.8 (95% confidence interval [CI]: 1.9 to 4.2), with a corresponding observational hazard ratio of 1.4 (95% CI: 1.3 to 1.5). For the ratio of nonfasting remnant cholesterol to HDL cholesterol, corresponding values were 2.9 (95% CI: 1.9 to 4.6) causal and 1.2 (95% CI 1.2 to 1.3) observational for a 1-U increase. However, for HDL cholesterol, corresponding values were 0.7 (95% CI: 0.4 to 1.4) causal and 1.6 (95% CI: 1.4 to 1.7) observational for a 1 mmol/l (39 mg/dl) decrease. Finally, for LDL cholesterol, corresponding values were 1.5 (95% CI: 1.3 to 1.6) causal and 1.1 (95% CI: 1.1 to 1.2) observational for a 1 mmol/l (39 mg/dl) increase.

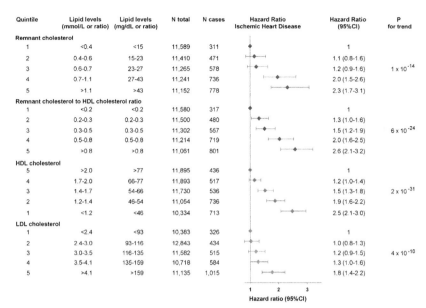

Quintile	Lipid levels (mmol/L or ratio)	Lipid levels (mg/dL or ratio)	N total	N cases	Hazard Ratio Ischemic Heart Disease	Hazard Ratio (95%CI)	P for trend
Remnant cholesterol							
1	<0.4	<15	11,589	311		1	
2	0.4-0.6	15-23	11,410	471		1.1 (0.8-1.6)	
3	0.6-0.7	23-27	11,265	578		1.2 (0.9-1.6)	1×10^{-14}
4	0.7-1.1	27-43	11,241	736		2.0 (1.5-2.6)	
5	>1.1	>43	11,152	778		2.3 (1.7-3.1)	
Remnant cholesterol to HDL cholesterol ratio							
1	<0.2	<0.2	11,580	317		1	
2	0.2-0.3	0.2-0.3	11,500	480		1.3 (1.0-1.6)	
3	0.3-0.5	0.3-0.5	11,302	557		1.5 (1.2-1.9)	6×10^{-24}
4	0.5-0.8	0.5-0.8	11,214	719		2.0 (1.6-2.5)	
5	>0.8	>0.8	11,061	801		2.6 (2.1-3.2)	
HDL cholesterol							
5	>2.0	>77	11,895	436		1	
4	1.7-2.0	66-77	11,893	517		1.2 (1.0-1.4)	
3	1.4-1.7	54-66	11,730	536		1.5 (1.3-1.8)	2×10^{-31}
2	1.2-1.4	46-54	11,054	736		1.9 (1.6-2.2)	
1	<1.2	<46	10,334	713		2.5 (2.1-3.0)	
LDL cholesterol							
1	<2.4	<93	10,383	326		1	
2	2.4-3.0	93-116	12,843	434		1.0 (0.8-1.3)	
3	3.0-3.5	116-135	11,582	515		1.2 (0.9-1.5)	4×10^{-10}
4	3.5-4.1	135-159	10,718	584		1.3 (1.0-1.6)	
5	>4.1	>159	11,135	1,015		1.8 (1.4-2.2)	

1   2   3
Hazard ratio (95%CI)

FIGURE 3.—Risk for ischemic heart disease: observational estimates. Risk for ischemic heart disease as a function of lipoprotein levels in quintiles in the prospective Copenhagen General Population Study, Copenhagen City Heart Study, and Copenhagen Ischemic Heart Disease Study controls combined. The *p* values are for trends across quintiles. CI = confidence interval; HDL = high-density lipoprotein; LDL = low-density lipoprotein. (Reprinted from the Journal of the American College of Cardiology. Varbo A, Benn M, Tybjærg-Hansen A, et al. Remnant cholesterol as a causal risk factor for ischemic heart disease. J Am Coll Cardiol. 2013;61:427-436, Copyright 2013, with permission from the American College of Cardiology.)

Conclusions.—A nonfasting remnant cholesterol increase of 1 mmol/l (39 mg/dl) is associated with a 2.8-fold causal risk for ischemic heart disease, independent of reduced HDL cholesterol. This implies that elevated cholesterol content of triglyceride-rich lipoprotein particles causes ischemic heart disease. However, because pleiotropic effects of the genetic variants studied cannot be totally excluded, these findings need to be confirmed using additional genetic variants and/or randomized intervention trials (Fig 3).

► When the triglyceride mass in chylomicrons and very low-density lipoproteins (VLDL) is incompletely digested by lipoprotein lipase, remnants of these lipoproteins are formed. It is controversial as to whether chylomicrons and their remnants are atherogenic. Chylomicrons, VLDLs, and their remnants are increased in the postprandial state, because these are the lipoproteins responsible for transporting lipids from enteric and hepatic sources, respectively. Evidence is building that apoB100-containing remnants (including small VLDL or VLDL3) and intermediate-density lipoproteins are associated with increased risk for atherosclerotic disease and such coronary artery disease events as myocardial infarction and death.

These authors explore the impact of nonfasting remnant cholesterol as a risk factor for ischemic heart disease (IHD) in 73 513 patients enrolled in the Copenhagen General Population Study, Copenhagen City Heart Study, and the Copenhagen Ischemic Heart Disease Study.[1] As might be expected, increased serum levels of triglycerides were highly correlated with increased levels of remnant cholesterol and reduced serum high-density lipoprotein cholesterol (HDL-C). Interquintile analyses of remnant cholesterol and remnant cholesterol/HDL-C showed progressive escalation of risk for IHD, with hazard ratios of 2.3 and 2.6, respectively, when comparing the fifth to the first quintile (Fig 3). Low serum levels of HDL-C correlated with an increased risk for IHD. Among patients with genotypes associated with increased remnant cholesterol, these authors also noted a causal odds ratio of 2.8 for every 39 mg/dL increase in serum remnant cholesterol.

In general, non-HDL-C is recognized as a better predictor of risk for IHD than is LDL-C.[2-4] Remnant lipoproteins are a component of non-HDL-C. It certainly makes considerable sense to lower all fractions of atherogenic lipoprotein burden, rather than focus on 1, namely LDL-C. Remnants warrant much more careful attention, but it will be some time before their specific measurement is incorporated into routine clinical practice. In the meantime, non-HDL-C is an important and easily calculated therapeutic target (ie, total cholesterol minus HDL-C) and its risk stratified target is simply LDL-C plus 30 mg/dL.

P. P. Toth, MD, PhD

References

1. Varbo A, Benn M, Tybjærg-Hansen A, Jørgensen AB, Frikke-Schmidt R, Nordestgaard BG. Remnant cholesterol as a causal risk factor for ischemic heart disease. *J Am Coll Cardiol.* 2013;61:427-436.
2. Liu J, Sempos CT, Donahue RP, Dorn J, Trevisan M, Grundy SM. Non-high-density lipoprotein and very-low-density lipoprotein cholesterol and their risk predictive values in coronary heart disease. *Am J Cardiol.* 2006;98:1363-1368.
3. Cui Y, Blumenthal RS, Flaws JA, et al. Non-high-density lipoprotein cholesterol level as a predictor of cardiovascular disease mortality. *Arch Intern Med.* 2001; 161:1413-1419.
4. Boekholdt SM, Arsenault BJ, Mora S, et al. Association of LDL cholesterol, non-HDL cholesterol, and apolipoprotein B levels with risk of cardiovascular events among patients treated with statins: a meta-analysis. *JAMA.* 2012;307:1302-1309.

Metabolic Syndrome

Low HDL Cholesterol and the Risk of Diabetic Nephropathy and Retinopathy: Results of the ADVANCE Study

Morton J, on Behalf of the Advance Collaborative Group (The Heart Res Inst, Sydney, New South Wales, Australia; et al)
Diabetes Care 35:2201-2206, 2012

Objective.—Although low HDL cholesterol (HDL-C) is an established risk factor for atherosclerosis, data on HDL-C and the risk of microvascular disease are limited. We tested the association between HDL-C and microvascular disease in a cohort of patients with type 2 diabetes.

Research Design and Methods.—A total of 11,140 patients with type 2 diabetes and at least one additional vascular risk factor were followed a median of 5 years. Cox proportional hazards models were used to assess the association between baseline HDL-C and the development of new or worsening microvascular disease, defined prospectively as a composite of renal and retinal events.

Results.—The mean baseline HDL-C level was 1.3 mmol/L (SD 0.45 mmol/L [range 0.1–4.0]). During follow-up, 32% of patients developed new or worsening microvascular disease, with 28% experiencing a renal event and 6% retinal event. Compared with patients in the highest third, those in the lowest third had a 17% higher risk of microvascular disease (adjusted hazard ratio 1.17 [95% CI 1.06–1.28], $P = 0.001$) after adjustment for potential confounders and regression dilution. This was driven by a 19% higher risk of renal events (1.19 [1.08–1.32], $P = 0.0005$). There was no association between thirds of HDL-C and retinal events (1.01 [0.82–1.25], $P = 0.9$).

Conclusions.—In patients with type 2 diabetes, HDL-C level is an independent risk factor for the development of microvascular disease affecting the kidney but not the retina.

▶ A common feature of diabetic dyslipidemia is a low serum level of high-density lipoprotein cholesterol (HDL-C). Insulin resistance initiates a broad range of biochemical changes at the level of the liver, adipose tissue, intravascular macrophages, and serum lipoprotein lipase activity that are associated with less HDL biogenesis and greater catabolism of this lipoprotein. Microangiopathy, including retinopathy, nephropathy, and neuropathy, is an important clinical sequela in the setting of inadequately controlled diabetes mellitus (DM). It is important to try to delineate more clearly whether derangements in lipid and lipoprotein metabolism contribute to the risk for diabetic microangiopathy.

Investigators from the ADVANCE study evaluated whether low serum levels of HDL-C correlate with risk for renal and retinal endpoints in 11 140 patients with type 2 DM over a median follow-up of 5 years. Twenty-eight percent of patients experienced a renal outcome, defined as microalbuminuria, macroalbuminuria, doubling of serum creatinine, renal-related death, and the need for renal replacement therapy. A retinal outcome occurred in 6% of patients and included the need for laser therapy for macular edema, proliferative retinopathy, and diabetes-related blindness. Comparing patients in the highest tertile of HDL-C with those in the lowest tertile, those in the lowest third had an 11% higher risk of adverse renal or retinal outcomes (Table 1 in the original article). Following multivariable adjustment (regression dilution, baseline age, gender, ethnicity, treatment groups, history of microvascular disease, smoking status, current drinking, hemoglobin A1c, body mass index, systolic blood pressure, diabetes duration, statin use, baseline creatinine, total cholesterol, and triglyceride levels), the risk was 17% higher. This increased risk was largely attributable to a 19% greater risk for developing some form of nephropathy. There was no apparent relationship between baseline tertiles of HDL-C and retinopathy.

The kidney plays an important role in HDL handling in that the cubulin-megalin system facilitates the renal metabolism and elimination of apoprotein A-I and small HDL particles. It is not possible to discern from these data if the low serum levels of HDL-C or the altered HDL proteome characteristic of diabetic dyslipidemia contributes to nephropathy. Based on these data no recommendation can be made to therapeutically increase HDL in an effort to reduce risk for developing diabetic nephropathy. However, this association should be studied further to more precisely determine whether HDL provides some type of nephroprotective or glomeruloprotective (perhaps through the antagonism of inflammation or oxidation or improved lipid handling) effect in patients with DM.

P. P. Toth, MD, PhD

Nutrition and Nutritional Supplements

Effects of *trans* fatty acids on glucose homeostasis: A meta-analysis of randomized, placebo-controlled clinical trials
Aronis KN, Khan SM, Mantzoros CS (VA Boston Healthcare System, MA; Beth Israel Deaconess Med Ctr, Boston, MA)
Am J Clin Nutr 96:1093-1099, 2012

Background.—Although evidence from cohort studies has suggested that *trans* fatty acid (TFA) consumption may be associated with insulin resistance and diabetes, randomized placebo-controlled trials (RCTs) have yielded conflicting results.

Objective.—In a meta-analysis, we combined all available RCTs that examined the role of TFA intake on glucose homeostasis.

Design.—A systematic review of PubMed was performed, and a total of 7 RCTs were included in the meta-analysis. Primary outcomes were glucose and insulin concentrations. Secondary outcomes were total, LDL-, and HDL-cholesterol and triglyceride concentrations. The pooled effect size (ES) was calculated through fixed- and random-effects meta-analyses. The potential existence of publication bias was evaluated by using funnel-plot analysis. Metaregression analysis was performed to evaluate for potential dose-response relations between the ES of outcomes and TFA intake.

Results.—Increased TFA intake did not result in significant changes in glucose or insulin concentrations. Increased TFA intake led to a significant increase in total and LDL-cholesterol [ES (95% CI): 0.28 (0.04, 0.51) and 0.36 (0.13, 0.60), respectively] and a significant decrease in HDL-cholesterol concentrations [ES (95% CI): −0.25 (−0.48, −0.01)]. Our analysis also showed the absence of publication bias and any dose-response relations between the ES and TFA intake.

Conclusions.—Increased TFA intake does not result in changes in glucose, insulin, or triglyceride concentrations but leads to an increase in total and LDL-cholesterol and a decrease in HDL-cholesterol concentrations. There

TABLE.—Characteristics of Studies Included in the Meta-Analysis[1]

Study	Year	Design	Sample Size (n)	Subjects	Duration (wk)	Control Diet	TFA Intake (% of Total Energy Intake)	Glucose (mmol/L) Control Group	Glucose (mmol/L) High-TFA Group	Insulin (μIU/mL) Control Group	Insulin (μIU/mL) High-TFA Group
Tardy et al (18)	2009	RCT	63	O	4	Isoenergetic substitution of TFAs with cis MUFAs	2.59	5.22 ± 0.01[2]	5.28 ± 0.01	10.00 ± 0.64	13.20 ± 1.19
Lovejoy et al (19)	2002	RCT-X	25	NO	4	Isoenergetic substitution of TFAs with oleic acid	9.0	4.90 ± 0.10	4.70 ± 0.10	26.2 ± 1.80	25.20 ± 1.8
Louheranta et al (20)	1999	RCT-X	14	NO	4	Isoenergetic substitution of TFAs with cis MUFAs	5.10	5.00 ± 0.10	5.00 ± 0.10	7.40 ± 0.50	8.10 ± 0.6
Lichtenstein et al (21)	2003	RCT-X	36	NO	5	Isoenergetic substitution of soybean oil with sticky margarine	7.83	5.06 ± 0.07	5.06 ± 0.09	11.20 ± 0.85	11.20 ± 0.81
Vega-López et al (23)	2006	RCT-X	15	HL	5	Isoenergetic substitution of TFAs with cis PUFAs	4.15	4.81 ± 0.10	4.94 ± 0.11	9.60 ± 0.97	11.50 ± 1.07
Sundram et al (22)	2007	RCT-X	30	NO	4	Isoenergetic substitution of partially hydrogenated soybean oil with palm olein	3.20	5.60 ± 0.01	5.90 ± 0.01	10.10 ± 0.15	9.10 ± 0.10
Bendsen et al (17)	2011	RCT	27C, 25T	OW, PM	16	Isoenergetic substitution of TFAs with oleic and palmitic acids	7.00	5.30 ± 0.02	5.20 ± 0.02	32.00 ± 2.07	33.00 ± 2.07

Editor's Note: Please refer to original journal article for full references.

[1] For all studies that had a crossover design, the sample size refers to the number of subjects who went through each phase of the study (ie, all subjects who completed a low–TFA-intake arm and a high–TFA-intake arm. For RCTs, the numbers of subjects who completed the low– and high–TFA-intake arms are given separately. C, control diet; HL, hyperlipidemic; NO, nonobese; O, obese; OW, overweight; PM, postmenopausal; RCT, randomized placebo-controlled trial; RCT-X, randomized placebo-controlled trial with crossover design; T, diet enriched with TFAs; TFA, trans fatty acid.

[2] Mean ± SEM (all such values).

is no evidence to support a potential benefit of the reduction of dietary TFA intake on glucose homeostasis (Table).

▶ Trans fatty acids (TFAs) are known to be associated with dyslipidemia, atherogenesis, and increased risk for cardiovascular morbidity and mortality. TFAs have become a sociopolitical issue, and the quantity of TFAs in foods is now explicitly included in its labeling. There has been significant suspicion that TFAs increase risk for insulin resistance and type 2 diabetes mellitus,[1,2] although testing this in a rigorous, prospective manner has been highly challenging.

These authors performed a meta-analysis of 7 randomized control trials (including 208 patients, average study size 30 patients) to evaluate the impact of TFAs on glucose and insulin concentrations and serum lipids. The average intake of TFAs was 2.6% to 7.8% of daily energy intake. The duration of studies varied from 4 to 16 weeks. These studies are summarized in Table 1. TFA consumption had no impact on either serum glucose or insulin levels (see Fig 1 in the original article). Increased TFA intake was significantly associated with increases in total cholesterol and low-density lipoprotein cholesterol (LDL-C), decreases in high-density lipoprotein cholesterol (HDL-C), and a nonsignificant trend for increasing serum triglycerides.

This meta-analysis provides the best attempt to date to evaluate whether TFAs have a dose—response relationship with risk for insulin resistance and type 2 diabetes mellitus. No correlation is demonstrable. It is, however, still important to curtail consumption of TFAs given the observation that they significantly increase LDL-C and reduce HDL-C. These changes contribute to the risk for all forms of atherosclerotic disease. The enrichment of food with TFAs remains a significant public health issue.

P. P. Toth, MD, PhD

References

1. Odegaard AO, Pereira MA. Trans fatty acids, insulin resistance, and type 2 diabetes. *Nutr Rev.* 2006;64:364-372.
2. Salmerón J, Hu FB, Manson JE, et al. Dietary fat intake and risk of type 2 diabetes in women. *Am J Clin Nutr.* 2001;73:1019-1026.

Pharmacologic Therapy

Efficacy and safety of a microsomal triglyceride transfer protein inhibitor in patients with homozygous familial hypercholesterolaemia: a single-arm, open-label, phase 3 study

Cuchel M, for the Phase 3 HoFH Lomitapide Study investigators (Univ of Pennsylvania, Philadelphia; et al)
Lancet 381:40-46, 2013

Background.—Patients with homozygous familial hypercholesterolaemia respond inadequately to existing drugs. We aimed to assess the efficacy and safety of the microsomal triglyceride transfer protein inhibitor lomitapide in adults with this disease.

TABLE.—Lipid and Lipoprotein Concentrations at Baseline and Weeks 26, 56, and 78 (End of Study)

	Baseline (n=29) Concentrations	Week 26 (n=23) Concentrations	Week 26 Change From Baseline (%)	Week 26 p Value†	Week 56 (n=23) Concentrations	Week 56 Change From Baseline (%)	Week 56 p value‡	Week 78 (n=23) Concentrations	Week 78 Change From Baseline (%)	Week 78 p Value‡
Total cholesterol, mmol/L	11.1 (3.5)	7.1 (3.7)	−46% (−56 to −35)	<0.0001	7.1 (3.7)	−39% (−51 to −27)	<0.0001	7.3 (3.9)	−35% (−48 to −22)	<0.0001
LDL cholesterol, mmol/L	8.7 (2.9)	5.1 (3.2)	−50% (−62 to −39)	<0.0001	5.1 (3.2)	−44% (−57 to −31)	<0.0001	5.4 (3.4)	−38% (−52 to −24)	0.0001
VLDL cholesterol, mmol/L	0.5 (0.3)	0.4 (0.4)	−45% (−61 to −29)	<0.0001	0.4 (0.4)	−28% (−48 to −10)	0.0185	0.4 (0.4)	−31% (−54 to −7)	0.0389
Non-HDL cholesterol, mmol/L	10.0 (3.4)	5.9 (3.6)	−50% (−61 to −39)	<0.0001	5.9 (3.6)	−44% (−57 to −31)	<0.0001	6.2 (3.8)	−39% (−53 to −25)	<0.0001
Triglycerides, mmol/L	1.0 (0.4 to 2.9)	0.7 (0.2 to 2.9)	−45% (−61 to −29)	<0.0001	0.7 (0.2 to 2.9)	−29% (−47 to −11)	0.0157	0.7 (0.2 to 4.1)	−31% (−54 to −8)	0.0368
ApoB, g/L	2.6 (0.8)	1.5 (0.8)	−49% (−60 to −38)	<0.0001	1.5 (0.8)	−45% (−57 to −33)	<0.0001	1.5 (0.9)	−43% (−56 to −29)	<0.0001
Lipoprotein (a), μmol/L	2.4 (0.6 to 21)	2.0 (0.5 to 8.6)	−15% (−30 to 0.9)	0.0003	2.0 (0.5 to 8.6)	−19% (−31 to −8)	0.0111	2.6 (0.6 to 7.0)	−1% (−17 to 6)	0.5827
HDL cholesterol, mmol/L	1.0 (0.4)	1.2 (0.4)	−12% (−20 to −4)	0.0001	1.1 (0.3)	1% (−13 to 15)	0.954	1.1 (0.3)	−5% (−13 to 3)	0.1396
ApoA-I, g/L	1.0 (0.2)	1.1 (0.3)	−14% (−17 to −4)	0.0003	1.1 (0.3)	1% (−11 to 13)	0.568	1.1 (0.3)	−4% (−10 to 3)	0.1155

Data are mean (SD), median (range) for triglycerides and lipoprotein (a) at baseline, weeks 26, 56, and 78, or mean (95% CI) for percent change.
†p values from mixed model.
‡p values from one-sample t test.

Methods.—We did a single-arm, open-label, phase 3 study of lomitapide for treatment of patients with homozygous familial hypercholesterolemia. Current lipid lowering therapy was maintained from 6 weeks before baseline through to at least week 26. Lomitapide dose was escalated on the basis of safety and tolerability from 5 mg to a maximum of 60 mg a day. The primary endpoint was mean percent change in levels of LDL cholesterol from baseline to week 26, after which patients remained on lomitapide through to week 78 for safety assessment. Percent change from baseline to week 26 was assessed with a mixed linear model.

Findings.—29 men and women with homozygous familial hypercholesterolaemia, aged 18 years or older, were recruited from 11 centres in four countries (USA, Canada, South Africa, and Italy). 23 of 29 enrolled patients completed both the efficacy phase (26 weeks) and the full study (78 weeks). The median dose of lomitapide was 40 mg a day. LDL cholesterol was reduced by 50% (95% CI −62 to −39) from baseline (mean 8·7 mmol/L [SD 2·9]) to week 26 (4·3 mmol/L [2·5]; $p < 0·0001$). Levels of LDL cholesterol were lower than 2·6 mmol/L in eight patients at 26 weeks. Concentrations of LDL cholesterol remained reduced by 44% (95% CI −57 to −31; $p < 0·0001$) at week 56 and 38% (−52 to −24; $p < 0·0001$) at week 78. Gastrointestinal symptoms were the most common adverse event. Four patients had aminotransaminase levels of more than five times the upper limit of normal, which resolved after dose reduction or temporary interruption of lomitapide. No patient permanently discontinued treatment because of liver abnormalities.

Interpretation.—Our study suggests that treatment with lomitapide could be a valuable drug in the management of homozygous familial hypercholesterolaemia (Table).

▶ Microsomal triglyceride transfer protein (MTTP) participates in the assembly of very low-density lipoproteins (VLDL) in hepatocytes. Patients with homozygous familial hypercholesterolemia (HoFH) have little-to-no functionality in their low-density lipoprotein (LDL) receptors and have severely compromised capacity to clear LDL cholesterol (LDL-C) from the central circulation.[1] This results in severe elevations of LDL-C of 500 to 1000 mg/dL. Homozygous FH occurs with a frequency of about 1 per million in the United States and is encountered throughout the world. HoFH is associated with severe premature-onset multivessel coronary artery disease and early mortality, with untreated patients frequently dying of myocardial infarction by the second or third decade of life. Lipid-lowering therapy with statins, ezetimibe, and bile acid—binding resins frequently do not work as well in patients with HoFH because of impaired LDL receptor functionality. Newer therapies have been sorely needed to help reduce the atherogenic lipoprotein burden in these patients.

Lomitapide is an orally administered MTTP inhibitor. Cuchel et al performed a single-arm, open-label, phase 3 study of lomitapide therapy in 23 patients with HoFH. Serum levels of total cholesterol, LDL-C, VLDL-C, apoprotein B100, and triglycerides were all reduced significantly at 26, 56, and 78 weeks (Table). Nine of 23 patients experienced elevations in their serum transaminases, but no one discontinued medication because of this. Elevations in serum transaminases were successfully treated by drug dose reduction or temporarily discontinuing drug therapy. Intrahepatic fat increased by approximately 8.6% as measured by magnetic resonance imaging (Fig 1 in the original article). The magnitude of reduction in atherogenic lipoproteins was attenuated over time likely because of reduced need for apheresis and adjustment in the doses of drugs given concomitantly with lomitapide.

Lomitapide is now approved for use in patients with HoFH. This MTTP inhibitor constitutes an important new intervention for patients with HoFH and reduces LDL-C and non—high-density lipoprotein cholesterol by up to 50% and VLDL-C by up to 45%. The accumulation of intrahepatic fat appears to plateau by week 26. Lomitapide has orphan drug status. It will be important to establish long-term safety with this medication, but it is an important alternative to LDL-C apheresis.

P. P. Toth, MD, PhD

Reference

1. Hopkins PN, Toth PP, Ballantyne CM, Rader DJ. Familial hypercholesterolemias: prevalence, genetics, diagnosis and screening recommendations from the National Lipid Association Expert Panel on Familial Hypercholesterolemia. *J Clin Lipidol.* 2011;5:S9-S17.

Effects of AMG 145 on Low-Density Lipoprotein Cholesterol Levels: Results From 2 Randomized, Double-Blind, Placebo-Controlled, Ascending-Dose Phase 1 Studies in Healthy Volunteers and Hypercholesterolemic Subjects on Statins

Dias CS, Shaywitz AJ, Wasserman SM, et al (Med Sciences, Amgen, Thousand Oaks, CA; Global Development, Amgen, Thousand Oaks, CA; et al)
J Am Coll Cardiol 60:1888-1898, 2012

Objectives.—The aim of this study was to evaluate the safety, tolerability, and effects of AMG 145 on low-density lipoprotein cholesterol (LDL-C) in healthy and hypercholesterolemic subjects on statin therapy.

Background.—Proprotein convertase subtilisin/kexin type 9 (PCSK9) down-regulates surface expression of the low-density lipoprotein receptor (LDL-R), increasing serum LDL-C. AMG 145, a fully human monoclonal antibody to PCSK9, prevents PCSK9/LDL-R interaction, restoring LDL-R recycling.

Methods.—Healthy adults (phase 1a) were randomized to 1 dose of AMG 145: 7, 21, 70, 210, or 420 mg SC; 21 or 420 mg IV; or matching placebo. Hypercholesterolemic adults (phase 1b) receiving low- to moderate-dose statins were randomized to multiple SC doses of AMG 145: 14 or 35 mg once weekly (QW) ×6, 140 or 280 mg every 2 weeks (Q2W) ×3, 420 mg every 4 weeks ×2, or matching placebo. Eleven subjects receiving high-dose statins and 6 subjects with heterozygous familial hypercholesterolemia were randomized to SC AMG 145 140 mg or placebo Q2W ×3.

A   Phase 1a: AMG 145 or Placebo, Single Ascending SC or IV Doses in Healthy Subjects

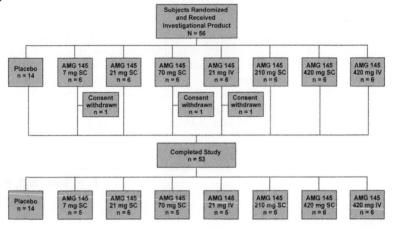

B   Phase 1b: AMG 145 or Placebo, Multiple Ascending SC Doses in Subjects with Hypercholesterolemia

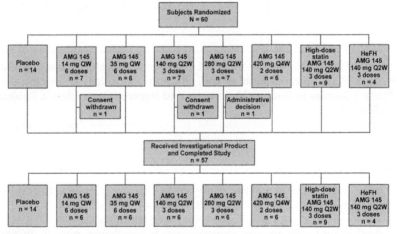

FIGURE 2.—Subject disposition. Three subjects in each study discontinued the studies, none because of adverse events. Abbreviations as in Figure 1. (Reprinted from the Journal of the American College of Cardiology. Dias CS, Shaywitz AJ, Wasserman SM, et al. Effects of AMG 145 on low-density lipoprotein cholesterol levels: results from 2 randomized, double-blind, placebo-controlled, ascending-dose phase 1 studies in healthy volunteers and hypercholesterolemic subjects on statins. *J Am Coll Cardiol.* 2012;60:1888-1898, Copyright 2012, with permission from the American College of Cardiology.)

Results.—In the trials (AMG 145 n = 85, placebo n = 28), AMG 145 reduced LDL-C up to 64% (*p* < 0.0001) versus placebo after 1 dose ≥ 21 mg and up to 81% (*p* < 0.001) with repeated doses ≥ 35 mg QW. No serious adverse events (AEs) occurred. Overall incidence of treatment-emergent AEs was similar in AMG 145 versus placebo groups: 69% versus 71% (phase 1a); 65% versus 64% (phase 1b).

Conclusions.—In phase 1 studies, AMG 145 significantly reduced serum LDL-C in healthy and hypercholesterolemic statin-treated subjects,

TABLE 2.—AMG 145 on Lipids: Mean Percentage Change

Healthy Subjects (Phase 1a): Change From Baseline at Nadir

Parameter	7 mg SC (n = 6)	21 mg SC (n = 6)	70 mg SC (n = 6)	210 mg SC (n = 6)	420 mg SC (n = 6)	21 mg IV (n = 6)	420 mg IV (n = 6)	Placebo (n = 14)
				AMG 145				
LDL-C								
Change from baseline, mean	−10%	−37%	−55%	−55%	−67%	−42%	−63%	−9%
Time to nadir, days	7	6	11	15	22	5	22	
Change vs. placebo, mean	−6%	−31%	−53%	−53%	−64%	−38%	−61%	
Time to nadir, days	4	5	11	15	22	5	22	
p value, change vs. placebo	0.4412	<0.0001	<0.0001	<0.0001	<0.0001	<0.0001	<0.0001	
Total cholesterol								
Change from baseline, mean	−10%	−29%	−38%	−40%	−44%	−28%	−47%	−10%
Time to nadir, days	8	5	11	15	22	5	22	
Change vs. placebo, mean	−3%	−21%	−32%	−36%	−40%	−21%	−43%	
Time to nadir, days	4	5	11	15	15	5	22	
p value, change vs. placebo	0.5287	<0.0001	<0.0001	<0.0001	<0.0001	<0.0001	<0.0001	
ApoB								
Change from baseline, mean	−16%	−31%	−48%	−49%	−57%	−34%	−56%	−15%
Time to nadir, days	8	5	11	15	22	5	22	
Change vs. placebo, mean	−6%	−25%	−42%	−45%	−55%	−28%	−53%	
Time to nadir, days	8	5	11	15	22	5	22	
p value, change vs. placebo	0.3446	<0.0001	<0.0001	<0.0001	<0.0001	<0.0001	<0.0001	

Subjects With Hypercholesterolemia (Phase 1b); Mean Percentage Change at End of Dosing Interval* and Mean Maximum Change

Parameter	Low- to Moderate-Dose Statins, Non-HeFH					High-Dose Statins 140 mg Q2W (3 doses) (n = 9)	HeFH 140 mg Q2W (3 doses) (n = 4)	Placebo[†] (n = 14)
	14 mg QW (6 doses) (n = 6)	35 mg QW (6 doses) (n = 6)	140 mg Q2W (3 doses) (n = 6)	280 mg Q2W (3 doses) (n = 6)	420 mg Q4W (2 doses) (n = 6)			
			AMG 145[†]					
LDL-C								
End of the dosing interval								
Change from baseline, mean	−24%	−55%	−73%	−75%	−63%	−65%	−66%	−2%
Change vs. placebo, mean	−22%	−54%	−73%	−75%	−66%	−63%	−65%	

(Continued)

TABLE 2.—(*Continued*)

Subjects With Hypercholesterolemia (Phase 1b): Mean Percentage Change at End of Dosing Interval* and Mean Maximum Change

Parameter	AMG 145†						High-Dose Statins 140 mg Q2W (3 doses) (n = 9)	HeFH 140 mg Q2W (3 doses) (n = 4)	Placebo† (n = 14)
	14 mg QW (6 doses) (n = 6)	Low- to Moderate-Dose Statins, Non-HeFH			420 mg Q4W (2 doses) (n = 6)				
		35 mg QW (6 doses) (n = 6)	140 mg Q2W (3 doses) (n = 6)	280 mg Q2W (3 doses) (n = 6)					
p value, change vs. placebo	0.14	<0.001	<0.001	<0.001	<0.001		<0.001	<0.001	
Maximum reduction at nadir									
Change from baseline, mean	−31%	−61%	−81%	−75%	−79%		−78%	−73%	−5%
Change vs. placebo, mean	−34%	−60%	−81%	−76%	−80%		−77%	−70%	
p value, change vs. placebo	0.015	0.001	<0.001	<0.001	<0.001		<0.001	<0.001	
Total cholesterol									
End of the dosing interval									
Change from baseline, mean	−15%	−35%	−46%	−41%	−41%		−36%	−41%	−2%
Change vs. placebo, mean	−14%	−34%	−45%	−40%	−45%		−35%	−42%	
p value, change vs. placebo	0.058	0.001	<0.001	<0.001	<0.001		<0.001	<0.001	
Maximum reduction									
Change from baseline, mean	−21%	−38%	−49%	−42%	−52%		−50%	−49%	−2%
Change vs. placebo, mean	−20%	−37%	−50%	−42%	−52%		−49%	−47%	
p value, change vs. placebo	0.006	0.001	<0.001	<0.001	<0.001		<0.001	<0.001	
ApoB									
End of the dosing interval									
Change from baseline, mean	−19%	−46%	−53%	−56%	−50%		−48%	−46%	−4%
Change vs. placebo, mean	−15%	−43%	−51%	−54%	−52%		−50%	−47%	

p value, change vs. placebo	0.096	<0.001	<0.001	<0.001	<0.001	<0.001	<0.001	
Maximum reduction at nadir								
Change from baseline, mean	−25%	−48%	−58%	−56%	−61%	−59%	−56%	
Change vs. placebo, mean	−25%	−48%	−59%	−56%	−59%	−59%	−57%	−6%
p value, change vs. placebo	0.004	<0.001	<0.001	<0.001	<0.001	<0.001	<0.001	
Lp(a)‡	n = 3	n = 4	n = 4	n = 2	n = 5	n = 7	n = 3	n = 13
End of the dosing interval								
Change from baseline, mean	−20%	−30%	−33%	−37%	−38%	−45%	−50%	
Change vs. placebo, mean	−16%	−27%	−30%	−34%	−35%	−43%	−50%	−4%
p value, change vs. placebo	0.28	0.033	0.016	0.027	0.001	<0.001	<0.001	
Maximum reduction at nadir								
Change from baseline, mean	−25%	−38%	−33%	−44%	−38%	−45%	−50%	−10%
Change vs. placebo, mean	−18%	−31%	−30%	−37%	−35%	−43%	−50%	
p value, change vs. placebo	0.21	0.011	0.016	0.015	0.001	<0.001	<0.001	

Data from subjects who withdrew early were excluded.
Abbreviations as in Table 1.
*The end of the dosing interval was day 43 for the QW and Q2W dose groups and day 57 for the Q4W dose group.
†In the study of hypercholesterolemic subjects (phase 1b), all doses of AMG 145 and placebo were SC.
‡The Lp(a) level was measured on day 43 for all cohorts. The analysis excluded subjects with screening or baseline Lp(a) values below the level of quantification and 1 subject whose baseline value seemed implausibly high compared with post-baseline values.

including those with heterozygous familial hypercholesterolemia or taking the highest doses of atorvastatin or rosuvastatin, with an overall AE profile similar to placebo (Fig 2, Table 2).

▶ Proprotein convertase subtilisin/kexin type 9 (PCSK9) is an important therapeutic target in patients with elevated serum low-density lipoprotein cholesterol (LDL-C). PCSK9 gain-of-function mutations associate with autosomal dominant hypercholesterolemia,[1] whereas loss-of-function mutations give rise to lifelong reductions in serum LDL-C and are associated with reduced risk for coronary heart disease.[2] PCSK9 function is something of a chaperone molecule, in that it binds the LDL receptor and the PCSK9-LDL receptor complex concentrate in clathrin-coated pits and is then taken up into the cell.[3] Once internalized, PCSK9 directs the LDL receptor to the endosomal compartment for degradation. Hence, any loss of function mutation or therapeutic intervention that limited the activity of PCSK9 would be associated with increased hepatocyte cell surface expression of LDL receptors, augmented capacity for LDL-C clearance, and reduced levels of serum cholesterol. Such an approach would be legitimate for patients capable of expressing functional LDL receptors, such as those with primary hyperlipidemia or heterozygous familial hypercholesterolemia. A novel approach to this is the development of human monoclonal antibodies that bind to PCSK9 and sterically hinder its interaction with LDL receptors.

AMG 145 is a human monoclonal antibody against PCSK9. The efficacy of this drug was tested in healthy humans on no medication. Patients on low-to-moderate-dose statin therapy, high-dose statin therapy, or patients with heterozygous hypercholesterolemia were randomly assigned to multiple weekly subcutaneous doses of AMG 145. Dose-dependent reductions were seen in LDL-C of up to 64%, total cholesterol of up to 40%, and apoprotein B of up to 55% compared with placebo. In patients on low-to-moderate-dose statin therapy, high-dose statin therapy, and those with heterozygous familial hypercholesterolemia, LDL-C decreased by up to 66%, 63%, and 65%, respectively (Fig 2, Table 2). AMG 145 also induced marked reductions in lipoprotein(a) (Lp[a]).

The inhibition of PCSK9 with monoclonal antibody therapy constitutes an important and novel approach to reducing the burden of atherogenic lipoproteins, including Lp(a). Safety studies of these agents to date suggest no undo risk for myopathy or hepatotoxicity. These agents are generally quite well tolerated. They will constitute an exciting new therapy for patients with primary hyperlipidemia, familial combined hyperlipidemia, and heterozygous familial hypercholesterolemia. They will provide a valued treatment alternative to statin-intolerant patients and will be a key adjuvant therapy for patients who cannot get their LDL-C level to goal on statin monotherapy.

P. P. Toth, MD, PhD

References

1. Abifadel M, Varret M, Rabès JP, et al. Mutations in PCSK9 cause autosomal dominant hypercholesterolemia. *Nat Genet.* 2003;34:154-156.
2. Cohen JC, Boerwinkle E, Mosley TH Jr, Hobbs HH. Sequence variations in PCSK9, low LDL, and protection against coronary heart disease. *N Engl J Med.* 2006;354:1264-1272.

3. Horton JD, Cohen JC, Hobbs HH. Molecular biology of PCSK9: its role in LDL metabolism. *Trends Biochem Sci.* 2007;32:71-77.

Efficacy and Safety of Eicosapentaenoic Acid Ethyl Ester (AMR101) Therapy in Statin-Treated Patients With Persistent High Triglycerides (from the ANCHOR Study)

Ballantyne CM, Bays HE, Kastelein JJ, et al (Baylor College of Medicine and the Methodist DeBakey Heart and Vascular Ctr, Houston, TX; Louisville Metabolic and Atherosclerosis Res Ctr, KY; Academic Med Ctr, Amsterdam, The Netherlands; et al)

Am J Cardiol 110:984-992, 2012

AMR101 is an ω-3 fatty acid agent containing ≥96% pure icosapentethyl, the ethyl ester of eicosapentaenoic acid. The efficacy and safety of AMR101 were evaluated in this phase 3, multicenter, placebo-controlled, randomized, double-blinded, 12-week clinical trial (ANCHOR) in high-risk statin-treated patients with residually high triglyceride (TG) levels

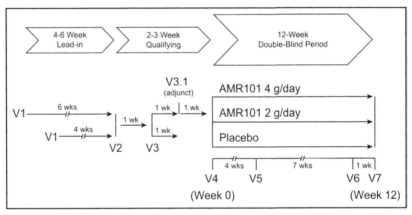

FIGURE 1.—Study design. The screening period consisted of a 4- to 6-week lead-in period during which patients underwent diet and lifestyle stabilization and nonstatin lipid-altering treatment washout if necessary. At the first screening visit, patients not taking a statin were initiated on statin therapy and likely to achieve a low-density lipoprotein cholesterol goal of <100 mg/dl and all patients received counseling on the National Cholesterol Education Program Therapeutic Lifestyle Changes diet.[2] Patients then entered a 2- to 3-week qualifying period. Lipid qualifications included an average fasting triglyceride level ≥200 and <500 mg/dl and an average fasting low-density lipoprotein cholesterol level ≥40 and <100 mg/dl based on the average (arithmetic mean) of 2 visits. If the average triglyceride and/or low-density lipoprotein cholesterol level was outside the required range, an additional measurement could be obtained at a third visit 1 week later, with eligibility determined based on the last 2 visits. Eligible patients were randomized 1 week later to AMR101 4 g/day (2 AMR101 1-g capsules 2 times/day), AMR101 2 g/day (1 AMR101 1-g capsule plus 1 matching placebo capsule 2 times/day), or placebo (2 matching placebo capsules 2 times/day). Investigators and patients were blinded to treatment assignment throughout the double-blinded, placebo-controlled, 12-week treatment period. Visit 1 (V1) was 6 weeks for patients requiring washout and 4 weeks for patients not requiring washout. V2 to V7 = visits 2 to 7. *Editor's Note:* Please refer to original journal article for full references. (Reprinted from the American Journal of Cardiology. Ballantyne CM, Bays HE, Kastelein JJ, et al. Efficacy and safety of eicosapentaenoic acid ethyl ester (AMR101) therapy in statin-treated patients with persistent high triglycerides (from the ANCHOR Study). *Am J Cardiol.* 2012;110:984-992, Copyright 2012, with permission from Elsevier.)

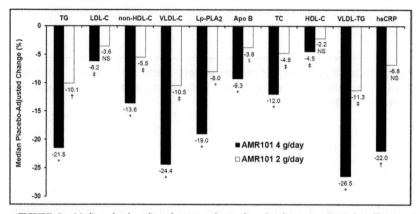

FIGURE 3.—Median placebo-adjusted percent change from baseline to week 12 for efficacy end points (intent-to-treat population). $*p < 0.0001$; $^{\dagger}p < 0.001$; $^{\ddagger}p < 0.01$; $^{\S}p < 0.05$. apo B = apolipoprotein B; HDL-C = high-density lipoprotein cholesterol; hsCRP = high-sensitivity C-reactive protein; LDL-C = low-density lipoprotein cholesterol; Lp-PLA$_2$ = lipoprotein-associated phospholipase A$_2$; non-HDL-C = non-high-density lipoprotein cholesterol; NS = not significant; TC = total cholesterol; TG = triglyceride; VLDL-C = very-low-density lipoprotein cholesterol; VLDL-TG = very-low-density lipoprotein triglyceride. (Reprinted from the American Journal of Cardiology. Ballantyne CM, Bays HE, Kastelein JJ, et al. Efficacy and safety of eicosapentaenoic acid ethyl ester (AMR101) therapy in statin-treated patients with persistent high triglycerides (from the ANCHOR Study). *Am J Cardiol*. 2012;110:984-992, Copyright 2012, with permission from Elsevier.)

(≥ 200 and < 500 mg/dl) despite low-density lipoprotein (LDL) cholesterol control (≥ 40 and < 100 mg/dl). Patients (n = 702) on a stable diet were randomized to AMR101 4 or 2 g/day or placebo. The primary end point was median percent change in TG levels from baseline versus placebo at 12 weeks. AMR101 4 and 2 g/day significantly decreased TG levels by 21.5% ($p < 0.0001$) and 10.1% ($p = 0.0005$), respectively, and non-high-density lipoprotein (non-HDL) cholesterol by 13.6% ($p < 0.0001$) and 5.5% ($p = 0.0054$), respectively. AMR101 4 g/day produced greater TG and non-HDL cholesterol decreases in patients with higher-efficacy statin regimens and greater TG decreases in patients with higher baseline TG levels. AMR101 4 g/day decreased LDL cholesterol by 6.2% ($p = 0.0067$) and decreased apolipoprotein B (9.3%), total cholesterol (12.0%), very-low-density lipoprotein cholesterol (24.4%), lipoprotein-associated phospholipase A$_2$ (19.0%), and high-sensitivity C-reactive protein (22.0%) versus placebo ($p < 0.001$ for all comparisons). AMR101 was generally well tolerated, with safety profiles similar to placebo. In conclusion, AMR101 4 g/day significantly decreased median placebo-adjusted TG, non-HDL cholesterol, LDL cholesterol, apolipoprotein B, total cholesterol, very-low-density lipoprotein cholesterol, lipoprotein-associated phospholipase A$_2$, and high-sensitivity C-reactive protein in statin-treated patients with residual TG elevations (Figs 1 and 3, Table 2).

▶ The omega-3 fish oils are highly effective agents for reducing serum levels of very low-density lipoproteins (VLDL) and triglycerides. In general, the omega-3

TABLE 2.—Changes in Efficacy End Points from Baseline to Week 12 (Intent-to-Treat Population)

| Variable | AMR101 Dose 4 g/day (n = 226) | | | AMR101 Dose 2 g/day (n = 234) | | | Placebo (n = 227) | | | Median Placebo-Adjusted Change From Baseline | | | |
	Baseline	End of Treatment	Change From Baseline (%)	Baseline	End of Treatment	Change From Baseline (%)	Baseline	End of Treatment	Change From Baseline (%)	AMR101 4 g/day vs Placebo (%)	p Value	AMR101 2 g/day vs Placebo (%)	p Value
Primary end point													
Triglycerides (mg/dl) (n = 226, 234, 227)	264.8 (93.0)	220.8 (92.0)	−17.5 (31.0)	254.0 (92.5)	244.3 (117.0)	−5.6 (34.5)	259.0 (81.0)	269.5 (149.5)	5.9 (44.9)	−21.5	<0.0001	−10.1	0.0005
Secondary end points													
Low-density lipoprotein cholesterol (mg/dl) (n = 225, 233, 226)	82.0 (25.0)	83.0 (31.0)	1.5 (26.6)	82.0 (24.0)	87.0 (27.0)	2.4 (26.1)	84.0 (27.0)	88.5 (31.0)	8.8 (31.0)	−6.2	0.0067	−3.6	0.0867
Non-high-density lipoprotein cholesterol (mg/dl) (n = 226, 234, 227)	128.0 (32.0)	122.0 (39.0)	−5.0 (21.3)	128.0 (33.0)	134.0 (41.0)	2.4 (26.1)	128.0 (34.0)	138.0 (43.0)	9.8 (27.6)	−13.6	<0.0001	−5.5	0.0054
Very-low-density lipoprotein cholesterol (mg/dl) (n = 225, 233, 226)	44.0 (21.0)	38.0 (22.0)	−12.1 (47.9)	43.0 (21.0)	44.0 (25.0)	1.6 (54.6)	42.0 (21.0)	49.0 (28.0)	15.0 (58.8)	−24.4	<0.0001	−10.5	0.0093
Lipoprotein-associated phospholipase A_2 (ng/ml) (n = 217, 224, 213)	180.0 (56.0)	160.0 (57.0)	−12.8 (18.5)	190.0 (55.5)	183.5 (57.5)	−1.8 (23.1)	185.0 (58.0)	200.0 (71.0)	6.7 (24.0)	−19.0	<0.0001	−8.0	<0.0001

(Continued)

TABLE 2.—(*Continued*)

Variable	AMR101 Dose 4 g/day (n = 226)			2 g/day (n = 234)			Placebo (n = 227)			Median Placebo-Adjusted Change From Baseline			
	Baseline	End of Treatment	Change From Baseline (%)	Baseline	End of Treatment	Change From Baseline (%)	Baseline	End of Treatment	Change From Baseline (%)	AMR101 4 g/day vs Placebo (%)	p Value	AMR101 2 g/day vs Placebo (%)	p Value
Apolipoprotein B (mg/dl) (n = 217, 227, 219)	93.0 (23.0)	90.0 (25.0)	−2.2 (16.4)	91.0 (22.0)	95.0 (24.0)	1.6 (20.7)	91.0 (24.0)	98.0 (25.0)	7.1 (23.2)	−9.3	<0.0001	−3.8	0.0170
Selected exploratory end points													
Total cholesterol (mg/dl) (n = 226, 234, 227)	167.0 (38.0)	162.0 (38.0)	−3.2 (16.8)	169.0 (34.0)	175.0 (44.0)	2.1 (19.6)	168.0 (38.0)	181.0 (46.0)	9.1 (20.8)	−12.0	<0.0001	−4.8	0.0019
High-density lipoprotein cholesterol (mg/dl) (n = 226, 234, 227)	37.0 (12.0)	37.0 (13.0)	−1.0 (18.2)	38.0 (13.0)	38.0 (11.0)	0.0 (19.5)	39.0 (12.0)	40.0 (14.0)	4.8 (22.0)	−4.5	0.0013	−2.2	0.1265
Very-low-density lipoprotein triglycerides (mg/dl) (n = 225, 233, 226)	190.0 (99.0)	147.0 (88.0)	−19.2 (46.2)	185.0 (86.0)	168.0 (98.0)	−2.1 (48.9)	183.0 (94.0)	196.0 (136.0)	8.9 (63.8)	−26.5	<0.0001	−11.3	0.0049
High-sensitivity C-reactive protein (mg/l) (n = 217, 227, 219)	2.2 (2.7)	2.0 (3.0)	−2.4 (62.8)	1.9 (2.9)	2.5 (3.4)	10.3 (88.6)	2.2 (4.0)	2.6 (4.7)	17.1 (108.0)	−22.0	0.0005	−6.8	0.2889

Data are presented as median (interquartile range) for end point values.

fish oils, eicosapentaenoic acid (EPA) and docosahexaenoic acid (DHA), induce these changes by promoting mitochondrial oxidation of fatty acid, inhibiting diacylglycerol acyltransferase-2 and triglyceride biosynthesis, decreasing VLDL secretion and increasing VLDL lipolysis by activating lipoprotein lipase.[1] EPA monotherapy was found to provide incremental reduction in risk for cardiovascular events over and above statin therapy in the JELIS trial.[2] One feature of fish oil therapy with EPA/DHA is that low-density lipoprotein cholesterol (LDL-C) tends to increase in proportion to the magnitude of VLDL and triglyceride reduction.

Ballantyne et al investigated the impact of multiple doses of the ethyl ester of EPA (AMR101 or Vascepa) on serum lipids and other markers of risk in the ANCHOR study. The study compared 2.0- and 4.0-g doses of AMR101 with placebo in patients with fasting triglycerides of 200 to 499 mg/dL and baseline LDL-C ≤100 mg/dL (Fig 1). Dose-dependent reductions in serum triglyceride, non−high-density lipoprotein cholesterol, apo B, and VLDL were observed, and LDL-C decreased slightly (Fig 3). In addition, the investigators found small but significant reductions in high-sensitivity C-reactive protein and lipoprotein-associated phospholipase A_2 levels, both important markers of inflammation and possible atherosclerotic plaque instability (Table 2).

Vascepa provides a therapeutic alternative to combination EPA/DHA therapy. It provides substantial reductions in triglycerides and atherogenic lipoprotein burden without inducing elevations in LDL-C. Moreover, these changes are significant when serum triglycerides are in the range of 200 to 499 mg/dL, not just > 500 mg/dL. The study showed excellent tolerability and no increased risk for liver or skeletal muscle toxicity.

P. P. Toth, MD, PhD

References

1. Toth PP, Dayspring TD, Pokrywka GS. Drug therapy for hypertriglyceridemia: fibrates and omega-3 fatty acids. *Curr Atheroscler Rep.* 2009;11:71-79.
2. Yokoyama M, Origasa H, Matsuzaki M, et al. Effects of eicosapentaenoic acid on major coronary events in hypercholesterolaemic patients (JELIS): a randomised open-label, blinded endpoint analysis. *Lancet.* 2007;369:1090-1098.

Effect of *Ezetimibe* on Major Atherosclerotic Disease Events and All-Cause Mortality
Hayek S, Canepa Escaro F, Sattar A, et al (Henry Ford Health System, Detroit, MI; et al)
Am J Cardiol 111:532-539, 2013

Despite ezetimibe's ability to reduce serum cholesterol levels, there are concerns over its vascular effects and whether it prevents or ameliorates atherosclerotic disease (AD). The aims of this study were to estimate the effect of ezetimibe use on major AD events and all-cause mortality and to compare these associations to those observed for hydroxymethylglutaryl coenzyme A reductase inhibitor (statin) use. A total of 367 new ezetimibe

TABLE 4.—Relation of Ezetimibe Monotherapy and Statin Monotherapy with the Primary Composite Outcome Stratified by Subgroups*

Outcome	Treatment	Number of Events	OR (95% CI)[†]	p Value	Wald Test p Value[‡]
Gender					
Male		81			0.188
	Ezetimibe		0.55 (0.15–2.04)	0.373	
	Statin		1.37 (0.61–3.07)	0.448	
Female		99			0.747
	Ezetimibe		0.25 (0.06–0.96)	0.043	
	Statin		0.31 (0.15–0.64)	0.001	
Race/ethnicity					
African American		33			0.343
	Ezetimibe		0.11 (0.01–2.19)	0.148	
	Statin		0.47 (0.12–1.79)	0.267	
White		145			0.745
	Ezetimibe		0.50 (0.19–1.36)	0.176	
	Statin		0.60 (0.33–1.08)	0.091	
History of AD[§]					
Yes		84			0.631
	Ezetimibe		0.56 (0.18–1.76)	0.324	
	Statin		0.42 (0.19–0.94)	0.034	
No		96			0.073
	Ezetimibe		0.11 (0.01–0.88)	0.037	
	Statin		0.75 (0.37–1.55)	0.441	
History of diabetes					
Yes		68			0.102
	Ezetimibe		0.15 (0.03–0.81)	0.027	
	Statin		0.61 (0.26–1.45)	0.263	
No		112			0.840
	Ezetimibe		0.59 (0.19–1.80)	0.353	
	Statin		0.67 (0.33–1.32)	0.245	
eGFR (ml/min/1.73 m^2)[‖]					
<60		52			—
	Ezetimibe		—	—	
	Statin		0.47 (0.15–1.48)	0.198	
≥60		123			0.429
	Ezetimibe		0.44 (0.14–1.38)	0.161	
	Statin		0.72 (0.36–1.41)	0.333	

Editor's Note: Please refer to original journal article for full references.

*The primary study outcome was a composite of all-cause death and major AD events (i.e., acute myocardial infarction, unstable angina, coronary revascularization procedures, cerebrovascular accidents, transient ischemic attacks, carotid revascularization, and peripheral vascular occlusive disease events).

[†]Ezetimibe use and statin use are estimated as CMMEs. However, statin use is weighted to account for differences in statin dose and preparation. Effect estimates represent the difference in going from no use to use of the maximal strength preparation every day.

[‡]The Wald test assesses differences in the effect estimates for ezetimibe and statins.

[§]Subjects were considered to have AD at baseline if they had previous diagnoses of coronary heart disease (i.e., myocardial infarction, unstable angina, or coronary revascularization), cerebrovascular disease (i.e., cerebrovascular accident, transient ischemic attack, or carotid revascularization), or peripheral vascular occlusive disease.

[‖]Estimated using the MDRD formula.[11]

users were identified from November 1, 2002, to December 31, 2009. These subjects were aged ≥ 18 years and had no previous statin use. One to 4 statin user matches were identified for each ezetimibe user, resulting in a total of 1,238 closely matched statin users. Pharmacy data and drug dosage information were used to estimate a moving window of ezetimibe and statin exposure for each day of study follow-up. The primary outcome was a composite of major AD events (coronary heart disease, cerebrovascular disease, and peripheral vascular disease events) and all-cause death. Ezetimibe use (odds ratio 0.33, 95% confidence interval 0.13 to 0.86) and statin use (odds ratio 0.61, 95% confidence interval 0.36 to 1.04) were associated with reductions in the likelihood of the composite outcome. These protective associations were most significant for cerebrovascular disease events and all-cause death. Subgroup analyses by gender, race or ethnicity, history of AD, diabetes status, and estimated renal function showed consistent estimates across strata, with no significant differences between ezetimibe and statin use. In conclusion, ezetimibe appeared to have a protective effect on major AD events and all-cause death that was not significantly different from that observed for statin use (Table 4).

▶ Since publication of the ENHANCE trial, doubt has lingered about the therapeutic efficacy of ezetimibe, an inhibitor of Niemann-pick C1-like 1 protein, a cholesterol transporter located along the jejunal enterocyte surface. It is likely that ezetimibe provided no incremental benefit in terms of carotid intima media thickness (CIMT) change over and above statin therapy because the starting CIMT of 0.69 mm was simply too low.[1] In the SANDS trial, ezetimibe did provide incremental capacity to regress CIMT when used in combination with simvastatin therapy in Native-American patients with diabetes mellitus.[2] CIMT regression correlated with magnitude of low-density lipoprotein cholesterol (LDL-C) reduction. Similarly in the SHARP trial, the treatment of patients with chronic kidney disease with simvastatin and ezetimibe reduced risk for the primary composite endpoint.[3] These investigators also showed that risk decreased in proportion to the magnitude of LDL-C reduction.

There are no prospective, randomized trials that compare ezetimibe monotherapy with statin therapy. Hayek et al performed an analysis of outcomes on patients from a health management organization database. These investigators compared the effect of ezetimibe (N = 367) and statin (N = 1238) therapy on major atherosclerotic disease events and all-cause mortality with an average follow-up of 51 months. When evaluating the impact of ezetimibe on the primary outcome of all-cause mortality, acute myocardial infarction, unstable angina, coronary and carotid revascularization, cerebrovascular accident, transient ischemic attacks, and peripheral vascular disease—related events, risk is reduced by 67% (P = .024). Risks for all-cause mortality and cerebrovascular disease were also significantly reduced as secondary endpoints, but coronary heart disease and peripheral vascular disease—related events were not (Table 4).

Although the sample size is relatively small and the study is retrospective and hypothesis generating, these results are reassuring. A weakness is that it did require a particularly broadly inclusive primary endpoint of hard and soft atherosclerotic disease—related endpoints to achieve significance. On the other hand, all-cause mortality as an independent endpoint did reach statistical significance.

P. P. Toth, MD, PhD

References

1. Toth PP, Maki KC. A commentary on the implications of the ENHANCE (Ezetimibe and Simvastatin in Hypercholesterolemia Enhances Atherosclerosis Regression) trial: should ezetimibe move to the "Back of the Line" as a therapy for dyslipidemia? *J Clin Lipidol.* 2008;2:313-317.
2. Fleg JL, Mete M, Howard BV, et al. Effect of statins alone versus statins plus ezetimibe on carotid atherosclerosis in type 2 diabetes: the SANDS (Stop Atherosclerosis in Native Diabetics Study) trial. *J Am Coll Cardiol.* 2008;52:2198-2205.
3. Baigent C, Landray MJ, Reith C, et al. The effects of lowering LDL cholesterol with simvastatin plus ezetimibe in patients with chronic kidney disease (Study of Heart and Renal Protection): a randomised placebo-controlled trial. *Lancet.* 2011;377:2181-2192.

Atorvastatin with or without an Antibody to PCSK9 in Primary Hypercholesterolemia

Roth EM, McKenney JM, Hanotin C, et al (Sterling Res Group, Cincinnati, OH; Virginia Commonwealth Univ and Natl Clinical Res, Richmond; Sanofi, Paris, France; et al)

N Engl J Med 367:1891-1900, 2012

Background.—Serum proprotein convertase subtilisin/kexin 9 (PCSK9) binds to low-density lipoprotein (LDL) receptors, increasing the degradation of LDL receptors and reducing the rate at which LDL cholesterol is removed from the circulation. REGN727/SAR236553 (designated here as SAR236553), a fully human PCSK9 monoclonal antibody, increases the recycling of LDL receptors and reduces LDL cholesterol levels.

Methods.—We performed a phase 2, multicenter, double-blind, placebo-controlled trial involving 92 patients who had LDL cholesterol levels of 100 mg per deciliter (2.6 mmol per liter) or higher after treatment with 10 mg of atorvastatin for at least 7 weeks. Patients were randomly assigned to receive 8 weeks of treatment with 80 mg of atorvastatin daily plus SAR236553 once every 2 weeks, 10 mg of atorvastatin daily plus SAR236553 once every 2 weeks, or 80 mg of atorvastatin daily plus placebo once every 2 weeks and were followed for an additional 8 weeks after treatment.

Results.—The least-squares mean ($\pm$ SE) percent reduction from baseline in LDL cholesterol was 73.2 $\pm$ 3.5 with 80 mg of atorvastatin plus SAR236553, as compared with 17.3 $\pm$ 3.5 with 80 mg of atorvastatin plus placebo ($P < 0.001$) and 66.2 $\pm$ 3.5 with 10 mg of atorvastatin plus SAR236553. All the patients who received SAR236553, as compared with 52% of those who received 80 mg of atorvastatin plus placebo, attained an LDL cholesterol level of less than 100 mg per deciliter, and at least 90% of the patients who received SAR236553, as compared with 17% who received 80 mg of atorvastatin plus placebo, attained LDL cholesterol levels of less than 70 mg per deciliter (1.8 mmol per liter).

Conclusions.—In a randomized trial involving patients with primary hypercholesterolemia, adding SAR236553 to either 10 mg of atorvastatin

TABLE 2.—Efficacy Outcomes in the Modified Intention-to-Treat Population*

Outcome	Atorvastatin, 80 mg, plus Placebo	Atorvastatin, 10 mg, plus SAR236553	Atorvastatin, 80 mg, plus SAR236553	P Value† Atorvastatin, 80 mg, plus SAR236553 vs. Atorvastatin, 80 mg, plus Placebo	P Value† Atorvastatin, 10 mg, plus SAR236553 vs. Atorvastatin, 80 mg, plus Placebo	P Value† Atorvastatin, 80 mg, plus SAR236553 vs. Atorvastatin, 10 mg, plus SAR236553
Mean least-squares percent change from baseline to week 8						
LDL cholesterol	−17.3 ± 3.5	−66.2 ± 3.5	−73.2 ± 3.5	<0.001	<0.001	0.16
HDL cholesterol	−3.6 ± 2.3	2.6 ± 2.3	5.8 ± 2.3	0.005	0.06	0.33
Apolipoprotein A1	−5.2 ± 2.3	0.4 ± 2.3	−2.2 ± 2.3	0.37	0.09	0.41
Median (interquartile range) percent change from baseline to week 8						
Triglycerides	−11.9 (−30.4 to 14.3)	−4.0 (−30.5 to 17.4)	−24.7 (−40.3 to −4.4)	0.03	0.84	0.02
Lipoprotein(a)	−2.7 (−19.5 to 16.7)	−34.7 (−50.0 to −24.7)	−31.0 (−50.0 to −15.4)	<0.001	<0.001	0.70
Total cholesterol	−16.6 (−25.1 to −3.2)	−40.5 (−44.8 to −36.0)	−47.2 (−51.5 to −37.8)	<0.001	<0.001	0.04
Non-HDL cholesterol	−22.3 (−31.4 to −3.7)	−58.3 (−63.9 to −50.2)	−63.9 (−73.9 to −56.1)	<0.001	<0.001	0.01
Apolipoprotein B	−12.0 (−23.6 to −3.5)	−54.4 (−60.2 to −48.3)	−58.0 (−67.1 to −46.1)	<0.001	<0.001	0.31

*Plus–minus values are means ± SE. The modified intention-to-treat population included all patients who underwent randomization and who had a primary end point that could be evaluated. Since the assumptions of normal distribution and equality of variances were not verified for apolipoprotein B, non-HDL cholesterol, total cholesterol, lipoprotein(a) and triglycerides, values for these variables are expressed as median (interquartile range).

†The P value for the difference in the percent change in LDL cholesterol between 80 mg of atorvastatin plus SAR236553 and 80 mg of atorvastatin plus placebo was calculated with the use of an analysis of covariance including terms for treatment and baseline value. No other P values have been adjusted for multiple comparisons and are included for descriptive purposes only.

or 80 mg of atorvastatin resulted in a significantly greater reduction in LDL cholesterol than that attained with 80 mg of atorvastatin alone. (Funded by Sanofi and Regeneron Pharmaceuticals; ClinicalTrials.gov number, NCT01288469.) (Table 2).

▶ It is currently believed that proprotein convertase subtilisin/kexin type 9 (PCSK9) attenuates the full capacity of statin therapy to increase the expression of the low-density lipoprotein (LDL) receptor; hence, it likely also reduces the magnitude of LDL reduction. Human monoclonal antibodies to PCSK9 may dampen this effect by preventing the interaction of PCSK9 with the LDL receptor, thereby increasing hepatocyte cell surface expression and systemic LDL cholesterol clearance.

These authors report the results of another PCSK9 monoclonal antibody (MAB; REGN727/SAR236553) and its effects on serum lipids in patients already being treated with high and low doses of atorvastatin. The addition of this MAB provided significant incremental reductions in LDL cholesterol, non−high-density lipoprotein cholesterol, apolipoprotein B, and lipoprotein(a) (Table 2). Interestingly, the incremental reduction of LDL-C induced by REGN727 to atorvastatin 10 or 80 mg was identical (see Fig 1 in the original article), suggesting that there is only so much additional LDL-C that can be stimulated by antagonizing LDL receptor clearance from the cell surface. The significant one-third reduction in serum lipoprotein(a) is striking and is postulated to occur secondary to increased availability of LDL receptor binding sites and less competition for receptor-dependent uptake from LDL particles. The incidence of liver and muscle toxicity was low, and the most frequent adverse event was injection site reaction (Table 2).

The MABs against PCSK9 will be a welcome addition to the lipid-lowering armamentarium at our disposal. These drugs will also provide a novel and important means by which to lower lipoprotein(a), thus making this important lipoprotein a target of future clinical trials to help us more fully explore its true impact on risk for coronary heart disease and whether therapeutic reduction of this lipoprotein beneficially impacts coronary heart disease risk in a meaningful and reproducible manner.

P. P. Toth, MD, PhD

Apolipoprotein B Synthesis Inhibition With Mipomersen in Heterozygous Familial Hypercholesterolemia: Results of a Randomized, Double-Blind, Placebo-Controlled Trial to Assess Efficacy and Safety as Add-On Therapy in Patients With Coronary Artery Disease
Stein EA, Dufour R, Gagne C, et al (Metabolic and Atherosclerosis Res Ctr, Cincinnati, OH; Clinical Res Inst of Montréal, Québec, Canada; Clinic of Lipid Disorders of Québec, Canada)
Circulation 126:2283-2292, 2012

Background.—Heterozygous familial hypercholesterolemia (HeFH) is a common genetic disorder leading to premature coronary artery disease. Despite statins and additional lipid-lowering therapies, many HeFH patients fail to achieve low-density lipoprotein cholesterol (LDL-C) goals. We evaluated mipomersen, an apolipoprotein B synthesis inhibitor, to further lower LDL-C in HeFH patients with coronary artery disease.

Methods and Results.—This double-blind, placebo-controlled, phase 3 trial randomized patients with HeFH and coronary artery disease on maximally tolerated statin and LDL-C ≥2.6 mmol/L (≥100 mg/dL) to weekly subcutaneous mipomersen 200 mg or placebo (2:1) for 26 weeks. The primary end point was percent change in LDL-C from baseline at week 28. Safety assessments included adverse events, laboratory tests, and magnetic resonance imaging assessment of hepatic fat. Of 124 randomized patients (41 placebo, 83 mipomersen), 114 (41 placebo, 73 mipomersen) completed treatment. Mean (95% confidence interval) LDL-C decreased significantly with mipomersen (−28.0% [−34.0% to −22.1%] compared with 5.2% [−0.5% to 10.9%] increase with placebo; $P < 0.001$). Mipomersen significantly reduced apolipoprotein B (−26.3%), total cholesterol (−19.4%), and lipoprotein(a) (−21.1%) compared with placebo (all $P < 0.001$). No significant change occurred in high-density lipoprotein cholesterol. Adverse events included injection site reactions and influenza-like symptoms. Five mipomersen patients (6%) had 2 consecutive alanine aminotransferase values ≥3 times the upper limit of normal at least 7 days apart; none were associated with significant bilirubin increases. Hepatic fat content increased a median of 4.9% with mipomersen versus 0.4% with placebo ($P < 0.001$).

Conclusions.—Mipomersen is an effective therapy to further reduce apolipoprotein B—containing lipoproteins, including LDL and lipoprotein(a), in HeFH patients with coronary artery disease on statins and other lipid-lowering therapy. The significance of hepatic fat and transaminase increases remains uncertain at this time (Fig 2, Tables 2 and 3).

▶ Mipomersen is an antisense 20-mer oligonucleotide that binds to a complementary region of messenger ribonucleic acid encoding the amino acid sequence for apoprotein B100 (apo B), thereby inhibiting ribosomal translation.[1] By inhibiting the biosynthesis of apo B, hepatic very low-density lipoprotein (VLDL) production and secretion are significantly reduced. With less VLDL secretion, there is less substrate for the formation of high-density lipoprotein (HDL) and LDL in serum. Mipomersen consists of a phosphorothioate backbone (an oxygen atom is substituted with a sulfur atom along the phosphate backbone), and it has 2'-O-(2-methoxytheyel)-modified ends, which enhances biological stability. Mipomersen is taken up by the liver following subcutaneous injection and is catabolized by a variety of endonuclei and exonuclei. Mipomersen is approved for use in patients with homozygous familial hypercholesterolemia.[2]

These authors evaluated the efficacy and safety of mipomersen therapy in patients with coronary artery disease and heterozygous familial hypercholesterolemia already on maximally tolerated doses of statins (HeFH). Mipomersen provided significant incremental reductions in apo B, VLDL cholesterol, LDL cholesterol, non-HDL cholesterol, lipoprotein(a), total cholesterol, and LDL cholesterol/HDL cholesterol ratio (Table 2). Maximal therapeutic effect on

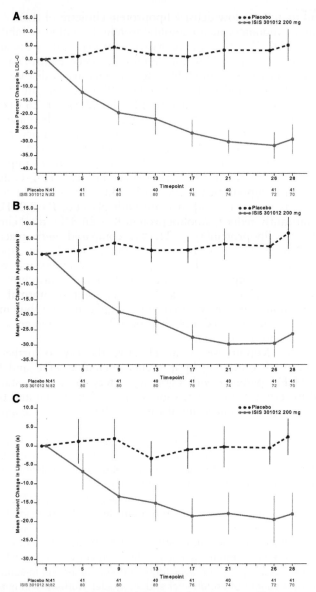

FIGURE 2.—Mean percent change from baseline (week 0) to primary efficacy time point for low-density lipoprotein cholesterol (LDL-C; **A**), apolipoprotein B (**B**), and lipoprotein(a) (**C**). Error bars indicate 95% confidence intervals. Placebo, n = 41; mipomersen (ISIS 301012) 200 mg weekly, n = 82. (Reprinted from Stein EA, Dufour R, Gagne C, et al. Apolipoprotein B synthesis inhibition with mipomersen in heterozygous familial hypercholesterolemia: results of a randomized, double-blind, placebo-controlled trial to assess efficacy and safety as add-on therapy in patients with coronary artery disease. *Circulation.* 2012;126:2283-2292, © 2012, American Heart Association, Inc.)

TABLE 2.—Baseline Lipid Concentrations and Effect of Treatment on Lipid and Inflammatory Parameters

	Placebo (n = 41)			Mipomersen (n = 82)			P
	Baseline	Primary Efficacy Time Point	% Change	Baseline	Primary Efficacy Time Point	% Change	
LDL-C	142.9 (51.6)	146.4 (43.4)	5.2 (−0.5, 10.9)	152.9 (48.7)	103.9 (33.0)	−28.0 (−34.0, −22.1)	<0.001
ApoB	126.8 (33.2)	133.8 (32.6)	7.02 (1.8, 12.2)	132.8 (33.9)	95.0 (29.7)	−26.3 (−31.2, −21.4)	<0.001
Total cholesterol	213.4 (54.6)	219.0 (49.0)	3.85 (−0.2, 7.9)	225.3 (51.5)	176.0 (35.9)	−19.4 (−23.7, −15.2)	<0.001
Non-HDL-C	165.3 (54.5)	168.2 (47.5)	3.74 (−1.3, 8.8)	175.5 (51.1)	125.2 (37.8)	−25.0 (−30.7, −19.4)	<0.001
HDL-C*	48 (41, 53)	51 (42, 58)	5.8 (0.0, 11.5)	47 (40, 58)	48 (40, 58)	2.5 (−10.3, 11.7)	0.207
Lipoprotein(a)*	53 (17, 108)	51 (18, 108)	0.0 (−8.0, 13.0)	45 (13, 93)	35 (9, 56)	−21.1 (−37.9, 0.0)	<0.001
Triglycerides*	100 (74, 137)	101 (76, 139)	0.50 (−16.2, 17.9)	107 (85, 137)	89 (70, 127)	−14.3 (−32.7, 9.7)	0.042
VLDL-C*	20 (15, 28)	20 (15, 28)	0.0 (−15.4, 15.0)	21 (17, 27)	18 (14, 25)	−13.8 (−33.3, 11.8)	0.023
ApoA1	146.1 (24.9)	151.5 (29.1)	3.71 (1.0, 6.4)	150.7 (28.1)	145.4 (27.9)	−2.4 (−5.6, 0.7)	0.004
LDL/HDL*	2.7 (2.5, 3.3)	3.0 (2.2, 3.5)	−2.8 (−13.1, 13.1)	3.0 (2.6, 4.0)	2.1 (1.5, 3.0)	−29.2 (−46.8, −13.7)	<0.001
hsCRP	0.8 (0.5, 1.8)	0.9 (0.5, 1.6)	0.0 (−0.4, 0.3)	0.8 (0.4, 1.6)	1.0 (0.5, 1.7)	0.1 (−0.1, 0.7)	NS

Data are provided as mg/dL for baseline and primary efficacy time point. Data are expressed as mean (SD) (baseline, primary efficacy time point) and mean (95% confidence interval) (percent change from baseline) for low-density lipoprotein cholesterol (LDL-C), apolipoprotein B (ApoB), total cholesterol, non–high-density lipoprotein cholesterol (HDL-C), and apolipoprotein A1 (ApoA1). Data are expressed as median with interquartile range for HDL-C, lipoprotein(a), triglycerides, very low-density lipoprotein cholesterol (VLDL-C), LDL/HDL ratio, and high-sensitivity C-reactive protein (hsCRP). To convert cholesterol (mg/dL) values to standard international units (mmol/L), multiply by 0.0259; to convert triglycerides to mmol/L, multiply by 0.0113; for ApoB, lipoprotein(a), and ApoA1, convert to g/L by multiplying by 0.01.

*The P value is for the between-group comparison of percent change from baseline to primary efficacy time point obtained via 2-sided t test when data for percent change from baseline were distributed normally or via Wilcoxon rank sum test when not distributed normally (parameters with *).

TABLE 3.—Adverse Events Reported in at Least 10% of Mipomersen-Treated Patients and Significant Laboratory Abnormalities

	Placebo (n = 41)		Mipomersen (n = 83)	
	Events No.	Patients No. (%)	Events No.	Patients No. (%)
Adverse events				
All events	269	38 (92.7)	1550	83 (100.0)
Injection site reaction	33	17 (41.5)	1013	77 (92.8)
Influenza-like symptoms*	24	13 (31.7)	129	41 (49.4)
Nausea	10	6 (14.6)	17	14 (16.9)
Headache	11	7 (17.1)	21	15 (18.1)
Diarrhea	7	5 (12.2)	9	9 (10.8)
Nasopharyngitis	3	3 (7.3)	10	9 (10.8)
Cough	2	2 (4.9)	9	9 (10.8)
Laboratory abnormalities				
ALT				
≥ULN and <2× ULN		14 (34.1)		34 (41.0)
≥2× ULN and <3× ULN		2 (4.9)		19 (22.9)
≥3× ULN and <5× ULN		1 (2.4)		9 (10.8)
≥5× ULN and <10× ULN		0		2 (2.4)
Maximum ALT ≥10× ULN		0		1 (1.2)
ALT ≥3× ULN with 2 consecutive results at least 7 d apart		0		5 (6.0)

ALT indicates alanine aminotransferase; ULN, upper limit of normal.
*Includes fatigue, influenza-like illness, pyrexia, chills, malaise, influenza, myalgia, and arthralgia.

atherogenic lipoproteins occurred within approximately 4 to 5 months (Fig 2). The most common adverse events were injection site reactions, influenza-like symptoms, and elevations in serum transaminases (Table 3). There was also an increased risk for elevations in intrahepatic fat of approximately 4.9% (median change not adjusted for placebo).

Mipomersen constitutes an important and innovative new approach for the reduction of atherogenic lipoprotein burden. This study shows that it is efficacious in patients with HeFH, a patient population in need of therapies adjuvant to established lipid lowering medications. Mipomersen, like the PCSK9 monoclonal antibodies, also provides a new approach for more fully evaluating the impact of Lp(a) on cardiovascular risk and whether Lp(a) reduction lowers this risk.

P. P. Toth, MD, PhD

References

1. Toth PP. Antisense therapy and emerging applications for the management of dyslipidemia. *J Clin Lipidol.* 2011;5:441-449.
2. Raal FJ, Santos RD, Blom DJ, et al. Mipomersen, an apolipoprotein B synthesis inhibitor, for lowering of LDL cholesterol concentrations in patients with homozygous familial hypercholesterolaemia: a randomised, double-blind, placebo-controlled trial. *Lancet.* 2010;375:998-1006.

The effects of lowering LDL cholesterol with statin therapy in people at low risk of vascular disease: meta-analysis of individual data from 27 randomised trials
Cholesterol Treatment Trialists' (CTT) Collaborators (Univ of Sydney, New South Wales, Australia)
Lancet 380:581-590, 2012

Background.—Statins reduce LDL cholesterol and prevent vascular events, but their net eff ects in people at low risk of vascular events remain uncertain.

Methods.—This meta-analysis included individual participant data from 22 trials of statin versus control (n=134 537; mean LDL cholesterol difference 1·08 mmol/L; median follow-up 4·8 years) and five trials of more versus less statin (n=39 612; difference 0·51 mmol/L; 5·1 years). Major vascular events were major coronary events (ie, non-fatal myocardial infarction or coronary death), strokes, or coronary revascularisations. Participants were separated into five categories of baseline 5-year major vascular event risk on control therapy (no statin or low-intensity statin) (<5%, ≥5% to <10%, ≥10% to <20%, ≥20% to <30%, ≥30%); in each, the rate ratio (RR) per 1·0 mmol/L LDL cholesterol reduction was estimated.

Findings.—Reduction of LDL cholesterol with a statin reduced the risk of major vascular events (RR 0·79, 95% CI 0·77–0·81, per 1·0 mmol/L reduction), largely irrespective of age, sex, baseline LDL cholesterol or previous vascular disease, and of vascular and all-cause mortality. The proportional reduction in major vascular events was at least as big in the two lowest risk categories as in the higher risk categories (RR per 1·0 mmol/L reduction from lowest to highest risk: 0·62 [99% CI 0·47–0·81], 0·69 [99% CI 0·60–0·79], 0·79 [99% CI 0·74–0·85], 0·81 [99% CI 0·77–0·86], and 0·79 [99% CI 0·74–0·84]; trend $p=0·04$), which reflected significant reductions in these two lowest risk categories in major coronary events (RR 0·57, 99% CI 0·36–0·89, $p = 0·0012$, and 0·61, 99% CI 0·50–0·74, $p < 0·0001$) and in coronary revascularisations (RR 0·52, 99% CI 0·35–0·75, and 0·63, 99% CI 0·51–0·79; both $p < 0·0001$). For stroke, the reduction in risk in participants with 5-year risk of major vascular events lower than 10% (RR per 1·0 mmol/L LDL cholesterol reduction 0·76, 99% CI 0·61–0·95, $p = 0·0012$) was also similar to that seen in higher risk categories (trend $p = 0·3$). In participants without a history of vascular disease, statins reduced the risks of vascular (RR per 1·0 mmol/L LDL cholesterol reduction 0·85, 95% CI 0·77–0·95) and all-cause mortality (RR 0·91, 95% CI 0·85–0·97), and the proportional reductions were similar by baseline risk. There was no evidence that reduction of LDL cholesterol with a statin increased cancer incidence (RR per 1·0 mmol/L LDL cholesterol reduction 1·00, 95% CI 0·96–1·04), cancer mortality (RR 0·99, 95% CI 0·93–1·06), or other non-vascular mortality.

Interpretation.—In individuals with 5-year risk of major vascular events lower than 10%, each 1 mmol/L reduction in LDL cholesterol produced an

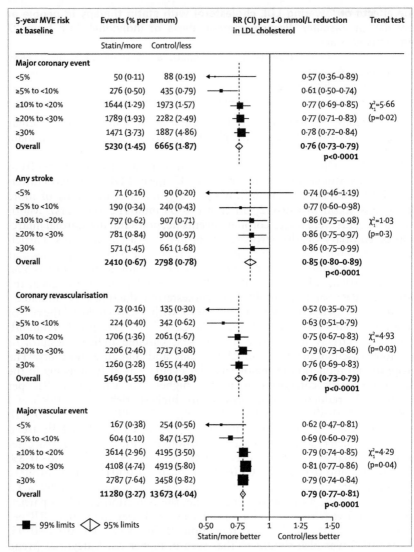

5-year MVE risk at baseline	Events (% per annum)		RR (CI) per 1·0 mmol/L reduction in LDL cholesterol	Trend test
	Statin/more	Control/less		
Major coronary event				
<5%	50 (0·11)	88 (0·19)	0·57 (0·36–0·89)	
≥5% to <10%	276 (0·50)	435 (0·79)	0·61 (0·50–0·74)	
≥10% to <20%	1644 (1·29)	1973 (1·57)	0·77 (0·69–0·85)	χ_1^2=5·66
≥20% to <30%	1789 (1·93)	2282 (2·49)	0·77 (0·71–0·83)	(p=0·02)
≥30%	1471 (3·73)	1887 (4·86)	0·78 (0·72–0·84)	
Overall	**5230 (1·45)**	**6665 (1·87)**	**0·76 (0·73–0·79)** p<0·0001	
Any stroke				
<5%	71 (0·16)	90 (0·20)	0·74 (0·46–1·19)	
≥5% to <10%	190 (0·34)	240 (0·43)	0·77 (0·60–0·98)	
≥10% to <20%	797 (0·62)	907 (0·71)	0·86 (0·75–0·98)	χ_1^2=1·03
≥20% to <30%	781 (0·84)	900 (0·97)	0·86 (0·75–0·97)	(p=0·3)
≥30%	571 (1·45)	661 (1·68)	0·86 (0·75–0·99)	
Overall	**2410 (0·67)**	**2798 (0·78)**	**0·85 (0·80–0·89)** p<0·0001	
Coronary revascularisation				
<5%	73 (0·16)	135 (0·30)	0·52 (0·35–0·75)	
≥5% to <10%	224 (0·40)	342 (0·62)	0·63 (0·51–0·79)	
≥10% to <20%	1706 (1·36)	2061 (1·67)	0·75 (0·67–0·83)	χ_1^2=4·93
≥20% to <30%	2206 (2·46)	2717 (3·08)	0·79 (0·73–0·86)	(p=0·03)
≥30%	1260 (3·28)	1655 (4·40)	0·76 (0·69–0·83)	
Overall	**5469 (1·55)**	**6910 (1·98)**	**0·76 (0·73–0·79)** p<0·0001	
Major vascular event				
<5%	167 (0·38)	254 (0·56)	0·62 (0·47–0·81)	
≥5% to <10%	604 (1·10)	847 (1·57)	0·69 (0·60–0·79)	
≥10% to <20%	3614 (2·96)	4195 (3·50)	0·79 (0·74–0·85)	χ_1^2=4·29
≥20% to <30%	4108 (4·74)	4919 (5·80)	0·81 (0·77–0·86)	(p=0·04)
≥30%	2787 (7·64)	3458 (9·82)	0·79 (0·74–0·84)	
Overall	**11280 (3·27)**	**13673 (4·04)**	**0·79 (0·77–0·81)** p<0·0001	

■— 99% limits ◇ 95% limits

0·50   0·75   1   1·25   1·50
Statin/more better   Control/less better

FIGURE 1.—Effects on major coronary events, strokes, coronary revascularisation procedures, and major vascular events per 1·0 mmol/L reduction in LDL cholesterol at different levels of risk MVE = major vascular event. RR = rate ratio. CI = confidence interval. (Reprinted from The Lancet Neurology. Cholesterol Treatment Trialists' [CTT] Collaborators. The effects of lowering LDL cholesterol with statin therapy in people at low risk of vascular disease: meta-analysis of individual data from 27 randomised trials. *Lancet.* 2012;380:581-590, Copyright 2012, with permission from Elsevier.)

absolute reduction in major vascular events of about 11 per 1000 over 5 years. This benefit greatly exceeds any known hazards of statin therapy. Under present guidelines, such individuals would not typically be regarded

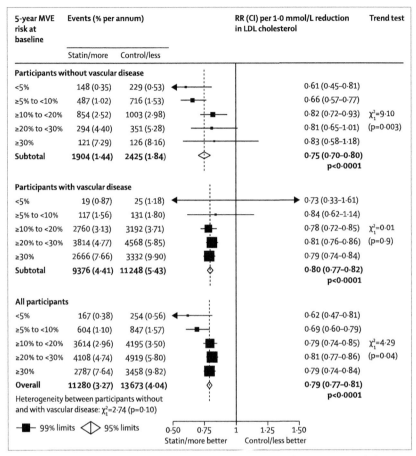

5-year MVE risk at baseline	Events (% per annum)		RR (CI) per 1·0 mmol/L reduction in LDL cholesterol	Trend test
	Statin/more	Control/less		
Participants without vascular disease				
<5%	148 (0·35)	229 (0·53)	0·61 (0·45–0·81)	
≥5% to <10%	487 (1·02)	716 (1·53)	0·66 (0·57–0·77)	
≥10% to <20%	854 (2·52)	1003 (2·98)	0·82 (0·72–0·93)	χ^2_1=9·10
≥20% to <30%	294 (4·40)	351 (5·28)	0·81 (0·65–1·01)	(p=0·003)
≥30%	121 (7·29)	126 (8·16)	0·83 (0·58–1·18)	
Subtotal	**1904 (1·44)**	**2425 (1·84)**	**0·75 (0·70–0·80)** p<0·0001	
Participants with vascular disease				
<5%	19 (0·87)	25 (1·18)	0·73 (0·33–1·61)	
≥5% to <10%	117 (1·56)	131 (1·80)	0·84 (0·62–1·14)	
≥10% to <20%	2760 (3·13)	3192 (3·71)	0·78 (0·72–0·85)	χ^2_1=0·01
≥20% to <30%	3814 (4·77)	4568 (5·85)	0·81 (0·76–0·86)	(p=0·9)
≥30%	2666 (7·66)	3332 (9·90)	0·79 (0·74–0·84)	
Subtotal	**9376 (4·41)**	**11248 (5·43)**	**0·80 (0·77–0·82)** p<0·0001	
All participants				
<5%	167 (0·38)	254 (0·56)	0·62 (0·47–0·81)	
≥5% to <10%	604 (1·10)	847 (1·57)	0·69 (0·60–0·79)	
≥10% to <20%	3614 (2·96)	4195 (3·50)	0·79 (0·74–0·85)	χ^2_1=4·29
≥20% to <30%	4108 (4·74)	4919 (5·80)	0·81 (0·77–0·86)	(p=0·04)
≥30%	2787 (7·64)	3458 (9·82)	0·79 (0·74–0·84)	
Overall	**11280 (3·27)**	**13673 (4·04)**	**0·79 (0·77–0·81)** p<0·0001	

Heterogeneity between participants without and with vascular disease: χ^2_1=2·74 (p=0·10)

■ 99% limits ◇ 95% limits

0·50   0·75   1   1·25   1·50
Statin/more better   Control/less better

FIGURE 2.—Effects on major vascular events per 1·0 mmol/L reduction in LDL cholesterol at different levels of risk, by history of vascular disease MVE = major vascular event. RR = rate ratio. CI = confidence interval. (Reprinted from The Lancet Neurology. Cholesterol Treatment Trialists' [CTT] Collaborators. The effects of lowering LDL cholesterol with statin therapy in people at low risk of vascular disease: meta-analysis of individual data from 27 randomised trials. *Lancet.* 2012;380:581-590, Copyright 2012, with permission from Elsevier.)

as suitable for LDL-lowering statin therapy. The present report suggests, therefore, that these guidelines might need to be reconsidered (Figs 1-3).

▶ There appears to be some periodicity to the resurgence of debate about whether statins should be prescribed to patients at low risk for coronary heart disease and those in the primary prevention setting in general. Although rigorous debate is generally a vital form of discourse in medicine, too often the debate centering around the use of statins in primary care reduces to personal opinion and does not necessarily reflect best evidence. Statin therapy in primary prevention works,[1-4] and attempts to minimize this constitute a distinct disservice to patients.

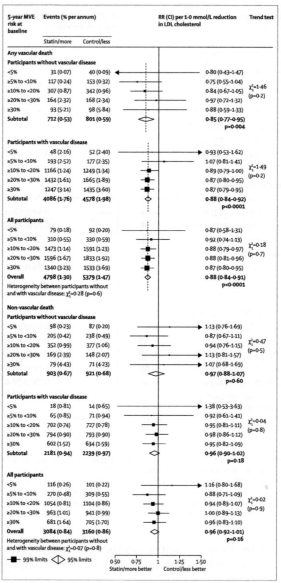

FIGURE 3.—Effects on vascular and non-vascular deaths per 1·0 mmol/L reduction in LDL cholesterol at different levels of risk, by history of vascular disease MVE = major vascular event. RR = rate ratio. CI = confidence interval. There were a further 179 (statin/more statin) versus 210 (control/less statin) deaths of unknown cause among participants without vascular disease and 309 (statin/more statin) versus 338 (control/less statin) deaths of unknown cause among participants with vascular disease. (Reprinted from The Lancet Neurology. Cholesterol Treatment Trialists' [CTT] Collaborators. The effects of lowering LDL cholesterol with statin therapy in people at low risk of vascular disease: meta-analysis of individual data from 27 randomised trials. *Lancet.* 2012;380:581-590, Copyright 2012, with permission from Elsevier.)

In the latest meta-analysis by the Cholesterol Treatment Trialists' Collaboration, the estimated benefit of statin therapy in patients with low risk for vascular events was evaluated based on 27 prospective randomized studies, including 174 149 patients. Patient-level data were used. Statin therapy reduced the risk of major vascular events by 21% per 39 mg/dL reduction in low-density lipoprotein cholesterol (LDL-C), with significant reductions observed in all risk groups, ranging from less than 5% to more than 30% (Fig 1). Uniform reductions were seen in major coronary events, stroke, and need for revascularization. The reduction in risk of major vascular events among the patients with lowest risk was attributable to a 43% reduction in major coronary events and a 48% reduction in coronary revascularization. Among patients without previous history of vascular disease, the lowest-risk patients derived as much benefit as higher-risk patients from statin therapy (Fig 2). Among all patients, there was a reduction in vascular mortality of 12% per 39 mg/dL reduction in LDL-C, which was principally because of a decrease in coronary deaths of 20% (Fig 3). There were too few deaths among the lower-risk participants to reliably quantify the impact of statin therapy on mortality.

This is the most rigorous analysis of its kind to evaluate the efficacy of statin therapy in low-risk patients. The results clearly support the use of statins in low-risk patients, consistent with such primary prevention trials as WOSCOPS (West of Scotland Coronary Prevention Study), AFCAPs/TexCAPs (the Air Force/Texas Coronary Atherosclerosis Prevention Study), and JUPITER (Justification for the Use of Statins in Primary Prevention: An Intervention Trial Evaluating Rosuvastatin). Important cardiovascular endpoints are reduced by statins irrespective of baseline risk stratification. Withholding therapy in eligible patients is inappropriate.

P. P. Toth, MD, PhD

References

1. Glynn RJ, Koenig W, Nordestgaard BG, Shepherd J, Ridker PM. Rosuvastatin for primary prevention in older persons with elevated C-reactive protein and low to average low-density lipoprotein cholesterol levels: exploratory analysis of a randomized trial. *Ann Intern Med.* 2010;152:488-496. W174.
2. Ridker PM, Macfadyen JG, Nordestgaard BG, et al. Rosuvastatin for primary prevention among individuals with elevated high-sensitivity c-reactive protein and 5% to 10% and 10% to 20% 10-year risk. Implications of the Justification for Use of Statins in Prevention: an Intervention Trial Evaluating Rosuvastatin (JUPITER) trial for "intermediate risk". *Circ Cardiovasc Qual Outcomes.* 2010;3: 447-452.
3. Downs JR, Clearfield M, Weis S, et al. Primary prevention of acute coronary events with lovastatin in men and women with average cholesterol levels: results of AFCAPS/TexCAPS. Air Force/Texas Coronary Atherosclerosis Prevention Study. *JAMA.* 1998;279:1615-1622.
4. Influence of pravastatin and plasma lipids on clinical events in the West of Scotland Coronary Prevention Study (WOSCOPS). *Circulation.* 1998;97:1440-1445.

Prevention of Atherosclerosis

Dysfunctional High-Density Lipoprotein in Patients on Chronic Hemodialysis

Yamamoto S, Yancey PG, Ikizler TA, et al (Vanderbilt Univ Med Ctr, Nashville, TN)

J Am Coll Cardiol 60:2372-2379, 2012

Objectives.—This study examined the functionality of high-density lipoprotein (HDL) in individuals with end-stage renal disease on dialysis (ESRD-HD).

Background.—The high rate of cardiovascular disease (CVD) in chronic kidney disease is not explained by standard risk factors, especially in patients with ESRD-HD who appear resistant to benefits of statin therapy. HDL is antiatherogenic because it extracts tissue cholesterol and reduces inflammation.

Methods.—Cellular cholesterol efflux and inflammatory response were assessed in macrophages exposed to HDL of patients with ESRD-HD or controls.

Results.—HDL from patients with ESRD-HD was dramatically less effective than normal HDL in accepting cholesterol from macrophages (median

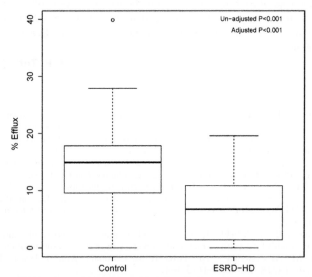

FIGURE 1.—Efflux to HDL from patients with ESRD-HD and controls with normal kidney function. Unadjusted p values from the Wilcoxon rank sum test. Adjusted p values from multivariable regression analysis with adjustment for age, sex, race, body mass index, diabetes, high-sensitivity C-reactive protein, total cholesterol, triglycerides, high-density lipoprotein (HDL), low-density lipoprotein, cardiovascular disease, and use of statins or angiotensin-converting enzyme inhibitors/angiotensin receptor blockers. ESRD-HD = end-stage renal disease on chronic hemodialysis. (Reprinted from the Journal of the American College of Cardiology. Yamamoto S, Yancey PG, Ikizler TA, et al. Dysfunctional high-density lipoprotein in patients on chronic hemodialysis. *J Am Coll Cardiol.* 2012;60:2372-2379, Copyright 2012, with permission from the American College of Cardiology.)

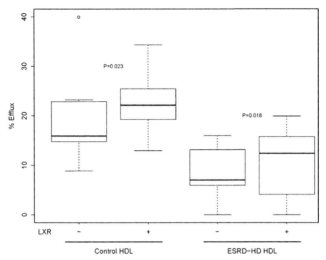

FIGURE 2.—Efflux with or without activation of ABC transporters by LXR agonist to HDL p values from the Wilcoxon rank sum test. ABC = ATP-binding cassette; LXR = liver X receptor; other abbreviations as in Figure 1. (Reprinted from the Journal of the American College of Cardiology. Yamamoto S, Yancey PG, Ikizler TA, et al. Dysfunctional high-density lipoprotein in patients on chronic hemodialysis. *J Am Coll Cardiol*. 2012;60:2372-2379, Copyright 2012, with permission from the American College of Cardiology.)

6.9%; interquartile range [IQR]: 1.4% to 10.2%) versus control (median 14.9%; IQR: 9.8% to 17.8%; $p < 0.001$). The profound efflux impairment was also seen in patients with ESRD-HD and diabetes compared with patients with diabetes without renal disease (median 8.1%; IQR: 3.3% to 12.9%) versus control (median 13.6%; IQR: 11.0% to 15.9%; $p = 0.009$). In vitro activation of cellular cholesterol transporters increased cholesterol efflux to both normal and uremic HDL. HDL of patients with ESRD-HD had reduced antichemotactic ability and increased macrophage cytokine response (tumor necrosis factor-alpha, interleukin-6, and interleukin-1-beta). HDL of patients with ESRD-HD on statin therapy had reduced inflammatory response while maintaining impaired cholesterol acceptor function. Interestingly, impaired HDL-mediated efflux did not correlate with circulating C-reactive protein levels or cellular inflammatory response.

Conclusions.—These findings suggest that abnormal HDL capacity to mediate cholesterol efflux is a key driver of excess CVD in patients on chronic hemodialysis and may explain why statins have limited effect to decrease CV events. The findings also suggest cellular cholesterol transporters as potential therapeutic targets to decrease CV risk in this population (Figs 1 and 2).

▶ High-density lipoprotein (HDL) cholesterol levels are highly predictive of risk for future cardiovascular events in both men and women.[1] The HDLs are believed to be protective by virtue of the beneficial effects exerted within the vasculature by specific enzymatic and apoprotein components of its proteome as well as its ability to carry bioactive sphingolipids and micro-ribonucleic acids.[2] Despite the data suggesting a protective effect by HDLs in prospective longitudinal observational cohorts, multiple clinical trials designed to ascertain the impact of increasing HDL therapeutically with either niacin or cholesterol ester transfer protein inhibitors have been negative to date.[3,4] This has prompted a much more detailed investigation of how HDL functionality may be affected by the genetic and metabolic milieu in which it circulates.

Reverse cholesterol transport is widely seen as one of the most important functions that HDL particles modulate. The capacity of an HDL particle to promote cholesterol efflux correlates with risk for coronary artery disease—related events.[5] Yamamoto et al evaluated the ability of HDLs extracted from patients with end-stage renal disease on hemodialysis (ESRD-HD) with or without diabetes mellitus to promote cholesterol efflux from macrophages. In both patient groups, efflux was significantly reduced compared with the HDL extracted from patients without renal disease or diabetes (Fig 1). Importantly, statin therapy did not improve efflux capacity. The HDLs from patients with ESRD had reduced capacity to inhibit the chemotaxis of macrophages and inhibit the elaboration of inflammatory cytokines, such as tumor necrosis factor—α and interleukin-1β and interleukin-6. Of great interest is the observation that treatment of cholesterol-loaded macrophages with the liver X receptor—α (LXR-α) agonist increased cell surface expression of ABCA1 and ABCG1 significantly and significantly increased the capacity of HDL to promote cholesterol efflux, although not to the level observed from control patients (Fig 2).

These findings confirm long-held suspicions that HDL functionality can be impaired by the metabolic milieu in which these lipoproteins are expressed. Cholesterol efflux capacity and the ability to attenuate the intensity of inflammatory mediator expression were markedly impaired in patients with ESRD. It is fascinating that treatment of macrophages with an LXR-α agonist successfully increased both adenosine-5'-triphosphate binding membrane cassette transport protein expression and cholesterol efflux capacity. Much work remains to be done in this area. Clearly, it would be premature to abandon research on the role of HDL in preventing cardiovascular disease.

P. P. Toth, MD, PhD

References

1. Toth PP. High-density lipoprotein: epidemiology, metabolism, and antiatherogenic effects. *Dis Mon.* 2001;47:369-416.
2. Toth PP. Activation of intracellular signaling systems by high-density lipoproteins. *J Clin Lipidol.* 2010;4:376-381.
3. Toth PP. CETP Inhibition: does the future look promising? *Curr Cardiol Rep.* 2011;13:559-565.
4. Boden WE, Probstfield JL, Anderson T, et al. Niacin in patients with low HDL cholesterol levels receiving intensive statin therapy. *N Engl J Med.* 2011;365: 2255-2267.
5. Khera AV, Cuchel M, de la Llera-Moya M, et al. Cholesterol efflux capacity, high-density lipoprotein function, and atherosclerosis. *N Engl J Med.* 2011;364: 127-135.

Altered Activation of Endothelial Anti-and Proapoptotic Pathways by High-Density Lipoprotein from Patients with Coronary Artery Disease: Role of High-Density Lipoprotein–Proteome Remodeling
Riwanto M, Rohrer L, Roschitzki B, et al (Univ Hosp Zurich, Switzerland; Univ of Zurich, Switzerland; Functional Genomics Ctr Univ and ETH, Zurich, Switzerland)
Circulation 127:891-904, 2013

Background.—Endothelial dysfunction and injury are thought to play an important role in the progression of coronary artery disease (CAD). High-density lipoprotein from healthy subjects ($HDL_{Healthy}$) has been proposed to exert endothelial antiapoptotic effects that may represent an important antiatherogenic property of the lipoprotein. The present study therefore aimed to compare effects of HDL_{CAD} and $HDL_{Healthy}$ on the activation of endothelial anti- and proapoptotic pathways and to determine which changes of the lipoprotein are relevant for these processes.

Methods and Results.—HDL was isolated from patients with stable CAD (HDL_{sCAD}), an acute coronary syndrome (HDL_{ACS}), and healthy subjects. $HDL_{Healthy}$ induced expression of the endothelial antiapoptotic Bcl-2 protein Bcl-xL and reduced endothelial cell apoptosis in vitro and in vivo in apolipoprotein E–deficient mice in vivo. In contrast, HDL_{sCAD} and HDL_{ACS} did not inhibit endothelial apoptosis, failed to activate endothelial Bcl-xL, and stimulated endothelial proapoptotic pathways, in particular, p38-mitogen-activated protein kinase–mediated activation of the proapoptotic Bcl-2 protein tBid. Endothelial antiapoptotic effects of $HDL_{Healthy}$ were observed after inhibition of endothelial nitric oxide synthase and after delipidation, but not completely mimicked by apolipoprotein A-I or reconstituted HDL, suggesting an important role of the HDL proteome. HDL proteomics analyses and subsequent validations and functional characterizations suggested a reduced clusterin and increased apolipoprotein C-III content of HDL_{sCAD} and HDL_{ACS} as mechanisms leading to altered effects on endothelial apoptosis.

Conclusions.—The present study demonstrates for the first time that HDL_{CAD} does not activate endothelial antiapoptotic pathways, but rather stimulates potential endothelial proapoptotic pathways. HDL-proteome remodeling plays an important role for these altered functional properties of HDL. These findings provide novel insights into mechanisms leading to altered vascular effects of HDL in coronary disease (Figs 2 and 5).

▶ High-density lipoprotein (HDL) in patients with coronary artery disease (CAD) is known to have a reduced capacity to inhibit the oxidation of lipids in low-density lipoprotein particles and inhibit the transmigration of monocytes into the subendothelial space.[1,2] The use of statin therapy and niacin has been shown to improve HDL functionality in patients with CAD.[3,4] An important function of HDL particles is to inhibit endothelial apoptosis and maintain normal endothelial barrier health.[5]

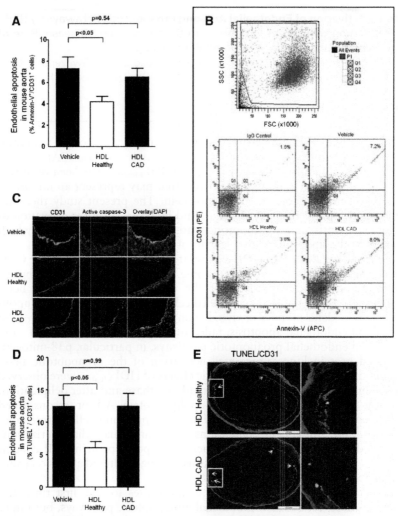

FIGURE 2.—Effects of HDL$_{Healthy}$, HDL$_{sCAD}$, or HDL$_{ACS}$ on endothelial apoptosis in vivo. (**A**) Administration of HDL$_{Healthy}$, but not HDL$_{CAD}$ (14 mg of HDL protein per kg body weight) to ApoE$-/-$ mice via tail-vein injection reduced endothelial apoptosis as detected in the aorta after 24 hours (n=8–9 per group) as measured by costaining of annexin-V+ and CD31+ with the use of FACS analysis. (**B**) Representative flow cytometric analyses using anti-CD31-PE/ annexin-V-APC costaining of cells harvested from mouse aortas. (**C**) Immunofluorescence staining showed reduced active caspase-3 staining of endothelial cells of mouse aortic sections after treatment with HDL$_{Healthy}$, but not with HDL$_{CAD}$. (**D and E**) TUNEL-FITC staining of mouse aortic sections costained with CD31-Texas red. The number of TUNEL+ cells/number of CD31+ cells was counted per high-power field and the average was taken from 5 fields. DAPI indicates 4′,6-diamidino-2-phenylindole; FACS, fluorescence-activated cell sorting; FITC, fluorescein isothiocyanate; HDL, high-density lipoprotein; HDL$_{ACS}$, HDL from patients with acute coronary syndrome; HDL$_{CAD}$, HDL from patients with coronary artery disease; HDL$_{Healthy}$, HDL from healthy subjects; HDL$_{sCAD}$, HDL from patients with stable coronary artery disease; and TUNEL, terminal deoxynucleotidyl transferasemediated dUTP-biotin nick-end labeling. For interpretation of the references to color in this figure legend, the reader is referred to web version of this article. (Reprinted from Riwanto M, Rohrer L, Roschitzki B, et al. Altered activation of endothelial anti-and proapoptotic pathways by high-density lipoprotein from patients with coronary artery disease: role of high–density lipoprotein-proteome remodeling. *Circulation*. 2013;127:891-904, © 2013, American Heart Association, Inc.)

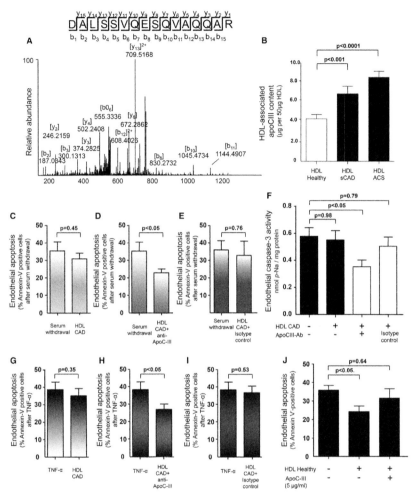

FIGURE 5.—Role of HDL-associated apoC-III for impaired endothelial antiapoptotic effects of HDL in patients with CAD. (**A**) Tandem mass spectrometry spectrum of a proteotypic peptide of apoC-III. (**B**) The amount of apoC-III in HDL$_{Healthy}$, HDL$_{sCAD}$, or HDL$_{ACS}$ was quantified with ELISA. (**C** through **E**) HDL$_{CAD}$ (50 μg/mL) was preincubated with specific blocking antibody against apoC-III (20 μg/mL or 1:50 dilution) or isotype control and the effects of HDL on serum withdrawal–induced endothelial apoptosis were analyzed with annexin-V staining with the use of FACS analysis and caspase-3 activity measurement (**F**). (**G** through **I**) Effects of HDL$_{CAD}$ preincubated with a specific blocking antibody against apoC-III or isotype control on TNF-α–induced endothelial apoptosis were analyzed with annexin-V staining with the use of FACS analysis. (**J**) Effects of HDL$_{Healthy}$ (50 μg/mL) on endothelial cell apoptosis in the presence of purified human apoC-III (5 μg/mL). CAD indicates coronary artery disease; ELISA, enzyme-linked immunosorbent assay; FACS, fluorescence-activated cell sorting; HDL, high-density lipoprotein; HDL$_{ACS}$, HDL from patients with acute coronary syndrome; HDL$_{CAD}$, HDL from patients with CAD; HDL$_{Healthy}$, HDL from healthy subjects; HDL$_{sCAD}$, HDL from patients with stable CAD; and TNF-α, tumor necrosis factor-α. (Reprinted from Riwanto M, Rohrer L, Roschitzki B, et al. Altered activation of endothelial anti-and proapoptotic pathways by high-density lipoprotein from patients with coronary artery disease: role of high–density lipoprotein-proteome remodeling. *Circulation.* 2013;127:891-904, © 2013, American Heart Association, Inc.)

In a fascinating study of HDL functionality, these authors evaluated the capacity of HDLs extracted from patients with established CAD or history of an acute coronary syndrome (ACS) to inhibit endothelial cell apoptosis compared with the HDL of healthy controls.[6] The HDLs of healthy controls promoted the expression of the endothelial antiapoptotic protein Bcl-xl via the phosphatidylinositol triphosphokinase/Akt pathway and inhibited endothelial cell apoptosis both in vitro and in an apoE knockout mouse model (Fig 2). Compared with intact HDLs, nonlipidated apoAI and recombinant HDLs had an attenuated impact on apoptosis prevention, suggesting the HDL proteome plays an important role in this process. In contrast, the HDLs from patients with CAD or ACS increased endothelial apoptosis by promoting p38-mitogen—activated protein kinase—driven expression of the proapoptotic protein tBid. The HDLs of patients with CAD or ACS had reduced clusterin content and increased levels of apoprotein CIII (apoCIII). These changes correlate significantly with HDL functionality. Antibody treatment of HDL from healthy controls against clusterin reduced antiapoptotic activity, while antibody neutralization of apoCIII led to a decrease in proapoptotic activity and caspase-3 activity, an enzyme that plays a critical role in the execution phase of apoptosis (Fig 5).

Once again, it is clear that the one-size-fits-all paradigm that has permeated thinking about HDL biochemistry and physiology is wrong. There is extraordinary complexity and functionality variation to HDL particles depending on their specific proteomic and lipidomic components and which specific bioactive lipids and microRNAs they are transporting. Considerable work remains to be done in any effort to therapeutically modulate HDL activity in a predictable and reliable way.

P. P. Toth, MD, PhD

References

1. Ansell BJ. A review of trials evaluating nonstatin lipid-lowering therapies. *Curr Atheroscler Rep.* 2009;11:64-66.
2. Ansell BJ, Fonarow GC, Fogelman AM. High-density lipoprotein: is it always atheroprotective? *Curr Atheroscler Rep.* 2006;8:405-411.
3. Ansell BJ, Navab M, Hama S, et al. Inflammatory/antiinflammatory properties of high-density lipoprotein distinguish patients from control subjects better than high-density lipoprotein cholesterol levels and are favorably affected by simvastatin treatment. *Circulation.* 2003;108:2751-2756.
4. Green PS, Vaisar T, Pennathur S, et al. Combined statin and niacin therapy remodels the high-density lipoprotein proteome. *Circulation.* 2008;118:1259-1267.
5. Nofer JR, Levkau B, Wolinska I, et al. Suppression of endothelial cell apoptosis by high density lipoproteins (HDL) and HDL-associated lysosphingolipids. *J Biol Chem.* 2001;276:34480-34485.
6. Singaraja RR, Sivapalaratnam S, Hovingh K, et al. The impact of partial and complete loss-of-function mutations in endothelial lipase on high-density lipoprotein levels and functionality in humans. *Circ Cardiovasc Genet.* 2013;6:54-62.

Stroke and Peripheral Artery Disease

Impact of low-density lipoprotein to high-density lipoprotein ratio on aortic arch atherosclerosis in unexplained stroke
Okuzumi A, Ueno Y, Shimada Y, et al (Juntendo Univ School of Medicine, Japan)
J Neurol Sci 326:83-88, 2013

The ratio of low- (LDL-C) to high- (HDL-C) density lipoprotein choles-terol serves as a positive predictor of atherosclerosis including coronary artery disease. We assessed the contribution of the LDL-C/HDL-C ratio to atheromatous aortic plaques (AAPs) in patients with unexplained ischemic stroke. One hundred thirty-seven patients (age, 65 ± 14 years; 87 male) with ischemic stroke underwent transesophageal echocardiography (TEE)

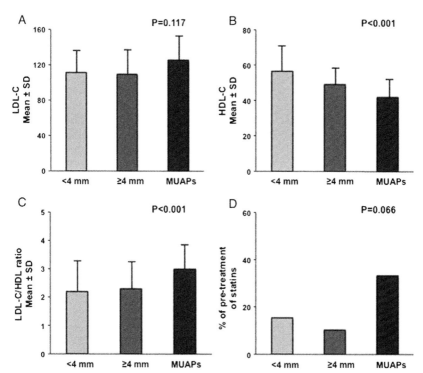

FIGURE 2.—Relationship between atheromatous aortic plaques and lipid profile. There was no signif-icant difference in low density lipoprotein cholesterol (LDL-C) among patients with atheromatous aortic plaques (AAPs) of <4 mm, ≥4 mm, and mobile and ulcerative aortic plaques (MUAPs) (A). Patients with MUAPs had significantly lower levels of high density lipoprotein cholesterol (HDL-C) (B) and higher levels of LDL-C/HDL-C ratio (C). Frequency of pre-treatment of statins were relatively higher in patients with MUAPs (D). (Reprinted from Journal of the Neurological Sciences. Okuzumi A, Ueno Y, Shimada Y, et al. Impact of low-density lipoprotein to high-density lipoprotein ratio on aortic arch atherosclerosis in unex-plained stroke. *J Neurol Sci.* 2013;326:83-88, Copyright 2013, with permission from Elsevier.)

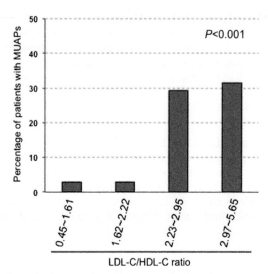

FIGURE 3.—Relationship between atheromatous aortic plaques and LDL-C/HDL-C ratio. Frequency of mobile and ulcerative aortic plaques (MUAPs) in stroke patients stratified by quartiles of LDL-C/HDL-C ratios. Percentages of MUAPs significantly increase in stroke patients with LDL-C/HDL-C ratios ≥ 2.23. (Reprinted from Journal of the Neurological Sciences. Okuzumi A, Ueno Y, Shimada Y, et al. Impact of low-density lipoprotein to high-density lipoprotein ratio on aortic arch atherosclerosis in unexplained stroke. *J Neurol Sci.* 2013;326:83-88, Copyright 2013, with permission from Elsevier.)

and enrolled to the study. Patients were classified based on TEE findings: (1) AAPs < 4 mm in thickness; (2) AAPs ≥ 4 mm; and (3) mobile or ulcerated aortic plaques (MUAPs). We assessed clinical characteristics and biochemical findings, and investigated the relationship between AAPs and the LDL-C/HDL-C ratio of stroke patients. 84 (61%) patients had AAPs < 4 mm, 29 (21%) had AAPs ≥ 4 mm, and 24 (18%) had MUAPs. Older age (OR: 1.18; 95% CI: 1.08 to 1.30; $p = 0.001$), and LDL-C/HDL-C ratio (OR: 2.94; 95% CI: 1.10 to 7.87; $p = 0.032$) were significantly associated with MUAPs. The incidence of MUAPs substantially increased in patients with LDL-C/HDL-C ratios of >2.23 ($p < 0.001$) when the ratios were divided into quartiles. The LDL-C/HDL-C ratio was closely associated with MUAPs. An elevated LDL-C/HDL-C ratio could be a positive predictor of aortogenic brain embolism (Figs 2 and 3).

▶ The low-density lipoprotein cholesterol (LDL-C) to high-density lipoprotein cholesterol (HDL-C) ratio is highly predictive of risk for both coronary and carotid atherosclerosis.[1,2] This is plausible based on the assumption that high LDL-C correlates with increased flux of atherogenic lipoprotein into the subendothelial space, whereas increased HDL-C presumptively correlates with higher capacity for reverse cholesterol transport. In the setting of ischemic stroke, it is standard of care to evaluate patients for the presence of carotid artery atherosclerosis and for the presence of mural thrombi in the left atrium and left ventricle. Although atherosclerotic plaque in the aorta can also be a source of thromboembolic phenomena,[3] evaluating the aorta via transesophageal echocardiography for computed tomography is less routinely undertaken.

In this retrospective case series of 137 patients (mean age, 65 years), Okuzumi et al evaluate the association between mobile and ulcerative aortic plaques (MUAPs) and unexplained embolic stroke. Low HDL-C and an increasing LDL-C/HDL-C ratio correlated significantly with the presence of MUAPs and risk of stroke (Figs 2 and 3). Eighteen percent of unexplained strokes were attributable to the presence of MUAPs.

MUAPs have complex morphology and frequently represent plaques that have undergone rupture (even repetitive rupture) with subsequent fibrosis and ulceration. Because of their instability and proclivity toward formation of overlying thrombus, they clearly pose a hazard for thromboembolic phenomena and occlusive stroke. This study highlights a high correlation between increasing LDL-C/HDL-C ratios and risk for aortic MUPAs and stroke. The threshold for elevated risk was approximately 2.33. In patients with unexplained stroke, evaluating the aorta for the presence of MUAPs appears warranted.

P. P. Toth, MD, PhD

References

1. Katakami N, Kaneto H, Osonoi T, et al. Usefulness of lipoprotein ratios in assessing carotid atherosclerosis in Japanese type 2 diabetic patients. *Atherosclerosis.* 2011;214:442-447.
2. Kimura T, Itoh T, Fusazaki T, et al. Low-density lipoprotein-cholesterol/high-density lipoprotein-cholesterol ratio predicts lipid-rich coronary plaque in patients with coronary artery disease—integrated-backscatter intravascular ultrasound study. *Circ J.* 2010;74:1392-1398.
3. Amarenco P, Duyckaerts C, Tzourio C, Hénin D, Bousser MG, Hauw JJ. The prevalence of ulcerated plaques in the aortic arch in patients with stroke. *N Engl J Med.* 1992;326:221-225.

3   Obesity

Introduction

This year, the subject of obesity continues to expand on concepts initiated by research over the last decade. Specifically, research in adipose tissue metabolism has elucidated that adipose cells in ectopic vs subcutaneous depots behave differently and that ectopic fat is more dysfunctional. It is possible that genetics control fat deposition. Those that can store copiously in subcutaneous fat tissue seem to evade obesity-related diseases and are considered "metabolically healthy" or insulin-sensitive obese. Those who cannot seem to store as much in subcutaneous depots then deposit fat "ectopically" in the liver, muscle, viscera, heart, and also in the pancreatic beta cells, and this tissue becomes inflamed. The inflammation causes dysfunction and leads to "metabolically unhealthy" or insulin-resistant obesity. There is still much to learn about inflamed adipose tissue and the pathways to insulin resistance and cardiovascular disease.

Bariatric surgical treatments are still the most successful treatment for extreme obesity, and research into the mechanism of bariatric surgery's effects on appetite and satiety has led to the discovery that the gut sends messages to the hypothalamus via ghrelin, Peptide YY, insulin, and GLP-1, among others, which govern and control the body set point. Bariatric surgery alters the secretion of these messages and is one of the main reasons for its tremendous success when compared to behavioral treatments. Weight loss by behavioral methods causes changes in gut hormone secretion that lead to more hunger and preoccupation with food than before weight was lost. Bariatric surgery causes alterations in gut hormone secretion which, in turn, causes more satiety with less food.

The gut microbiome is altered with bariatric surgery and, thus, adds to the reasoning that a change in the gut microflora is necessary for a change in the body set point, such that the microbiome interacts with gut hormones. Or is it that the microflora change brings about gut hormone alterations?

More work into adipose tissue has identified that adult humans have locales of brown adipose tissue (BAT), and that some white adipose tissue can be stimulated to become "beige" or "brite" adipose tissue with properties similar to BAT and enhanced nonshivering thermogenesis. This avenue of research may be the antidote for the deposition of ectopic dysfunctional fat, if indeed stimulating brown fat in adult humans is possible, and that the stimulation of BAT leads to enhanced oxidation of lipids and carbohydrates altering energy balance.

Despite the increasing prevalence of obesity worldwide, malnutrition and failure to thrive is still present in various parts of the world, and work in this area documents changes in prevalence of malnutrition with industrialization of the country, as well as novel treatment strategies to combat malnutrition.

Caroline M. Apovian, MD

Diet and Obesity

A Trial of Sugar-Free or Sugar-Sweetened Beverages and Body Weight in Children
de Ruyter JC, Olthof MR, Seidell JC, et al (VU Univ Amsterdam, the Netherlands)
N Engl J Med 367:1397-1406, 2012

Background.—The consumption of beverages that contain sugar is associated with overweight, possibly because liquid sugars do not lead to a sense of satiety, so the consumption of other foods is not reduced. However, data are lacking to show that the replacement of sugar-containing beverages with noncaloric beverages diminishes weight gain.

Methods.—We conducted an 18-month trial involving 641 primarily normal-weight children from 4 years 10 months to 11 years 11 months of age. Participants were randomly assigned to receive 250 ml (8 oz) per day of a sugar-free, artificially sweetened beverage (sugar-free group) or a similar sugar-containing beverage that provided 104 kcal (sugar group). Beverages were distributed through schools. At 18 months, 26% of the children had stopped consuming the beverages; the data from children who did not complete the study were imputed.

Results.—The z score for the body-mass index (BMI, the weight in kilograms divided by the square of the height in meters) increased on average by 0.02 SD units in the sugar-free group and by 0.15 SD units in the sugar group; the 95% confidence interval (CI) of the difference was −0.21 to −0.05. Weight increased by 6.35 kg in the sugar-free group as compared with 7.37 kg in the sugar group (95% CI for the difference, −1.54 to −0.48). The skinfold-thickness measurements, waist-to-height ratio, and fat mass also increased significantly less in the sugar-free group. Adverse events were minor. When we combined measurements at 18 months in 136 children who had discontinued the study with those in 477 children who completed the study, the BMI z score increased by 0.06 SD units in the sugar-free group and by 0.12 SD units in the sugar group ($P = 0.06$).

Conclusions.—Masked replacement of sugar-containing beverages with noncaloric beverages reduced weight gain and fat accumulation in normal-weight children. (Funded by the Netherlands Organization for Health Research and Development and others; DRINK ClinicalTrials.gov number, NCT00893529.)

▶ To contrast this study with the study by Ebbeling et al also commented on in this section, this is a study looking at an intervention in normal-weight children as opposed to those already overweight or obese. In addition, the study design was different from the one conducted by Ebbeling et al in that both groups here received beverages to consume, 1 receiving sugar-sweetened and the other sugar-free beverages. In this study, the effects of sugar-sweetened liquids as opposed to sugar-free liquids consumption was studied in normal-weight children, and it was found that noncaloric beverages reduced weight gain as well as fat accumulation in these children. Once again, this study can be used to support efforts to restrict the consumption of sugar-sweetened beverages as a public health method to curtail the obesity epidemic in the United States and elsewhere around the world. This study, as opposed to that of Ebbeling et al, suggests that sugar-sweetened beverage consumption causes fat accumulation in normal-weight children—a directly causative relationship as opposed to simply exacerbating the problem in the overweight and obese population. It plants the seed of causality because the relationship of sugar-sweetened beverages and the prevalence of obesity and the increase in this prevalence as it is being seen to be causative in normal-weight children, and not just in those already overweight or obese.

The study also leaves open to conjecture the premise that the consumption of sugar-sweetened beverages and other sugars, for that matter, can be habituating. This study supports the work of Schwartz et al that shows that sugar and fat consumption causes an inflammatory pattern in the hypothalamus such that body-weight regulation is impaired.[1] More research needs to be performed to show that, indeed, sugar consumption is causing this impairment of body-weight regulation resulting from inflammation in the hypothalamus.

C. Apovian, MD

Reference

1. Thaler JP, Yi CX, Schur EA, et al. Obesity is associated with hypothalamic injury in rodents and humans. *J Clin Invest*. 2012;122:153-162.

A Randomized Trial of Sugar-Sweetened Beverages and Adolescent Body Weight
Ebbeling CB, Feldman HA, Chomitz VR, et al (Boston Children's Hosp, MA; Inst for Community Health, Cambridge, MA; et al)
N Engl J Med 367:1407-1416, 2012

Background.—Consumption of sugar-sweetened beverages may cause excessive weight gain. We aimed to assess the effect on weight gain of an intervention that included the provision of noncaloric beverages at home for overweight and obese adolescents.

Methods.—We randomly assigned 224 overweight and obese adolescents who regularly consumed sugar-sweetened beverages to experimental and control groups. The experimental group received a 1-year intervention designed to decrease consumption of sugar-sweetened beverages, with follow-up for an additional year without intervention. We hypothesized that the experimental group would gain weight at a slower rate than the control group.

Results.—Retention rates were 97% at 1 year and 93% at 2 years. Reported consumption of sugar-sweetened beverages was similar at baseline in the experimental and control groups (1.7 servings per day), declined to nearly 0 in the experimental group at 1 year, and remained lower in the experimental group than in the control group at 2 years. The primary outcome, the change in mean body-mass index (BMI, the weight in kilograms divided by the square of the height in meters) at 2 years, did not differ significantly between the two groups (change in experimental group minus change in control group, -0.3; $P = 0.46$). At 1 year, however, there were significant between-group differences for changes in BMI (-0.57, $P = 0.045$) and weight (-1.9 kg, $P = 0.04$). We found evidence of effect modification according to ethnic group at 1 year ($P = 0.04$) and 2 years ($P = 0.01$). In a prespecified analysis according to ethnic group, among Hispanic participants (27 in the experimental group and 19 in the control group), there was a significant between-group difference in the change in BMI at 1 year (-1.79, $P = 0.007$) and 2 years (-2.35, $P = 0.01$), but not among non-Hispanic participants ($P > 0.35$ at years 1 and 2). The change in body fat as a percentage of total weight did not differ significantly between groups at 2 years (-0.5%, $P = 0.40$). There were no adverse events related to study participation.

Conclusions.—Among overweight and obese adolescents, the increase in BMI was smaller in the experimental group than in the control group after a 1-year intervention designed to reduce consumption of sugar-sweetened beverages, but not at the 2-year follow-up (the prespecified primary outcome). (Funded by the National Institute of Diabetes and Digestive and Kidney Diseases and others; ClinicalTrials.gov number, NCT00381160.)

▶ This study focuses on adolescents who are already overweight or obese and who regularly consume sugar-sweetened beverages. In a randomized, controlled trial, the researchers showed that a 1-year intervention designed to decrease consumption of sugar-sweetened beverages actually works. That is, compared with a control group, those in the experimental group gained less weight than those in the control group. However, at 2 years, there was no difference in the rate of weight gain in both groups. It is interesting that 1 year out of the intervention, there was no change in the weight gain trajectory of the 2 groups. This effect could occur because once the intervention ceased, adolescents were exposed to the same environmental cues to consume sugar-sweetened beverages as before, and, in fact, the data do corroborate this.

This study elegantly confirms hypotheses that a decrease in sugar-sweetened beverage consumption carried out by replacement by diet sodas or water can decrease weight gain seen in adolescents who are overweight or obese and who are on a trajectory of weight gain.

This study also confirms the utility of a suggested public health policy to restrict consumption of sugar-sweetened beverages in an effort to halt or curtail the obesity epidemic.

Studies have suggested mechanisms of action for the single effect of sugar-sweetened liquids to increase body weight. Food intake studies have found that ingestion of sugar-sweetened liquids does not result in a decrease in food intake to compensate for liquid calories, suggesting that sugar intake in the form of liquids does not cause satiation in the hypothalamus to the same extent as does solid food of similar caloric content.[1]

The political ramifications of a study such as this can be striking, such as a mandated tax on sugar-sweetened beverages or other forms of restriction that can be even more striking, as evidenced by the policies mandated by governments to successfully decrease tobacco use in the United States and elsewhere. The outcomes of this study support the claim that a decrease in sugar-sweetened beverage intake can single-handedly decrease the trajectory of increase in body weight compared with intake of water or diet beverages in the same quantity in obese adolescents. Other supportive facts are that sugar-sweetened beverages do not contribute to the nutritional quality of the diet in any form except to provide fluid intake, which can be replaced solely by water.

C. Apovian, MD

Reference

1. Cassady BA, Considine RV, Mattes RD. Beverage consumption, appetite, and energy intake: what did you expect? *Am J Clin Nutr.* 2012;95:587-593.

Natural killer T cells in adipose tissue prevent insulin resistance
Schipper HS, Rakhshandehroo M, van de Graaf SFJ, et al (Univ Med Ctr Utrecht, the Netherlands; et al)
J Clin Invest 122:3343-3354, 2012

Lipid overload and adipocyte dysfunction are key to the development of insulin resistance and can be induced by a high-fat diet. CD1d-restricted invariant natural killer T (iNKT) cells have been proposed as mediators between lipid overload and insulin resistance, but recent studies found decreased iNKT cell numbers and marginal effects of iNKT cell depletion on insulin resistance under high-fat diet conditions. Here, we focused on the role of iNKT cells under normal conditions. We showed that iNKT cell—deficient mice on a low-fat diet, considered a normal diet for mice, displayed a distinctive insulin resistance phenotype without overt adipose tissue inflammation. Insulin resistance was characterized by adipocyte dysfunction, including adipocyte hypertrophy, increased leptin, and decreased adiponectin levels. The lack of liver abnormalities in CD1d-null mice together with the enrichment of CD1d-restricted iNKT cells in both mouse and human adipose tissue indicated a specific role for adipose tissue—resident iNKT cells in the development of insulin resistance. Strikingly, iNKT cell function was directly modulated by adipocytes, which acted as lipid antigen-presenting cells in a CD1d-mediated fashion. Based on these findings, we propose that, especially under low-fat diet conditions, adipose

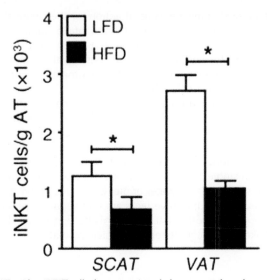

FIGURE 2.—AT-resident iNKT cells show an activated phenotype and are downregulated on a long-term HFD. **(F)** Number of iNKT cells per gram of SCAT and VAT of WT mice on LFD and HFD regimens. $n = 10$ mice per group; total 20 mice. *$P < 0.05$. (Reprinted from Schipper HS, Rakhshandehroo M, van de Graaf SFJ, et al. Natural killer T cells in adipose tissue prevent insulin resistance. *J Clin Invest.* 2012;122:3343-3354, © 2012, American Society of Clinical Investigation.)

tissue-resident iNKT cells maintain healthy adipose tissue through direct interplay with adipocytes and prevent insulin resistance (Fig 2F).

▶ The last few years in adipose tissue (AT) research has led to the realization that excess fat accumulation in certain types of adipose cells leads to dysfunction, which is crucial to development of an inflammatory response in AT. This activates the inflammasome and the release of free fatty acids and adipocytokines, which impairs insulin receptor signaling and is the cascade that ultimately leads to dysmetabolic syndrome, type 2 diabetes, and atherosclerosis. More research has found that control of this inflammation by immune homeostasis is imparted by Treg cells in addition to eosinophils, which serve to counteract the influx into AT of M1 macrophages, CD8 T cells, CD4 T cells, and B cells, and prevent AT inflammation and insulin resistance. This article by Schipper et al serves to implicate natural killer T (iNKT) cells in controlling AT inflammation and insulin resistance. The researchers found that iNKT cell–deficient mice on a low-fat diet (normal diet for mice) showed an insulin resistance phenotype without developing AT inflammation first.

Interestingly, in wild type mice fed a high fat diet, a decrease in iNKT numbers in visceral and subcutaneous AT was observed (Fig 2F).

The authors proposed, based on the findings, that AT resident iNKT cells maintain healthy adipose tissue by direct interaction with adipose tissue and that inflammation may be heralded by AT itself, modulating itself via the action of cells such as natural killer T cells. In addition, the authors conclude that iNKT cell function seems to depend on the composition of the diet and duration of the diet (ie, high fat vs low fat), which is a direct link from the diet to inflammation starting with AT. In addition, other work has shown that not only does immune function depend on diet composition but also possibly on the gut microbiota.[1] Thus, iNKT cells can be seen as protective of the health of the AT as well as of the entire host. The protective role of iNKT cells appears most pronounced under long-term low-fat diet ingestion and in lean mice. Therefore, if these results can be extrapolated to human AT, the development of insulin resistance and metabolic syndrome may be delayed or impaired by iNKT cells, and they may be able to do this job best under conditions of a lean phenotype and/or a low-fat healthy diet. More research in the area of AT inflammation and development of insulin resistance should focus on composition of long-term diet as well as interactions between the diet, gut microbiota, and AT inflammation both in visceral and subcutaneous human adipose tissue.

C. Apovian, MD

Reference

1. Cani PD, Delzenne NM. Interplay between obesity and associated metabolic disorders: new insights into the gut microbiota. *Curr Opin Pharmacol.* 2009;9:737-743.

History of weight cycling does not impede future weight loss or metabolic improvements in postmenopausal women
Mason C, Foster-Schubert KE, Imayama I, et al (Fred Hutchinson Cancer Res Ctr, Seattle, WA; Univ of Washington, Seattle, WA; Univ of Illinois at Chicago, IL; et al)
Metabolism 62:127-136, 2013

Objective.—Given that the repetitive loss and regain of body weight, termed weight cycling, is a prevalent phenomenon that has been associated with negative physiological and psychological outcomes, the purpose of this study was to investigate weight change and physiological outcomes in women with a lifetime history of weight cycling enrolled in a 12-month diet and/or exercise intervention.

Methods.—439 overweight, inactive, postmenopausal women were randomized to: i) dietary weight loss with a 10% weight loss goal (N = 118); ii) moderate-to-vigorous intensity aerobic exercise for 45 min/ day, 5 days/week (n = 117); iii) both dietary weight loss and exercise (n = 117); or iv) control (n = 87). Women were categorized as non-, moderate- (≥3 losses of ≥4.5 kg), or severe-cyclers (≥3 losses of ≥9.1 kg). Trend tests and linear regression were used to compare adherence and changes in weight, body composition, blood pressure, insulin, C-peptide, glucose, insulin resistance (HOMA-IR), C-reactive protein, leptin, adiponectin, and interleukin-6 between cyclers and non-cyclers.

Results.—Moderate (n = 103) and severe (n = 77) cyclers were heavier and had less favorable metabolic profiles than non-cyclers at baseline. There were, however, no significant differences in adherence to the lifestyle interventions. Weight-cyclers (combined) had a greater improvement in HOMA-IR compared to non-cyclers participating in the exercise only intervention ($P = .03$), but no differences were apparent in the other groups.

Conclusion.—A history of weight cycling does not impede successful participation in lifestyle interventions or alter the benefits of diet and/or exercise on body composition and metabolic outcomes.

▶ The prevalence of overweight and obesity is high, and in many Western countries it exceeds 50% of the population. Lifestyle modification, including a low-calorie diet, physical activity, and behavioral treatment, is the main stem of therapy. Unfortunately, success with such approaches is disappointing, and up to 95% of individuals losing weight will regain part or the whole amount of weight lost. Weight cycling is, therefore, common in overweight or obese subjects and is associated with a negative psychological and physiological outcome; for instance, it is known that in the process of weight gain, there is an increase in fat mass compared with lean mass, which will decrease resting energy expenditure and promote weight gain over time. Hormonal changes such as an increase in ghrelin levels have also been reported in cyclers compared to noncyclers.

These authors randomly assigned 439 postmenopausal women to 4 different groups: calorie-reduced diet, aerobic exercise, aerobic exercise and calorie-reduced diet, and a control group. A history of weight cycling was assessed in the participants of the study. Women were characterized as noncyclers, moderate cyclers if they had more than 3 cycles of diet with a weight loss greater than 4.5 kg, or severe cyclers if they had more than 3 cycles in which they achieved a weight loss of greater than 9.1 kg. Moderate and severe cyclers were heavier and had a larger waist circumference and percentage of body weight as fat. Nevertheless, the adherence to the different lifestyle modalities and weight loss was similar among the groups. Concerning homeostatic hormones (leptin, insulin, adiponectin), no differences were found between cyclers and noncyclers after 12 months of diet with or without exercise.

Unsuccessful weight loss should not preclude further weight loss attempts.

R. Ness-Abramof, MD

Translating the Diabetes Prevention Program Lifestyle Intervention for Weight Loss Into Primary Care: A Randomized Trial
Ma J, Yank V, Xiao L, et al (Palo Alto Med Foundation Res Inst, CA; et al)
JAMA Intern Med 173:113-121, 2013

Background.—The Diabetes Prevention Program (DPP) lifestyle intervention reduced the incidence of type 2 diabetes mellitus (DM) among high-risk adults by 58%, with weight loss as the dominant predictor. However, it has not been adequately translated into primary care.

Methods.—We evaluated 2 adapted DPP lifestyle interventions among overweight or obese adults who were recruited from 1 primary care clinic and had pre-DM and/or metabolic syndrome. Participants were randomized to (1) a coach-led group intervention (n = 79), (2) a self-directed DVD intervention (n = 81), or (3) usual care (n = 81). During a 3-month intensive intervention phase, the DPP-based behavioral weight-loss curriculum was delivered by lifestyle coach—led small groups or home-based DVD. During the maintenance phase, participants in both interventions received lifestyle change coaching and support remotely—through secure email within an electronic health record system and the American Heart Association Heart360 website for weight and physical activity goal setting and self-monitoring. The primary outcome was change in body mass index (BMI) (calculated as weight in kilograms divided by height in meters squared) from baseline to 15 months.

Results.—At baseline, participants had a mean (SD) age of 52.9 (10.6) years and a mean BMI of 32.0 (5.4); 47% were female; 78%, non-Hispanic white; and 17%, Asian/Pacific Islander. At month 15, the mean ± SE change in BMI from baseline was −2.2 ± 0.3 in the coach-led group vs −0.9 ± 0.3 in the usual care group (P < .001) and −1.6 ± 0.3 in the self-directed group vs usual care (P = .02). The percentages of participants who achieved the 7% DPP-based weight-loss goal were 37.0% (P = .003) and 35.9% (P = .004) in the coach-led and self-directed groups, respectively, vs 14.4% in the usual care group. Both interventions also achieved greater net improvements in waist circumference and fasting plasma glucose level.

Conclusion.—Proven effective in a primary care setting, the 2 DPP-based lifestyle interventions are readily scalable and exportable with potential for substantial clinical and public health impact.

▶ Obesity is a major health problem and the main culprit for the increasing prevalence of type 2 diabetes mellitus (T2DM) worldwide. T2DM was shown to be delayed or prevented by lifestyle changes, including weight loss and exercise. The Diabetes Preventions Program (DPP) enrolled and randomized 3232 patients with impaired glucose tolerance to intensive lifestyle changes (including a weight loss of 7% of original body weight and at least 150 minutes of physical activity per week), metformin therapy, or placebo. The incidence of T2DM was reduced by 58% in the lifestyle intervention group and by 31% in the metformin group compared with the placebo group.[1] A 10-year follow-up trial showed a protective effect of lifestyle change and metformin therapy in the incidence of T2DM.[2]

The main question is whether intensive lifestyle changes delivered by specialized staff may be adapted and incorporated into primary care practices with the same success.

This study recruited overweight and obese adults with prediabetes, metabolic syndrome, or both and evaluated 2 adapted DPP lifestyle interventions: a coach-led personal intervention group, a self-directed DVD intervention, and a usual care group and followed these patients over 15 months. In the coach-led group, 37% achieved a weight loss of at least 7%, in the self-directed group 35.9%, and in the usual care group 14.4%. Fasting blood glucose was lowered in the 2 intervention groups and both had a decrease in waist circumference. Weight loss was more pronounced in the coached-based program compared with the DVD program. Women responded better to the coach-based intervention, while men responded equally to both (see Fig 2 in the original article).

Although this study was not designed to evaluate prevention of diabetes, its strength is in the adaptation of a complex lifestyle change program in a primary care clinic and even to a self-directed approach through DVD sessions. Although promising, the study, as mentioned by the authors, was done with a relatively well-educated population, and its implementation in lower socioeconomic classes needs to be evaluated. Nevertheless, this study brings the commendable DPP study to clinical practice.

R. Ness-Abramof, MD

References

1. Knowler WC, Barrett-Connor E, Fowler SE, et al. Diabetes Prevention Program Research Group. Reduction in the incidence of type 2 diabetes with lifestyle intervention or metformin. *N Engl J Med.* 2002;346:393-403.
2. Diabetes Prevention Program Research Group. Knowler WC, Fowler SE, Hamman RF, et al. 10-year follow-up of diabetes incidence and weight loss in the Diabetes Prevention Program Outcomes Study. *Lancet.* 2009;374:1677-1686.

Epidemiology and Complications of Obesity

Metabolically healthy obesity and risk of all-cause and cardiovascular disease mortality
Hamer M, Stamatakis E (Univ College London, UK)
J Clin Endocrinol Metab 97:2482-2488, 2012

Context.—Previous studies have identified an obese phenotype without the burden of adiposity-associated cardiometabolic risk factors, although the health effects remain unclear.

Objective.—This study examined the association between metabolically healthy obesity and risk of cardiovascular disease (CVD) and all-cause mortality.

Research Design and Methods.—This was an observational study with prospective linkage to mortality records in community-dwelling adults from the general population in Scotland and England. A total of 22,203 men and women [aged 54.1 (SD 12.7 yr), 45.2% men] without known history of CVD at baseline. Participants were classified as metabolically healthy (0 or 1 metabolic abnormality) or unhealthy (two or more metabolic abnormalities) based on blood pressure, high-density lipoprotein-cholesterol, diabetes diagnosis, waist circumference, and low-grade inflammation (C-reactive protein ≥ 3 mg/liter). Obesity was defined as a body mass index of 30 kg/m^2 or greater. Study members were followed up, on average, more than 7.0 ± 3.0 yr for cause-specific mortality. Cox proportional hazards models were used to examine the association of metabolic health/obesity categories with mortality.

Results.—There were 604 CVD and 1868 all-cause deaths, respectively. Compared with the metabolically healthy nonobese participants, their obese counterparts were not at elevated risk of CVD [hazard ratio (HR) 1.26, 95% confidence interval (CI) 0.74–2.13], although both nonobese (HR 1.59, 95% CI 1.30–1.94) and obese (HR 1.64, 95% CI 1.17–2.30) participants with two or more metabolic abnormalities were at elevated risk. Metabolically unhealthy obese participants were at elevated risk of all-cause mortality compared with their metabolically healthy obese counterparts (HR 1.72, 95% CI 1.23–2.41).

Conclusion.—Metabolically healthy obese participants were not at increased risk of CVD and all-cause mortality over 7 yr.

▶ This is a large epidemiologic study of 22 203 subjects in England and Scotland. The study looked the development of cardiovascular disease (CVD) and all-cause mortality in healthy and unhealthy obese compared with nonobese subjects for an average of 7 years. The findings from this study show that obesity is not an independent risk factor for development of CVD; rather, the presence of 2 or more metabolic syndrome characteristics is needed. On the mutually adjusted models, diabetes had the highest hazard ratio (1.77, 95% confidence interval [CI], 1.33–2.35) associated with CVD, followed by low-grade inflammation, C-reactive protein greater than 3 mg/L (1.67, 95% CI, 1.42–1.97), and hypertension (1.55, 95% CI, 1.30–1.84). There was no difference in the risk of CVD when comparing the metabolic healthy obese with the metabolic healthy nonobese. These findings contradict those in some other studies,[1] including the one previously mentioned (Lee and Seung Ku, Korean epidemiology study). The inconsistency in results is likely due to the time that the patients were followed up and its endpoints. This study only looks at mortality related to obesity in a 7 ± 3-years period and not at morbidity. Participants who are obese may take years to have metabolic syndrome characteristics that would eventually affect the cardiovascular system leading to death. In addition, the metabolic healthy participants were younger than the metabolic unhealthy, which may also affect the results—a higher percentage of the metabolic unhealthy had higher CVD mortality. Another possible confounding factor is the use of overweight participants with body mass index from 25 to 29.9 kg/m^2 and one metabolic risk factor in the control group. Although the authors of this study address this issue by doing a sensitivity analysis, it may affect the interpretation of the results because there may be no difference between the healthy nonobese to the healthy obese. There may also be an overestimation of the healthy participants because fasting glucose levels and triglycerides were not checked. Those labeled as healthy may actually have insulin resistance, which is a significant risk factor for CVD development. Another problem with the study was that only one evaluation was done at baseline, and participants' metabolic profiles possibly changed over the 7 years from healthy to unhealthy. Although this was a large epidemiologic study with an appropriate population sample, there are confounding factors and flaws in the study design that could have affected the interpretation of the results. The study does raise some interesting questions about the effects of inflammation in the development of CVD; however, given the conflicting results from other studies on the independent effect of obesity on CVD, more large-scale prospective studies with multiple endpoints need to be done to conclude whether obesity is an independent risk factor in the development of CVD. We can then use these results to target our clinical practices.

J. Simonetti, MD

Reference

1. Després JP. What is "metabolically healthy obesity"?: from epidemiology to pathophysiological insights. *J Clin Endocrinol Metab.* 2012;97:2283-2285.

Myths, Presumptions, and Facts about Obesity

Casazza K, Fontaine KR, Astrup A, et al (Univ of Alabama at Birmingham; Univ of Copenhagen, Denmark; et al)
N Engl J Med 368:446-454, 2013

Background.—Many beliefs about obesity persist in the absence of supporting scientific evidence (presumptions); some persist despite contradicting evidence (myths). The promulgation of unsupported beliefs may yield poorly informed policy decisions, inaccurate clinical and public health

TABLE 1.—Seven Myths about Obesity*

Myth	Basis of Conjecture
Small sustained changes in energy intake or expenditure will produce large, long-term weight changes	National health guidelines and reputable websites advertise that large changes in weight accumulate indefinitely after small sustained daily lifestyle modifications (e.g., walking for 20 minutes or eating two additional potato chips)
Setting realistic goals in obesity treatment is important because otherwise patients will become frustrated and lose less weight	According to goal-setting theory, unattainable goals impair performance and discourage goal-attaining behavior; in obesity treatment, incongruence between desired and actual weight loss is thought to undermine the patient's perceived ability to attain goals, which may lead to the discontinuation of behaviors necessary for weight loss
Large, rapid weight loss is associated with poorer long-term weight outcomes than is slow, gradual weight loss	This notion probably emerged in reaction to the adverse effects of nutritionally insufficient very-low-calorie diets (<800 kcal per day) in the 1960s; the belief has persisted, has been repeated in textbooks and recommendations from health authorities, and has been offered as a rule by dietitians
Assessing the stage of change or diet readiness is important in helping patients who seek weight-loss treatment	Many believe that patients who feel ready to lose weight are more likely to make the required lifestyle changes
Physical-education classes in their current format play an important role in preventing or reducing childhood obesity	The health benefits of physical activity of sufficient duration, frequency, and intensity are well established and include reductions in adiposity
Breast-feeding is protective against obesity	The belief that breast-fed children are less likely to become obese has persisted for more than a century and is passionately defended
A bout of sexual activity burns 100 to 300 kcal for each person involved	Many sources state that substantial energy is expended in typical sexual activity between two adults

*We define myths as beliefs held true despite substantial evidence refuting them. A list of articles in which these myths are espoused is provided in the Supplementary Appendix.

TABLE 2.—Presumptions about Obesity*

Presumption	Basis for Conjecture
Regularly eating (vs. skipping) breakfast is protective against obesity	Skipping breakfast purportedly leads to overeating later in the day
Early childhood is the period during which we learn exercise and eating habits that influence our weight throughout life	Weight-for-height indexes, eating behaviors, and preferences that are present in early childhood are correlated with those later in life
Eating more fruits and vegetables will result in weight loss or less weight gain, regardless of whether one intentionally makes any other behavioral or environmental changes	By eating more fruits and vegetables, a person presumably spontaneously eats less of other foods, and the resulting reduction in calories is greater than the increase in calories from the fruit and vegetables
Weight cycling (i.e., yo-yo dieting) is associated with increased mortality	In observational studies, mortality rates have been lower among persons with stable weight than among those with unstable weight
Snacking contributes to weight gain and obesity	Snack foods are presumed to be incompletely compensated for at subsequent meals, leading to weight gain
The built environment, in terms of sidewalk and park availability, influences obesity	Neighborhood-environment features may promote or inhibit physical activity, thereby affecting obesity

*We define presumptions as unproved yet commonly espoused propositions. A list of articles in which these presumptions are implied is provided in the Supplementary Appendix.

recommendations, and an unproductive allocation of research resources and may divert attention away from useful, evidence-based information.

Methods.—Using Internet searches of popular media and scientific literature, we identified, reviewed, and classified obesity-related myths and presumptions. We also examined facts that are well supported by evidence, with an emphasis on those that have practical implications for public health, policy, or clinical recommendations.

Results.—We identified seven obesity-related myths concerning the effects of small sustained increases in energy intake or expenditure, establishment of realistic goals for weight loss, rapid weight loss, weight-loss readiness, physical-education classes, breast-feeding, and energy expended during sexual activity. We also identified six presumptions about the purported effects of regularly eating breakfast, early childhood experiences, eating fruits and vegetables, weight cycling, snacking, and the built (i.e., human-made) environment. Finally, we identified nine evidence-supported facts that are relevant for the formulation of sound public health, policy, or clinical recommendations.

Conclusions.—False and scientifically unsupported beliefs about obesity are pervasive in both scientific literature and the popular press. (Funded by the National Institutes of Health.) (Tables 1-3).

▶ The 3 tables in this review of the literature identify 7 myths of obesity, 6 presumptions of obesity, and 9 evidence-supported facts that should be used to move forward with public policy and clinical guidelines to combat the obesity epidemic.

TABLE 3.—Facts about Obesity*

Fact	Implication
Although genetic factors play a large role, heritability is not destiny; calculations show that moderate environmental changes can promote as much weight loss as the most efficacious pharmaceutical agents available[26]	If we can identify key environmental factors and successfully influence them, we can achieve clinically significant reductions in obesity
Diets (i.e., reduced energy intake) very effectively reduce weight, but trying to go on a diet or recommending that someone go on a diet generally does not work well in the long-term[27]	This seemingly obvious distinction is often missed, leading to erroneous conceptions regarding possible treatments for obesity; recognizing this distinction helps our understanding that energy reduction is the ultimate dietary intervention required and approaches such as eating more vegetables or eating breakfast daily are likely to help only if they are accompanied by an overall reduction in energy intake
Regardless of body weight or weight loss, an increased level of exercise increases health[28]	Exercise offers a way to mitigate the health-damaging effects of obesity, even without weight loss
Physical activity or exercise in a sufficient dose aids in long-term weight aintenance[28,29]	Physical-activity programs are important, especially for children, but for physical activity to affect weight, there must be a substantial quantity of movement, not mere participation
Continuation of conditions that promote weight loss promotes maintenance of lower weight[30]	Obesity is best conceptualized as a chronic condition, requiring ongoing management to maintain long-term weight loss
For overweight children, programs that involve the parents and the home setting promote greater weight loss or maintenance[31]	Programs provided only in schools or other out-of-home structured settings may be convenient or politically expedient, but programs including interventions that involve the parents and are provided at home are likely to yield better outcomes
Provision of meals and use of meal-replacement products promote greater weight loss[32]	More structure regarding meals is associated with greater weight loss, as compared with seemingly holistic programs that are based on concepts of balance, variety, and moderation
Some pharmaceutical agents can help patients achieve clinically meaningful weight loss and maintain the reduction as long as the agents continue to be used[33]	While we learn how to alter the environment and individual behaviors to prevent obesity, we can offer moderately effective treatment to obese persons
In appropriate patients, bariatric surgery results in long-term weight loss and reductions in the rate of incident diabetes and mortality[34]	For severely obese persons, bariatric surgery can offer a life-changing, and in some cases lifesaving, treatment

Editor's Note: Please refer to original journal article for full references.
*We classify the listed propositions as facts because there is sufficient evidence to consider them empirically proved.

These myths and presumptions have been promulgated by the media but also by the difficulty that medicine and public health have had combating the consistent increase in prevalence of overweight and obesity since the early 1970s in this country and abroad.

C. Apovian, MD

Trends in mild, moderate, and severe stunting and underweight, and progress towards MDG 1 in 141 developing countries: a systematic analysis of population representative data
Stevens GA, on behalf of Nutrition Impact Model Study Group (Child Growth) (WHO, Geneva, Switzerland; et al)
Lancet 380:824-834, 2012

Background.—There is little information on country trends in the complete distributions of children's anthropometric status, which are needed to assess all levels of mild to severe undernutrition. We aimed to estimate trends in the distributions of children's anthropometric status and assess progress towards the Millennium Development Goal 1 (MDG 1) target of halving the prevalence of weight-for-age Z score (WAZ) below -2 between 1990 and 2015 or reaching a prevalence of $2 \cdot 3\%$ or lower.

Methods.—We collated population-representative data on height-for-age Z score (HAZ) and WAZ calculated with the 2006 WHO child growth standards. Our data sources were health and nutrition surveys, summary statistics from the WHO Global Database on Child Growth and Malnutrition, and summary statistics from reports of other national and international agencies. We used a Bayesian hierarchical mixture model to estimate Z-score distributions. We quantified the uncertainty of our estimates, assessed their validity, compared their performance to alternative models, and assessed sensitivity to key modelling choices.

Findings.—In developing countries, mean HAZ improved from -1.86 (95% uncertainty interval $-2 \cdot 01$ to $-1 \cdot 72$) in 1985 to $-1 \cdot 16$ ($-1 \cdot 29$ to $-1 \cdot 04$) in 2011; mean WAZ improved from $-1 \cdot 31$ ($-1 \cdot 41$ to $-1 \cdot 20$) to $-0 \cdot 84$ ($-0 \cdot 93$ to $-0 \cdot 74$). Over this period, prevalences of moderate-and-severe stunting declined from $47 \cdot 2\%$ ($44 \cdot 0$ to $50 \cdot 3$) to $29 \cdot 9\%$ ($27 \cdot 1$ to $32 \cdot 9$) and underweight from $30 \cdot 1\%$ ($26 \cdot 7$ to $33 \cdot 3$) to $19 \cdot 4\%$ ($16 \cdot 5$ to $22 \cdot 2$). The largest absolute improvements were in Asia and the largest relative reductions in prevalence in southern and tropical Latin America. Anthropometric status worsened in sub-Saharan Africa until the late 1990s and improved thereafter. In 2011, 314 (296 to 331) million children younger than 5 years were mildly, moderately, or severely stunted and 258 (240 to 274) million were mildly, moderately, or severely underweight. Developing countries as a whole have less than a 5% chance of meeting the MDG 1 target; but 61 of these 141 countries have a 50–100% chance.

Interpretation.—Macroeconomic shocks, structural adjustment, and trade policy reforms in the 1980s and 1990s might have been responsible for worsening child nutritional status in sub-Saharan Africa. Further progress in the improvement of children's growth and nutrition needs equitable economic growth and investment in pro-poor food and primary care programmes, especially relevant in the context of the global economic crisis (Fig 5).

▶ With overnutrition on the increase in industrialized countries, a concern still exists in many developing countries regarding undernutrition and stunting in

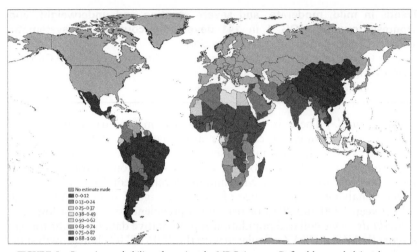

FIGURE 5.—Posterior probability of meeting the MDG 1 target. Defined here as halving the preva-lence of WAZ below −2 between 1990 and 2015 or reaching a prevalence 2·3% or lower if post-2000 trend continues. WAZ = weight-for-age Z score. (Reprinted from The Lancet. Stevens GA, on behalf of Nutrition Impact Model Study Group [Child Growth]. Trends in mild, moderate, and severe stunting and underweight, and progress towards MDG 1 in 141 developing countries: a systematic analysis of pop-ulation representative data. *Lancet.* 2012;380:824-834, Copyright 2012, with permission from Elsevier.)

children side by side with overnutrition in older children and adults. This system-atic analysis of population representative data evaluates stunting and under-weight children in 141 developing countries between 1985 and 2011. With all developing countries taken together, the data show that children's anthropo-metric status improved between 1985 and 2011 but did not reach the optimum nutritional status as defined by the World Health Organization growth standards. In addition, there were differences in trends across regions and countries and in current nutritional status. There were vast improvements in the nutritional status of children in Asian and the Latin Americas and Caribbean regions compared with stagnation or deterioration in nutritional status of children in Oceania and sub-Saharan Africa. Therefore, results show that children in some countries of sub-Saharan Africa and south Asia are extremely undernourished. In the Latin American region, Caribbean, central Asia, Middle East, north Africa, and east Asia children are, for the most part, fulfilling their growth potential. Even though this is promising, more than half of the developing countries have less than a 50% chance of meeting the Millennium Development Goal target of children fulfilling growth potential (Fig 5).

Children's growth depends on lowering infection rates and improving nutrition in challenged countries. Food insufficiency, poor water and sanitation, and restricted access to high-quality primary care are all associated with poverty and lead to poor growth outcomes. This article noted that reductions in stunting and underweight prevalence were caused by an improvement in all the items listed above. Growth in national income needs to be coupled with equitable income distribution and investments in health care, agriculture, and government programs that improve access to food. Sub-Saharan Africa saw reforms in the

1980s and 1990s that led to adverse effects on nutrition that were the largest in poorer households because they led to lower spending on agriculture and health care. The authors suggest that child nutrition is best improved through policies that improve agricultural productivity and earnings of smallholder farmers and proper primary care and food programs. Taken in the context of the worldwide obesity epidemic, these are similar programs that have been targeted to combat obesity—improvement by offering access to fresh fruits and vegetables through subsidized farming, among other public policy efforts.

C. Apovian, MD

Sugar-Sweetened Beverages and Genetic Risk of Obesity
Qi Q, Chu AY, Kang JH, et al (Harvard School of Public Health, Boston, MA; Brigham and Women's Hosp and Harvard Med School, Boston, MA)
N Engl J Med 367:1387-1396, 2012

Background.—Temporal increases in the consumption of sugar-sweetened beverages have paralleled the rise in obesity prevalence, but whether the intake of such beverages interacts with the genetic predisposition to adiposity is unknown.

Methods.—We analyzed the interaction between genetic predisposition and the intake of sugar-sweetened beverages in relation to body-mass index (BMI; the weight in kilograms divided by the square of the height in meters) and obesity risk in 6934 women from the Nurses' Health Study (NHS) and in 4423 men from the Health Professionals Follow-up Study (HPFS) and also in a replication cohort of 21,740 women from the Women's Genome Health Study (WGHS). The genetic-predisposition score was calculated on the basis of 32 BMI-associated loci. The intake of sugar-sweetened beverages was examined prospectively in relation to BMI.

Results.—In the NHS and HPFS cohorts, the genetic association with BMI was stronger among participants with higher intake of sugar-sweetened beverages than among those with lower intake. In the combined cohorts, the increases in BMI per increment of 10 risk alleles were 1.00 for an intake of less than one serving per month, 1.12 for one to four servings per month, 1.38 for two to six servings per week, and 1.78 for one or more servings per day ($P < 0.001$ for interaction). For the same categories of intake, the relative risks of incident obesity per increment of 10 risk alleles were 1.19 (95% confidence interval [CI], 0.90 to 1.59), 1.67 (95% CI, 1.28 to 2.16), 1.58 (95% CI, 1.01 to 2.47), and 5.06 (95% CI, 1.66 to 15.5) ($P = 0.02$ for interaction). In the WGHS cohort, the increases in BMI per increment of 10 risk alleles were 1.39, 1.64, 1.90, and 2.53 across the four categories of intake ($P = 0.001$ for interaction); the relative risks for incident obesity were 1.40 (95% CI, 1.19 to 1.64), 1.50 (95% CI, 1.16 to 1.93), 1.54 (95% CI, 1.21 to 1.94), and 3.16 (95% CI, 2.03 to 4.92), respectively ($P = 0.007$ for interaction).

Conclusions.—The genetic association with adiposity appeared to be more pronounced with greater intake of sugar-sweetened beverages. (Funded by the National Institutes of Health and others.)

▶ This study is an epidemiologic complimentary article to the other 2 interventional articles commented on in this section on sugar-sweetened beverages and risk of obesity.

This study utilizes data from both the Nurses' Health Study and the Health Professionals follow-up study to obtain data from both men and women on genetic predisposition to obesity and intake of sugar-sweetened beverages. The other 2 studies support a causal relationship among the consumption of sugar-sweetened beverages, weight gain, and the risk of obesity.

This study shows that the genetic effects on adiposity are stronger in persons with higher intake of sugar-sweetened beverages than those with lower intake of those beverages. Put another way, the impact of one serving of sugar-sweetened beverages per day on body mass index (BMI) varies according to how many obesity predisposition genes are present. Fig 2 in the original article taken from the report and reproduced here illustrates this visually in several different cohorts of persons. The increased consumption might contribute to the obesity epidemic by interacting with a genetic predisposition to elevated BMI. Or perhaps persons with a greater genetic predisposition may be more susceptible to obesity-inducing effects of sugar-sweetened beverages. The consumption of sugar-sweetened liquids most likely causes or contributes to obesity because of incomplete compensation for liquid calories by decreasing intake of solid food calories. However, there may be an additional contribution of sugar intake to inflammation in the hypothalamus as has been seen with high-fat feeding in mice and rats. This causes a dysfunction in the appetite and satiety regulation, and the mice and rats continue to eat beyond their body set point. This needs to be shown to be the case in humans, although magnetic resonance imaging of obese persons does show hypothalamic inflammation.

It may be a stretch to attribute the effects of high-fat feeding in mice to overfeeding fat and then assume that high-sugar feeding would exert the same effect on the hypothalamus in humans. However, it remains a fact that sugar-sweetened beverages make up at least 7% of daily caloric intake in Americans and that the increase in prevalence of obesity parallels the increase in consumption of sugar-sweetened beverages in the United States. It is just too easy a target for public policy makers to leave alone, and the eradication of sugar-sweetened beverages would not affect nutritional quality in the least.

C. Apovian, MD

Obesity phenotype and incident hypertension: a prospective community-based cohort study

Lee SK, Kim SH, Cho GY, et al (Korea Univ Ansan Hosp)
J Hypertens 31:145-151, 2013

Objective.—This is a prospective investigation of the association between the obesity phenotype (healthy vs. unhealthy obese) and the incidence of hypertension.

Research Design and Methods.—2352 participants, aged 40-69 years at baseline, with normal blood pressure (BP) from the Ansan cohort and the Ansung cohort of the Korean Genome Epidemiology Study. Participants were divided into six groups based on BMI and the metabolic syndrome (MetS) components: healthy (none of the five MetS components) normal weight (BMI 2), unhealthy (one or more MetS component) normal weight, healthy overweight (BMI 23-24.9 kg/m^2), unhealthy overweight, healthy obesity (BMI >=25 kg/m^2), and unhealthy obesity. The incidence of hypertension was identified by biennial health examinations during the 8-year follow-up.

Results.—After adjusting for age, sex, cohort, physical activity, smoking, alcohol consumption, and family history of hypertension and cardiovascular diseases, an increased risk for hypertension in combined cohort was observed in the healthy obesity [hazard ratio (HR): 2.20, 95% confidence interval (CI): 1.34-3.60], unhealthy overweight (HR: 1.47, 95% CI: 1.00-2.14), and unhealthy obesity (HR:2.45, 95% CI: 1.79-3.37), compared with the healthy normal weight group. In each cohort, the healthy obesity was still associated with a higher incidence of hypertension (HR 2.20, 95% CI 1.11-4.36 for the Ansan cohort and HR 2.21, 95% CI 1.01-4.83 for the Ansung cohort).

Conclusion.—These findings provide evidence that the metabolically healthy obese phenotype may not be a benign condition.

▶ It is well established that obesity increases the risk of cardiovascular morbidity and mortality; however, there are studies that negate this risk factor in patients who are obese and lack metabolic syndrome characteristics (central obesity, hypertriglyceridemia, low high density lipoprotein cholesterol, hypertension, and insulin resistance).[1,2] These subjects are often called the healthy obese.

This study tries to establish whether obesity is an independent risk factor from metabolic syndrome in the development of hypertension. Subjects are followed for 8 years and even after adjusting for potential cofounders, the results show that both the "healthy" and the "unhealthy" obese have a higher incident of hypertension when compared with the normal weight subjects (see Fig 2 in the original article). The presence of metabolic syndrome characteristics, in addition to obesity, leads to higher incidences of hypertension. The study also shows a significant change in the obese phenotype from healthy (no metabolic syndrome characteristics) to unhealthy obese (presence of at least 1 characteristic of metabolic syndrome, excluding hypertension) over the 8-year period. The authors suggest that if overweight and obese patients were followed for a long enough period of time, they would eventually develop hypertension and metabolic syndrome, therefore leading to an increased risk of cardiovascular disease. There is a lag time in obese patients for changes in the metabolic phenotype and associated morbidity related to cardiovascular disease. Although this was a large study and subjects were followed for 8 years, it has significant limitations. First, its results cannot be applied to the general population, given that this was a study that looked at a homogeneous population in South Korea. The study also uses different numbers for body mass index and waist circumferences, which reflect World Health Organization diagnoses of obesity in the Asian population. The study used blood pressure readings from one day, measured biannually, which could give an inaccurate diagnosis of hypertension. In summary, this study poses the question of whether obesity is an independent risk factor for cardiovascular disease; however, more long-term prospective studies need to be done in a heterogeneous population.

J. Simonetti, MD

References

1. Blüher M. The distinction of metabolically 'healthy' from 'unhealthy' obese individuals. *Curr Opin Lipidol.* 2010;21:38-43.
2. de Gusmão Correia ML. Is 'metabolically healthy' obesity a benign condition? *J Hypertens.* 2013;31:39-41.

Bariatric Surgery Results in Cortical Bone Loss

Stein EM, Carrelli A, Young P, et al (Columbia Univ of Physicians and Surgeons, NY; et al)
J Clin Endocrinol Metab 98:541-549, 2013

Background.—Bariatric surgery results in bone loss at weight-bearing sites, the mechanism of which is unknown.

Methods.—Twenty-two women (mean body mass index 44 kg/m²; aged 45 years) who underwent Roux-en-Y gastric bypass (n = 14) and restrictive procedures (n = 8) had measurements of areal bone mineral density by dual-energy x-ray absorptiometry at the lumbar spine, total hip (TH), femoral neck (FN), and one third radius and trabecular and cortical volumetric bone mineral density and microstructure at the distal radius and tibia by high-resolution peripheral quantitative computed tomography (HR-pQCT) at baseline and 12 months postoperatively.

Results.—Mean weight loss was 28 ± 3 kg ($P < .0001$). PTH rose 23% ($P < .02$) and 25-hydroxyvitamin D was stable. C-telopeptide increased by 144% ($P < .001$). Bone-specific alkaline phosphatase did not change. Areal bone mineral density declined at TH (-5.2%; $P < .005$) and FN (-4.5%; $P < .005$). By HR-pQCT, trabecular parameters were stable, whereas cortical bone deteriorated, particularly at the tibia: cortical area (-2.7%; $P < .01$); cortical thickness (-2.1%; $P < .01$); total density (-1.3%; $P < .059$); cortical density (-1.7%; $P < .01$). In multivariate regression, bone loss at the TH and FN were predicted by weight loss. In contrast, only PTH increase predicted cortical deterioration at the tibia. Roux-en-Y gastric bypass patients lost more weight, had more bone loss by dual-energy x-ray absorptiometry and HR-pQCT than those with restrictive procedures, and had declines in cortical load share estimated by finite element analysis.

Conclusions.—After bariatric surgery, hip bone loss reflects skeletal unloading and cortical bone loss reflects secondary hyperparathyroidism. This study highlights deterioration of cortical bone loss as a novel mechanism for bone loss after bariatric surgery.

▶ The prevalence of obesity has increased significantly worldwide. Obesity is related to increased comorbid conditions, such as cardiovascular disease, type 2 diabetes mellitus, obstructive sleep apnea, and more, but osteoporosis and fractures were not a concern until recently. Epidemiologic studies link excess body weight to increased bone mass, but this relation is not so simple. The deleterious effect of excess fat has been recently studied; for instance, obese women have lower rates of bone formation, and according to recent literature, there is a correlation between visceral fat and marrow fat, explaining a possible link between obesity and the risk for osteoporosis.[1]

Bariatric surgery is the most effective way to promote long-term weight loss in moderate and severe obese patients who failed lifestyle changes. The 2 main surgical categories include the diversionary-malabsorptive procedures, in which the Roux-en-Y bypass is the most popular, and the restrictive procedures, including the laparoscopic adjustable gastric band or sleeve gastrectomy. There are many plausible mechanisms by which these procedures may induce bone loss, which was found mainly on the weight-bearing sites (total hip and femoral neck). First, the weight loss may promote bone adaptation to skeletal unloading. Other possible mechanisms include vitamin D deficiency, which is common in obese patients and may be exacerbated by malabsorption and low intake of vitamins and minerals, leading to secondary hyperparathyroidism and further bone loss.

This study is innovative because of the assessment of bone microarchitecture with high-resolution peripheral quantitative computed tomography (HR-pQCT) and not just by dual-energy x-ray absorptiometry. In the present study, there was a decrease in hip bone mineral density (BMD), possibly due to unloading of the skeleton. Spine BMD did not decline. HR-pQCT showed a decrease in cortical area, while the trabecular bone tended to increase. This change correlated to parathyroid hormone levels, a hormone known to promote cortical bone resorption. According to this study, skeletal unloading and secondary hyperparathyroidism are the 2 main culprits for the deterioration of cortical bone mass in bariatric patients. Further studies are needed to better define and prevent the cortical bone loss observed in this population.

R. Ness-Abramof, MD

Reference

1. Brzozowska MM, Sainsbury A, Eisman JA, Baldock PA, Center JR. Bariatric surgery, bone loss, obesity and possible mechanisms. *Obes Rev.* 2013;14:52-67.

The Effect of Excess Weight Gain With Intensive Diabetes Mellitus Treatment on Cardiovascular Disease Risk Factors and Atherosclerosis in Type 1 Diabetes Mellitus: Results From the Diabetes Control and Complications Trial/Epidemiology of Diabetes Interventions and Complications Study (DCCT/EDIC) study

Purnell JQ, for the DCCT/EDIC Research Group (Oregon Health and Science Univ, Portland; et al)
Circulation 127:180-187, 2013

Background.—Intensive diabetes mellitus therapy of type 1 diabetes mellitus reduces diabetes mellitus complications but can be associated with excess weight gain, central obesity, and dyslipidemia. The purpose of this study was to determine whether excessive weight gain with diabetes mellitus therapy of type 1 diabetes mellitus is prospectively associated with atherosclerotic disease.

Methods and Results.—Subjects with type 1 diabetes mellitus (97% white, 45% female, mean age 35 years) randomly assigned to intensive or conventional diabetes mellitus treatment during the Diabetes Control and Complications Trial (DCCT) underwent intima-media thickness (n = 1015) and coronary artery calcium score (n = 925) measurements during follow-up in the Epidemiology of Diabetes Interventions and Complications (EDIC) Study. Intensive treatment subjects were classified by quartile of body mass index change during the DCCT. Excess gainers (4th quartile, including conventional treatment subjects meeting this threshold) maintained greater body mass index and waist circumference, needed more insulin, had greater intima-media thickness (+5%, $P < 0.001$ EDIC year 1, $P = 0.003$ EDIC year 6), and trended toward greater coronary

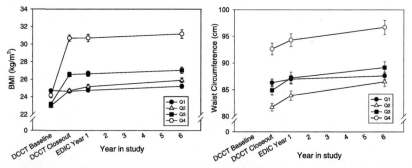

FIGURE 1.—Body mass index (BMI; left graph) and waist circumference (right graph) of subjects treated intensively in the Diabetes Control and Complications Trial/Epidemiology of Diabetes Interventions and Complications Study (DCCT/EDIC) cohort during the DCCT and study years 1 and 6 of EDIC. $P < 0.001$ for both BMI and waist circumference comparing the fourth quartile of weight gain during the DCCT (Q4, excess gainers; n = 122) vs quartiles Q1–Q3 (n = 394, minimal-gainers, shown in graphs separately) at each study time point by Mann–Whitney rank sum test. Waist circumference not measured at DCCT baseline. Results are mean ± SE. (Reprinted from Purnell JQ, for the DCCT/EDIC Research Group. The effect of excess weight gain with intensive diabetes mellitus treatment on cardiovascular disease risk factors and atherosclerosis in type 1 diabetes mellitus: results from the Diabetes Control and Complications Trial/Epidemiology of Diabetes Interventions and Complications Study (DCCT/EDIC) study. *Circulation.* 2013;127:180-187, © 2013, American Heart Association, Inc.)

artery calcium scores (odds ratio, 1.55; confidence interval, 0.97 to 2.49; $P = 0.07$) than minimal gainers. DCCT subjects meeting metabolic syndrome criteria for waist circumference and blood pressure had greater intima-media thickness in both EDIC years ($P = 0.02$ to < 0.001); those meeting high-density lipoprotein criteria had greater coronary artery calcium scores (odds ratio, 1.6; confidence interval, 1.1 to 2.4; $P = 0.01$) during follow-up. Increasing frequency of a family history of diabetes mellitus, hypertension, and hyperlipidemia was associated with greater intima-media thickness with intensive but not conventional treatment.

Conclusions.—Excess weight gain in DCCT is associated with sustained increases in central obesity, insulin resistance, dyslipidemia and blood pressure, as well as more extensive atherosclerosis during EDIC.

Clinical Trial Registration.—URL for DCCT: http://clinicaltrials.gov; Unique identifier: NCT00360815. URL for EDIC: http://clinicaltrials.gov; Unique identifier: NCT00360893 (Fig 1).

▶ Intensive insulin therapy for the treatment of type 1 diabetes mellitus (T1DM), either through multiple daily injections or through a continuous infusion via a pump, is the cornerstone therapy for T1DM. In the Diabetes Control and Complications Trial (DCCT), 1441 patients with T1DM were randomized to conventional or intensive therapy.[1] The intensive therapy group, treated with at least 3 daily injections of insulin or through an insulin pump, achieved an A1C of 7% while the conventional therapy group (that had 1 or 2 daily injections of insulin) achieved an A1C of 9%. The improvement in glucose control was accompanied by a substantial reduction in the incidence and progression of microvascular complications (nephropathy, retinopathy, and neuropathy). The better control was not without side effects, and the intensive therapy group had more hypoglycemic episodes and gained more weight. Concerning macrovascular complications, because of the young age of the participants (mean age 27 at enrollment), no statistical difference in macrovascular complications was detected, but there was a decrease in risk factors for macrovascular complications, coronary artery calcium, and intima-media thickness (IMT). Greater than 90% of the DCCT initial participants continued in an observational study with annual follow-up, through the Diabetes Control and Complications Trial/Epidemiology of Diabetes Intervention and Complications study (DCCT/EDIC). The DCCT/EDIC was able to demonstrate a continuous effect of intensive therapy in reducing kidney disease and a 42% risk reduction for nonfatal myocardial infarction and stroke, which was statistically significant. The intensive insulin therapy group also had reduced subclinical measures of atherosclerosis (IMT and CCA).

These authors used the DCCT/EDIC data up to 6 years after the completion of the study and examined the subgroups who gained the most weight in both the conventional and the intensive therapy groups. The groups were divided into quartiles of body mass index change (excess gainers are defined as an increase of body mass index by at least 4.39 kg/m^2). Excessive gainers in the intensive group had an increase in total and low-density cholesterol, triglycerides, non-high-density cholesterol, and systolic and diastolic blood pressure, and more patients fulfilled the criteria for metabolic syndrome and had an increase in IMT compared with minimal gainers. Similar changes were not observed in the conventional group (Fig 1).

According to this study, intensively treated patients with T1DM who markedly gained weight acquired features of metabolic syndrome similar to type 2 diabetes patients and had an increase in cardiovascular risk factors and of subclinical measures of atherosclerosis. It is possible that in the future combination therapies combining insulin and incretins may decrease weight gain and cardiovascular risk factors. In the meantime, it is important to prevent excess weight in intensively treated patients with T1DM.

R. Ness-Abramof, MD

Reference

1. The effect of intensive treatment of diabetes on the development and progression of long-term complications in insulin-dependent diabetes mellitus. The Diabetes Control and Complications Trial Research Group. *N Engl J Med.* 1993;329: 977-986.

New Developments in Obesity

AMP-Activated Protein Kinase α1 Protects Against Diet-Induced Insulin Resistance and Obesity

Zhang W, Zhang X, Wang H, et al (Univ of Minnesota, Minneapolis; et al)
Diabetes 61:3114-3125, 2012

AMP-activated protein kinase (AMPK) is an essential sensor of cellular energy status. Defects in the α2 catalytic subunit of AMPK (AMPKα1) are associated with metabolic syndrome. The current study investigated the role AMPKα1 in the pathogenesis of obesity and inflammation using male AMPKα1-deficent (AMPKα1$^{-/-}$) mice and their wild-type (WT) littermates. After being fed a high-fat diet (HFD), global AMPKα1$^{-/-}$ mice gained more body weight and greater adiposity and exhibited systemic insulin resistance and metabolic dysfunction with increased severity in their adipose tissues compared with their WT littermates. Interestingly, upon HFD feeding, irradiated WT mice that received the bone marrow of AMPKα1$^{-/-}$ mice showed increased insulin resistance but not obesity, whereas irradiated AMPKα1$^{-/-}$ mice with WT bone marrow had a phenotype of metabolic dysregulation that was similar to that of global AMPKα1$^{-/-}$ mice. AMPKα1 deficiency in macrophages markedly increased the macrophage proinflammatory status. In addition, AMPKα1 knockdown enhanced adipocyte lipid accumulation and exacerbated the inflammatory response and insulin resistance. Together, these data show that AMPKα1 protects mice from diet-induced obesity and insulin resistance, demonstrating that AMPKα1 is a promising therapeutic target in the treatment of the metabolic syndrome.

▶ Nutrient excess, such as is seen in obesity, leads to insulin resistance in many animal and human tissues. Adenosine 5′-monophosphate-activated protein kinase (AMPK) is a fuel-sensing enzyme that is decreased in this process and this leads to impaired fatty acid oxidation among other downstream outcomes. In this article, the authors aim to define the physiologic role of AMPalpha1 (a catalytic subunit of AMPK) in energy homeostasis. To do this, they administered a high-fat diet (HFD) to AMPKalpha1$^{-/-}$ mice and then evaluated diet-induced obesity and insulin resistance. They also used bone marrow transplantation to characterize the roles of AMPKalpha1 in macrophages and adipocytes in the regulation of diet-induced inflammatory response and insulin resistance. The results showed that AMPKalpha1$^{-/-}$ mice fed a low-fat diet increased body weight compared with AMPKalpha$^{+/+}$ mice (wild-type [WT]). AMPKalpha1$^{-/-}$ mice fed a HFD gained more body weight than did AMPKalpha$^{+/+}$ mice (Fig 1 in the original article). Levels of glucose and insulin were higher in the AMPKalpha$^{-/-}$ mice than in WT, and insulin resistance and glucose intolerance were more severe than in WT mice. Significant levels of AMPKalpha1 were detected in the adipose tissue of the WT mice but not in the AMPKalpha$^{-/-}$ mice (Fig 2 in the original article). Also, there was a greater number of macrophages in the adipose tissue of the AMPKalpha$^{-/-}$ mice than in the WT. This indicates that AMPKalpha1 deficiency causes an increase in the accumulation of proinflammatory macrophages in the adipose tissue.

The next set of studies using bone marrow transplantation of cells in AMPKalpha$^{-/-}$ mice vs WT mice demonstrated that macrophage AMPKalpha1 deficiency compromises macrophage infiltration into adipose tissue and that transferring AMPKalpha1-deficient bone marrow cells into WT mice causes insulin resistance. The authors also showed that adipocyte AMPKalpha1 is crucial for the protection from diet-induced insulin resistance and obesity.

Why is this study important?

Numerous studies have already shown that decreased AMPK activity is associated with inflammation, oxidative stress, and apoptosis. Decreased AMPK activity has been shown in adipose tissue of rodents with obesity and insulin resistance. In human studies, Gauthier and Xu et al[1,2] have reported decreased AMPK activity and an increase in inflammatory cells in adipose tissue of obese persons who are insulin-resistant. So these studies have shown that AMPK-decreased activity is a critical factor in inflammation, diabetes, and obesity. The study here shows that AMPKalpha1 is a viable therapeutic target in the treatment of metabolic syndrome and obesity.

C. Apovian, MD

References

1. Gauthier MS, O'Brien EL, Bigornia S, et al. Decreased AMP-activated protein kinase activity is associated with increased inflammation in visceral adipose tissue and with whole-body insulin resistance in morbidly obese humans. *Biochem Biophys Res Commun.* 2011;404:382-387.
2. Xu XJ, Gauthier MS, Hess DT, et al. Insulin sensitive and resistant obesity in humans: AMPK activity, oxidative stress, and depot-specific changes in gene expression in adipose tissue. *J Lipid Res.* 2012;53:792-801.

Short-Term Caloric Restriction Normalizes Hypothalamic Neuronal Responsiveness to Glucose Ingestion in Patients With Type 2 Diabetes

Teeuwisse WM, Widya RL, Paulides M, et al (Leiden Univ Med Ctr, the Netherlands)
Diabetes 61:3255-3259, 2012

The hypothalamus is critically involved in the regulation of feeding. Previous studies have shown that glucose ingestion inhibits hypothalamic neuronal activity. However, this was not observed in patients with type 2 diabetes. Restoring energy balance by reducing caloric intake and losing weight are important therapeutic strategies in patients with type 2 diabetes. We hypothesized that caloric restriction would have beneficial effects on the hypothalamic neuronal response to glucose ingestion. Functional magnetic resonance imaging was performed in 10 male type 2 diabetic patients before and after a 4-day very-low-calorie diet (VLCD) at a 3.0 Tesla scanner using a blood oxygen level–dependent technique for measuring neuronal activity in the hypothalamus in response to an oral glucose load. Hypothalamic signals were normalized to baseline value, and differences between the pre- and postdiet condition were tested using paired *t* tests. Pre-VLCD scans showed no response of the hypothalamus to glucose intake (i.e., no signal decrease after glucose intake was observed). Post-VLCD scans showed a prolonged signal decrease after glucose ingestion. The results of the current study demonstrate that short-term caloric restriction readily normalizes hypothalamic responsiveness to glucose ingestion in patients with type 2 diabetes.

▶ The hypothalamus plays a crucial role in the regulation of feeding. Hypothalamic neurons are involved in glucose metabolism. Glucose ingestion inhibits hypothalamic neuronal activity, but this effect was not observed in type 2 diabetic patients. It is known that caloric restriction improves insulin sensitivity and lowers blood glucose even before any appreciable weight loss. A previous study has shown that diabetic patients fail to inhibit hypothalamic neuronal activity after a glucose load compared with controls.[1]

The present study evaluated whether a very low calorie diet (VLCD) containing a total of 450 kcal per day for 4 days in 10 patients with type 2 diabetes treated by diet or metformin would have a beneficial effect on neuronal hypothalamic response by blood oxygen level-dependent, functional magnetic resonance imaging. The scan, after a short-term VLCD, showed a normalized hypothalamic response to glucose ingestion. This short period of caloric restriction promoted a significant weight loss (3 kg) and a decrease in fasting glucose and the homeostasis model assessment parameter of insulin resistance. This study was conducted in well-controlled patients with a relatively short duration of diabetes. It will be interesting to evaluate whether the same changes will be induced in a less-controlled group with long-standing type 2 diabetes mellitus.

R. Ness-Abramof, MD

Reference

1. Vidarsdottir S, Smeets PA, Eichelsheim DL, et al. Glucose ingestion fails to inhibit hypothalamic neuronal activity in patients with type 2 diabetes. *Diabetes.* 2007; 56:2547-2550.

Surgical Treatment of Obesity

Alterations in Gastrointestinal, Endocrine, and Metabolic Processes After Bariatric Roux-en-Y Gastric Bypass Surgery

Anderwald C-H, Tura A, Promintzer-Schifferl M, et al (Natl Res Council (ISIB-CNR), Padua, Italy; Med Univ of Vienna, Austria; et al)
Diabetes Care 35:2580-2587, 2012

Objective.—Obesity leads to severe long-term complications and reduced life expectancy. Roux-en-Y gastric bypass (RYGB) surgery induces excessive and continuous weight loss in (morbid) obesity, although it causes several abnormal anatomical and physiological conditions.

Research Design and Methods.—To distinctively unveil effects of RYGB surgery on β-cell function and glucose turnover in skeletal muscle, liver, and gut, nondiabetic, morbidly obese patients were studied before (pre-OP, five female/one male, BMI: 49 ± 3 kg/m^2, 43 ± 2 years of age) and 7 ± 1 months after (post-OP, BMI: 37 ± 3 kg/m^2) RYGB surgery, compared with matching obese (CON$_{ob}$, five female/one male, BMI: 34 ± 1 kg/m^2, 48 ± 3 years of age) and lean controls (CON$_{lean}$, five female/one male, BMI: 22 ± 0 kg/m^2, 42 ± 2 years of age). Oral glucose tolerance tests (OGTTs), hyperinsulinemic-isoglycemic clamp tests, and mechanistic mathematical modeling allowed determination of whole-body insulin sensitivity (M/I), OGTT and clamp test β-cell function, and gastrointestinal glucose absorption.

Results.—Post-OP lost ($P < 0.0001$) 35 ± 3 kg body weight. M/I increased after RYGB, becoming comparable to CON$_{ob}$, but remaining markedly lower than CON$_{lean}$ ($P < 0.05$). M/I tightly correlated ($\tau = -0.611$, $P < 0.0001$) with fat mass. During OGTT, post-OP showed $\geq 15\%$ reduced plasma glucose from 120 to 180 min (≤ 4.5 mmol/L), and 29-fold elevated active glucagon-like peptide-1 (GLP-1) dynamic areas under the curve, which tightly correlated ($r = 0.837$, $P < 0.001$) with 84% increased β-cell secretion. Insulinogenic index (0—30 min) in post-OP was $\geq 29\%$ greater ($P < 0.04$). At fasting, post-OP showed approximately halved insulin secretion ($P < 0.05$ vs. pre-OP). Insulin-stimulated insulin secretion in post-OP was 52% higher than before surgery, but 1—2 pmol/min^2 lower than in CON$_{ob}$/CON$_{lean}$ ($P < 0.05$). Gastrointestinal glucose absorption was comparable in pre-OP and post-OP, but 9—26% lower from 40 to 90 min in post-OP than in CON$_{ob}$/CON$_{lean}$ ($P < 0.04$).

Conclusions.—RYGB surgery leads to decreased plasma glucose concentrations in the third OGTT hour and exaggerated β-cell function, for which increased GLP-1 release seems responsible, whereas gastrointestinal glucose absorption remains unchanged but lower than in matching controls.

▶ There is much debate over the effects of roux-en-y gastric bypass surgery (RYGB) on amelioration of type 2 diabetes. Is it because of the weight loss or is it from a change in hormonal milieu in the gut? Studies, so far, are equivocal. This study purports to extend previously published data by in-depth analysis of the effects of RYGB on insulin sensitivity, insulin secretion from β cells during oral glucose tolerance tests (OGTT) and clamp test, gastrointestinal glucose absorption using modeling analyses, hepatic glucose production with hepatic insulin sensitivity, and GLP-1 release. The authors hypothesized that after RYGB surgery, the decrease in glycemia after a glucose load would result from alterations in insulin and GLP-1 release, gut glucose absorption, and/or hepatic glucose production (HGP). Six nondiabetic persons underwent testing pre- and 7 months postoperative RYGB surgery. Nondiabetics were required to exclude the effects of glucose toxicity on whole body insulin sensitivity and β-cell function. These subjects were compared with 6 matching obese and 6 lean controls. Patients underwent OGTTs, hyperinsulinemic-isoglycemic clamp tests, and mathematical modeling for determination of whole body insulin sensitivity, OGTT and clamp test β-cell function, and gastrointestinal glucose absorption. It was found that the first-phase β-cell secretion postoperatively is accompanied by an increased secretion of GLP-1 that closely correlates to C-peptide area under the curve. It also showed that insulin secretion during hyperglycemia during a clamp improves after weight loss after RYGB, but it is still lower than in matching obese controls. In addition, basal hepatic insulin sensitivity improves after surgery, whereas insulin-mediated HGP suppression remains impaired. In addition, gastrointestinal glucose absorption is similar after surgery when compared with conditions before, but it is lower within the second OGTT hour when compared with both control groups. The authors concluded that RYGB surgery leads to decreased plasma glucose concentration in the third OGTT hour and exaggerated β-cell function, for which increased GLP-1 release seems responsible. Gastrointestinal glucose absorption remains unchanged but lower than in matching controls.

What is the importance of these conclusions?

Gastric bypass surgery leads to a weight loss of approximately 32% or roughly 35 kg within 9 to 12 months; this is accompanied by improved whole body insulin sensitivity and lower glucose concentrations between 2 and 3 hours after a glucose load for which GLP-1 may be responsible. The predominant mediator of the observed effects of RYGB seems to be GLP-1 release and also mediated via improvement in hepatic insulin sensitivity with reduced fasting insulin secretion. More work is needed to elucidate the extent of these effects in obese persons with type 2 diabetes. However, if it can be extrapolated to those with type 2 diabetes mellitus, the major effect on glycemic control and improvement in insulin sensitivity seems to be GLP-1—mediated. This has ramifications for a pharmacotherapeutic option for those obese type 2 diabetics who seek amelioration of their weight and comorbidities. It also raises more questions than answers for research in GLP-1 agonists because these agents do not seem to create the extent of the amelioration in type 2 diabetes that is seen with RYGB. It could be the other minor factors, such as glucose absorption or hepatic glucose production or simply the effect of the massive weight loss along with GI P-1 effects.

This study contrasts with Bradley et al,[1] published in 2012, in which it was concluded that marked weight loss itself is primarily responsible for the effects of RYGB as well as the laparoscopic adjustable gastric band on insulin sensitivity, β-cell function, and oral glucose tolerance in nondiabetic obese subjects. This article did not, however, compare effects in a lean or obese control population.

C. Apovian, MD

Reference

1. Bradley D, Conte C, Mittendorfer B, et al. Gastric bypass and banding equally improve insulin sensitivity and β cell function. *J Clin Invest*. 2012;122:4667-4674.

4 Thyroid

Introduction

A number of studies in the "Thyroid Section" of the 2013 YEAR BOOK OF ENDOCRINOLGY are likely to have an important bearing on the understanding of endocrine mechanisms as well as on endocrine practice. Two of the most important studies, at least in my eyes, were published in *Nature* and in *The New England Journal of Medicine*, and I would now like to introduce them.

The aim of the study by Antonica et al published in *Nature* was to generate thyroid follicular cells (TFCs) generated from murine embryonic stem cells (ESCs). The authors overexpressed two transcription factors (NKX2-1 and PAX8) which led to the generation of TFCs and subsequently to the self-formation of thyroid follicles. The authors could demonstrate that ESC-derived thyroid cells show full morphological and functional maturation and that these cells are able to form thyroid follicles in mice (under the kidney capsule where cells were injected). Importantly, the generated thyroid worked under the control of TSH (secreted by the pituitary gland) resulting in an increase of T4 and a rise in body temperature (in comparison to hypothyroid mice without transplantation). In my eyes, this is certainly one of the most important studies published in the thyroid field in the last couple of years. The authors clearly demonstrated the generation of a completely functional thyroid from ESC. Based on that protocol, functional thyroids might be generated sometime in the future for patients with dysfunctional or dysplastic thyroids.

Another important study was published in the *New England Journal of Medicine* by Alexander et al describing the validation of a gene-expression classifier designed to characterize thyroid nodules in a large population of fine-needle aspirates with indeterminate cytologic findings. Based on gene expression analyses, the authors were able to distinguish benign from malignant thyroid nodules with a high sensitivity and specificity. From the clinical point of view, this study has a direct clinical consequence, as this method might be used in the future in clinical routines for distinguishing benign from malignant thyroid nodules.

Matthias Schott, MD, PhD

Autoimmunity

Thyroid Dysfunction and Autoantibodies in Early Pregnancy Are Associated with Increased Risk of Gestational Diabetes and Adverse Birth Outcomes

Karakosta P, Alegakis D, Georgiou V, et al (Univ of Crete, Heraklion, Greece; et al)
J Clin Endocrinol Metab 97:4464-4472, 2012

Context.—Maternal thyroid dysfunction, especially in early pregnancy, may lead to pregnancy complications and adverse birth outcomes. Few population-based prospective studies have evaluated these effects and results are discrepant.

Objective.—We examined the association of thyroid function and autoimmunity in early pregnancy with adverse pregnancy and birth outcomes.

Setting and Participants.—The study used data from the prospective mother-child cohort "Rhea" study in Crete, Greece. A total of 1170 women with singleton pregnancies participated in this analysis. Maternal serum samples in the first trimester of pregnancy were tested for thyroidhormones (TSH, free T_4, and free T_3) and thyroid antibodies (thyroid peroxidase antibody and thyroglobulin antibody). Multivariable log-Poisson regression models were used adjusting for confounders.

Main Outcome Measures.—Outcomes included gestational diabetes, gestational hypertension/preeclampsia, cesarean section, preterm delivery, low birth weight, and small-for-gestational-age neonates.

Results.—The combination of high TSH and thyroid autoimmunity in early pregnancy was associated with a 4-fold increased risk for gestational diabetes [relative risk (RR) 4.3, 95% confidence interval (CI) 2.1−8.9)] and a 3-fold increased risk for low birth weight neonates (RR 3.1, 95% CI 1.2−8.0) after adjustment for several confounders. Women positive for thyroid antibodies without elevated TSH levels in early pregnancy were at high risk for spontaneous preterm delivery (RR 1.7, 95% CI 1.1−2.8), whereas the combined effect of high TSH and positive thyroid antibodies did not show an association with preterm birth.

Conclusions.—High TSH levels and thyroid autoimmunity in early pregnancy may detrimentally affect pregnancy and birth outcomes (Table 3).

▶ It has already been proposed that thyroid antibodies have an influence on the pregnancy outcome. The aim of the present study was to examine the association of thyroid function and autoimmunity in early pregnancy with adverse pregnancy and birth outcomes. A total of 1170 women with singleton pregnancies participated in this analysis. The authors demonstrated that high thyroid-stimulating hormone (TSH) levels and thyroid autoimmunity in early pregnancy may detrimentally affect pregnancy and birth outcomes (Table 3).

What might be the reasons for these phenomena? As discussed by the authors, thyroid antibodies could be associated with a subtle decrease of thyroid function or may reflect a generalized activation of the immune system and, specifically, a deregulated activity of the immune system at the fetal-maternal interface. Because pregnancy represents an inflammatory process with a shift in the regulation of

TABLE 3.—Associations of Thyroid Autoimmunity and High TSH Values in Early Pregnancy with Preterm Birth, Low Birth Weight, and SGA Neonates (n = 1170), Rhea Birth Cohort, CRETE, 2007–2009

| | Preterm Birth | | | | | | Low Birth Weight | | | | SGA | | | |
| | All (n = 133) | | Spontaneous (n = 99) | | Medically Indicated (n = 34) | | All (n = 60) | | Preterm Excluded (n = 25) | | All (n = 56) | | Preterm Excluded (n = 48) | |
	n	RR (95% CI)[a]	n	RR (95% CI)[a]	n	RR (95% CI)[a]	n	RR (95% CI)[b]	n	RR (95% CI)[b]	n	RR (95% CI)[c]	n	RR (95% CI)[c]
Clinical entities[d]														
Normal TSH/Abs (−) (n = 914)	103	Reference	75	Reference	28	Reference	44	Reference	16	Reference	44	Reference	38	Reference
Normal TSH/Abs (+) (n = 148)	24	1.3 (0.8, 2.1)	22	**1.7 (1.1, 2.8)**	2	NA	7	0.9 (0.5, 1.9)	2	0.4 (0.1, 2.7)	7	0.9 (0.3, 2.2)	6	1.1 (0.4, 2.7)
High TSH/Abs (−) (n = 47)	3	0.7 (0.2, 2.1)	1	0.3 (0.1, 2.4)	2	1.6 (0.4, 7.0)	4	**2.6 (1.1, 5.9)**	3	**2.7 (1.0, 7.3)**	3	1.5 (0.5, 4.4)	3	1.1 (0.3, 4.1)
High TSH/Abs (+) (n = 32)	3	0.8 (0.2, 3.0)	1	0.5 (0.9, 3.4)	2	1.6 (0.2, 10.9)	5	**3.1 (1.2, 8.0)**	4	**3.7 (1.4, 9.7)**	2	0.7 (0.1, 4.9)	1	0.9 (0.1, 5.5)

All models are adjusted for maternal age, maternal education, and parity. NA, Not applicable; Abs, antibodies. *Bold* indicates statistically significant difference (*P* < 0.05).

[a] Also adjusted for prepregnancy BMI and sleeping duration.

[b] Also adjusted for smoking during pregnancy, physical activity before pregnancy, and gestational age.

[c] Also adjusted for smoking during pregnancy and physical activity before pregnancy.

[d] TSH reference limits: 0.05–2.53 μIU/ml for the first trimester and 0.18–2.73 μIU/ml for the second trimester; Abs(+): TPO-Ab 35 IU/ml or greater and/or TG-Ab greater than 40 IU/ml.

cytokine networks within the local placental-decidual environment, a deregulation of the local inflammatory processes can be associated with miscarriage and premature delivery. Supporting our results, a recent meta-analysis showed that maternal thyroid autoimmunity increased 2-fold the risk of preterm delivery in women with biochemically normal thyroid function.[1] Another explanation might be the hormone status itself. Thyroid hormones are essential for infant growth and maturation of many target tissues, including the brain, bone, and skeleton, through the actions of growth hormone and insulin growth factor-1. More specifically, insufficient T4 supply to the fetus may negatively affect the development of the pituitary-thyroid axis of the newborn and interfere with normal vascular responsiveness and cardiovascular homeostasis in utero. The present data show a 10% increased risk of overall cesarean sections in women with high TSH values in early pregnancy. This increase could be attributed to coexisting pregnancy complications (ie, gestational diabetes) or fetal distress and fetal growth restriction as supported by our results.

As discussed in the article, there is 1 limitation in the present study: Pregnant and lactating women may require additional iodine intake to eliminate iodine deficiency disorders. Unfortunately, the authors did not have available data on possible dietary iodine supplementation, nor did they measure urinary iodine excretion to test for individual iodine status. Nonetheless, it is a well-performed study suggesting a direct role of thyroid antibodies in preterm delivery and other complications.

M. Schott, MD, PhD

Reference

1. Thangaratinam S, Tan A, Knox E, Kilby MD, Franklyn J, Coomarasamy A. Association between thyroid autoantibodies and miscarriage and preterm birth: meta-analysis of evidence. *BMJ.* 2011;342:d2616.

A TSHR-LH/CGR Chimera that Measures Functional Thyroid-Stimulating Autoantibodies (TSAb) Can Predict Remission or Recurrence in Graves' Patients Undergoing Antithyroid Drug (ATD) Treatment

Giuliani C, Cerrone D, Harii N, et al (Univ "G. D'Annunzio" and Aging Res Ctr, Chieti-Pescara, Italy; Ohio Univ, Athens; et al)
J Clin Endocrinol Metab 97:E1080-E1087, 2012

Context.—A functional thyroid-stimulating autoantibodies (TSAb) assay using a thyroid-stimulating hormone receptor chimera (Mc4) appears to be clinically more useful than the commonly used assay, a binding assay that measures all the antibodies binding to the thyroid-stimulating hormone receptor without functional discrimination, in diagnosing patient with Graves' disease (GD).

Objective.—The objective of the study was to investigate whether an Mc4 assay can predict relapse/remission of hyperthyroidism after antithyroid drug (ATD) treatment in patients with GD.

TABLE 3.—PPV, NPV, Sensitivity, Specificity, and Accuracy for the Different Assays

Assay	Number of Patients	PPV (%)	NPV (%)	Sensitivity (%)	Specificity (%)	Accuracy (%)
Mc4	55	95.4	81.8	77.8	96.4	87.3
Thyretain	42	84.2	82.6	80.0	86.4	83.3
M22	42	87.5	76.9	70.0	90.9	80.9

Design.—An Mc4 assay was used to prospectively track TSAb activity in GD patients treated with ATD over a 5-yr period.

Setting and Patients.—GD patients from the Chieti University participated in this study.

Interventions.—Interventions included the assessment of patients' sera using the Mc4 assay, the Mc4-derivative assay (Thyretain), and a human monoclonal thyroid-stimulating hormone receptor antibody, M22 assay.

Main Outcome Measures.—The Mc4 assay, a sensitive index of remission and recurrence, was used in this study.

Results.—The TSAb levels significantly decreased only in the remitting group as evidenced by Mc4 assay values at the end of ATD (0.96 ± 1.47, 10.9 ± 26.6. and 24.7 ± 37.5 arbitrary units for the remitting, relapsing, and unsuspended therapy groups, respectively). Additional prognostic help was obtained by thyroid volume measurements at the end of treatment. Although not statistically significant, the Mc4 assay has a trend toward improved positive predictive value (95.4 *vs.* 84.2 or 87.5%), specificity (96.4 *vs.* 86.4 and 90.9%), and accuracy (87.3 *vs.* 83.3 and 80.9%) comparing the Mc4, Thyretain, and M22 assays, respectively. Thyretain has a trend toward improved negative predictive value (82.6 *vs.* 81.8 and 76.9%) and sensitivity (80 *vs.* 77.8 and 70%) comparing Thyretain, Mc4, and M22 assays, respectively.

Conclusion.—The Mc4 assay is a clinically useful index of remission and relapse in patients with GD. Larger studies are required to confirm these findings (Table 3).

▶ Graves' disease (GD) is characterized by the presence of thyroid-stimulating hormone receptor (TSHr) autoantibodies (TSAb). These antibodies can be detected in different ways, mostly in terms of the presence of antibodies. These assays, however, can not distinguish blocking from stimulating antibodies. Another clinical problem is related to the high possibility of relapse of GD 12–18 months after completion of oral antithyroid drug (ATD) treatment. Currently there is no index that is able to identify the fate of the patients. The absence of a fate-predicting index can affect the therapeutic modality of choice when the endocrinologist has to face a newly diagnosed GD patient. The aim of the present study was to create a bioassay by using cells stably transfected with a TSHr chimera (Mc4) that measured only TSAb functional activity and had a clear cutoff between GD patients and controls. The Mc4 chimera retains an agonist-sensitive TSAb epitope on the N-terminal portion of the extracellular domain of the TSHr but replaces a TSAb epitope on the C-terminal portion with amino acids 261–329 from the rat luteinizing hormone/chorionic gonadotropin receptor. The data from Giuliani et al show that the use of cells transfected with the Mc4 chimera improves sensitivity and specificity for the detection of TSAb (Table 3). Furthermore, there are early indications of a trend that the Mc4 assay is a better indicator of Graves' prognosis, compared with the TSH receptor antibody assay and even the most recent M22 monoclonal antibody assay; however, larger studies are required to demonstrate a difference conclusively. A commercially available kit form of the Mc4 assay (Thyretain) makes the assay simple, significantly faster, and useful for many laboratories not experienced with TSAb measurements. The clinical utility of the Mc4 assay, as demonstrated herein, is a proof-of-principle test of the epitope assignments and delineates its usefulness in tracking disease remission and relapse with oral ATD, particularly when used in conjunction with measurements of thyroid volume.

M. Schott, MD, PhD

Efficacy and Safety of Three Different Cumulative Doses of Intravenous Methylprednisolone for Moderate to Severe and Active Graves' Orbitopathy

Bartalena L, for the European Group on Graves' Orbitopathy (Univ of Insubria, Varese, Italy; et al)
J Clin Endocrinol Metab 97:4454-4463, 2012

Background.—Optimal doses of iv glucocorticoids for Graves' orbitopathy (GO) are undefined.

Methods.—We carried out a multicenter, randomized, double-blind trial to determine efficacy and safety of three doses of iv methylprednisolone in 159 patients with moderate to severe and active GO. Patients were randomized to receive a cumulative dose of 2.25, 4.98, or 7.47 g in 12 weekly infusions. Efficacy was evaluated objectively at 12 wk by blinded ophthalmologists and subjectively by blinded patients (using a GO specific quality of life questionnaire). Adverse events were recorded at each visit.

Results.—Overall ophthalmic improvement was more common using 7.47 g (52%) than 4.98 g (35%; $P = 0.03$) or 2.25 g (28%; $P = 0.01$). Compared with lower doses, the high-dose regimen led to the most improvement in objective measurement of ocular motility and in the Clinical Activity Score. The Clinical Activity Score decreased in all groups and to the least extent with 2.25 g. Quality of life improved most in the 7.47-g group, although not reaching statistical significance. No significant differences occurred in exophthalmos, palpebral aperture, soft tissue changes, and subjective diplopia score. Dysthyroid optic neuropathy developed in several patients in all groups. Because of this, differences among the three groups were no longer apparent at the exploratory 24-wk visit. Major adverse events were slightly more frequent using the highest dose but occurred also using the lowest dose. Among patients whose GO improved at 12 wk, 33% in the 7.47-group, 21% in the 4.98-group, and 40% in the 2.25-group had relapsing orbitopathy after glucocorticoid withdrawal at the exploratory 24-wk visit.

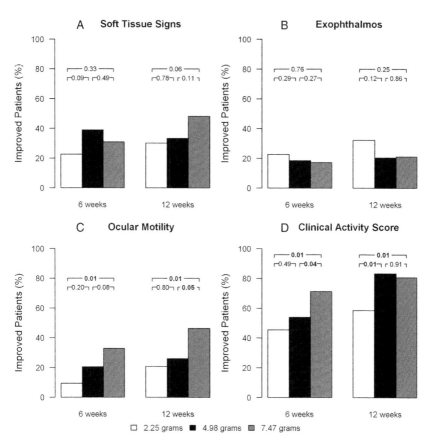

FIGURE 3.—Improvement at 6 and 12 wk in soft tissue signs (A), exophthalmos (B), ocular motility (C), and CAS (D) in the three treatment groups. Improvement was defined according to predefined criteria. *Numbers about the bars represent the P values.* (Reprinted from Bartalena L, for the European Group on Graves' Orbitopathy. Efficacy and safety of three different cumulative doses of intravenous methylprednisolone for moderate to severe and active Graves' orbitopathy. *J Clin Endocrinol Metab.* 2012;97:4454-4463, © 2012, with permission from the Author[s] and The Endocrine Society.)

Conclusions.—The 7.47-g dose provides short-term advantages over lower doses. However, this benefit is transient and associated with slightly greater toxicity. The use of a cumulative dose of 7.47 g of methylprednisolone provides short-term advantage over lower doses. This may suggest that an intermediate-dose regimen be used in most cases and the high-dose regimen be reserved to most severe cases of GO (Fig 3).

▶ Medical treatment of Graves' ophthalmopathy (GO) is challenging. In this large, randomized control trial (RCT), 3 different cumulative doses of intravenous methylprednisolone (MP) were evaluated (high dose [HD]: 7.47 g; middle dose: 4.98 g; low dose: 2.25 g). Improvement of GO occurred in a significantly higher proportion of HD patients (Fig 3). However, improvement was lower than in 2 previous major RCTs (77%-88%).[1,2] This difference may be caused by several factors. Higher MP doses (9-12 g) combined with orbital radiotherapy were used in 1 study.[1] Although the greater efficacy of this combined treatment has been proven using only oral glucocorticoids (GCs), the combination of intravenous GCs with orbital radiotherapy may be more effective than intravenous GCs alone. In the other study (MP as monotherapy, cumulative dose: 4.5 g), the duration of GO was shorter (median, 4 months) and the disease more severe than reported here.[2] The strength of the study is that it is the first multicenter, double-blind, RCT evaluating the efficacy and safety of 3 different doses of intravenous MP for GO. This is particularly relevant because enrollment of large numbers of patients with a rare disease is extremely difficult.

A recent study from Denmark reported an incidence of moderate-to-severe and active GO of 15.5 per million per year.[3] This study shows that both intermediate and high cumulative doses of MP reduce inflammation more effectively and earlier than low doses. High doses, at least in the short term, are more efficacious on eye motility. The fact that the duration of GO was slightly longer in the HD group may have underestimated differences between HD group and other groups. High doses carry a slightly higher risk of major adverse events, which are, however, also encountered with low doses. The risk of relapses, in particular the risk of dysthyroid optic neuropathy, is not completely eliminated, even by high doses, despite the initial favorable response.

This study also has limitations. The response rates were lower than expected, and differences between the high and the intermediate doses were modest. This is possibly because of the exclusion of patients with very severe GO and the inclusion of some patients with relatively long duration of GO (as stated by the authors). In conclusion, the use of a cumulative dose of 7.47 g of MP provides a short-term advantage over lower doses. However, this benefit is transient and is associated with slightly greater toxicity, suggesting that an intermediate dose regimen may be used in most cases and the high-dose regimen should be reserved for the most severe cases of GO.

M. Schott, MD, PhD

References

1. Marcocci C, Bartalena L, Tanda ML, et al. Comparison of the effectiveness and tolerability of intravenous or oral glucocorticoids associated with orbital radiotherapy in the management of severe Graves' ophthalmopathy: results of a prospective, single-blind, randomized study. *J Clin Endocrinol Metab.* 2001;86: 3562-3567.
2. Kahaly GJ, Pitz S, Hommel G, Dittmar M. Randomized, single blind trial of intravenous versus oral steroid monotherapy in Graves' orbitopathy. *J Clin Endocrinol Metab.* 2005;90:5234-5240.
3. Laurberg P, Berman DC, Bülow Pedersen I, Andersen S, Carlé A. Incidence and clinical presentation of moderate to severe Graves' orbitopathy in a Danish population before and after iodine fortification of salt. *J Clin Endocrinol Metab.* 2012;97:2325-2332.

Thyroid Cancer

Serum Antithyroglobulin Antibodies Interfere with Thyroglobulin Detection in Fine-Needle Aspirates of Metastatic Neck Nodes in Papillary Thyroid Carcinoma

Jeon MJ, Park JW, Han JM, et al (Univ of Ulsan College of Medicine, Seoul, Korea)
J Clin Endocrinol Metab 98:153-160, 2013

Context.—It is recommended to measure thyroglobulin (Tg) levels in the needle washout fluids from fine-needle aspirations (FNAs) in patients with papillary thyroid carcinoma (PTC) who have ultrasonographically suspicious metastatic lymph nodes (LNs). However, it is not clear whether serum anti-Tg antibodies (TgAbs) interfere with the detection of Tg in needle washout fluids from FNAs (FNA-Tg).

Objective.—The objective of the study was to evaluate the influence of serum TgAbs on FNA-Tg detection.

Design and Settings.—This retrospective observational cohort study enrolled 207 patients with conventional PTC in whom FNA-Tg values had been measured. All patients initially underwent total thyroidectomy and remnant ablation. FNA-Tg levels were measured from ultrasonographically suspicious metastatic LNs of 0.5 cm or greater in the longest diameter.

Results.—From 207 patients, 263 LNs were evaluated. Final histopathology was available for 92 LNs, of which 88 (96%) were malignant. FNA-Tg levels were lower in the LNs from serum TgAb-positive patients than in those from TgAb-negative patients ($P < 0.001$). In four of 13 metastatic LNs from TgAb-positive patients, the FNA-Tg levels were below 10 μg/liter including one in which both FNA-Tg and serum-stimulated Tg levels were below 1 μg/liter and stained positively for Tg in pathology. There was also one malignant LN with negative for FNA-Tg, serum-stimulated Tg, and serum TgAb but that nonetheless stained intensely for Tg. However, there were no malignant LNs with both negative cytology and negative FNA-Tg. A diagnosis based on FNA-Tg had a lower sensitivity and negative predictive value in the TgAb-positive group than in the TgAb-negative group.

Conclusion.—FNA-Tg measurement is highly reliable in the diagnosis of neck metastases in PTC patients, even in cases of negative-stimulated Tg or positive TgAb. However, high-serum TgAb levels could interfere with FNA-Tg measurements and thereby result in falsely low FNA-Tg levels.

▶ This study describes that fine-needle aspiration (FNA) thyroglobulin (Tg) measurement is highly reliable in the diagnosis of neck metastases in papillary thyroid cancer (PTC) patients, even in cases of negative-stimulated Tg or positive Tg antibodies (TgAb). However, high-serum TgAb levels could interfere with FNA-Tg measurements and thereby result in falsely low FNA-Tg levels. Details of this study are given in Fig 2 of the original article. In most of the metastatic lymph nodes (LNs) examined in this study, FNA-Tg values exceeded 10 g/L.

However, the FNA-Tg levels were significantly lower in LNs from patients with positive serum TgAb than in LNs from patients with negative TgAb. Moreover, the finding of a metastatic LN in a TgAb-positive patient with undetectable FNA-Tg but strong Tg staining in the pathology suggests that high serum TgAb levels interfere with FNA-Tg measurement and thereby cause false-negative FNA-Tg results. High TgAb levels were also associated with a significantly lower sensitivity and negative predictive value of FNA-Tg. This study has a direct clinical consequence. FNA-based Tg measurement helps to assure the existence of a PTC; however, TgAb positivity may lead to false-negative results.

M. Schott, MD, PhD

Correlation between the Number of Lymph Node Metastases and Lung Metastasis in Papillary Thyroid Cancer
Machens A, Dralle H (Martin Luther Univ Halle-Wittenberg, Halle (Saale), Germany)
J Clin Endocrinol Metab 97:4375-4382, 2012

Context.—A prognostic classification system based on aggregate numbers of lymph node metastases may better estimate the risk of distant metastasis.

Objective.—This investigation sought to evaluate a papillary thyroid cancer (PTC) patient's risk of distant metastasis.

Design.—This was a retrospective analysis.

Setting.—The setting was a tertiary referral center.

Patients.—Included were 972 PTC patients.

Intervention.—The intervention was compartment-oriented surgery.

Main Outcome Measure.—The main outcome measure was lung, bone, and liver metastasis.

Results.—Eighty-seven (9.0%) of the 972 PTC patients had distant metastases to lung (79 patients), bone (16 patients), liver (two patients), brain and skin (one patient each). For distant metastasis, more than 20 lymph node metastases had a specificity of 90.8% and a negative predictive value of 92.7%, whereas sensitivity and positive predictive value were low (27.6 and 22.9%). On multivariate logistic regression, 1−5, 6−10, and 11−20 involved nodes denoted a moderate risk of lung metastasis [odds ratio (OR), 9.9, 10.6, and 13.8; $P \leq 0.004$], whereas more than 20 involved nodes indicated a high risk of lung metastasis (OR, 25.0; $P < 0.001$). Mediastinal lymph node metastasis carried a moderate risk of lung metastasis (OR, 7.5; $P = 0.001$). When these numeric categories of lymph node metastases were exchanged for current tumor node metastasis (TNM) N categories, the OR decreased from 25.0 (for >20 lymph node metastases) to 16.4 (N1b), and from 9.9−13.8 (for 1−20 lymph node metastases) to 4.7 (N1a).

Conclusion.—In PTC, categories of 0, 1–20, and more than 20 lymph node metastases correlate better with lung metastasis than current TNM N categories N0, N1a, and N1b.

▶ Papillary thyroid cancer (PTC), a follicular cell—derived parenchymal cancer, also commonly spreads to neck nodes. The clinical relevance of occult lymph node metastases is unclear, given the absence of natural history data. In 2005, Leboulleux et al[1] introduced a risk classification system based on the number of involved lymph nodes, with less than 5, 6–10, and more than 10 nodes signifying low, intermediate, and high risks of tumor persistence and recurrence, respectively. The uptake of this risk stratification scheme has been poor in an environment eschewing routine lymph node dissections because of concerns regarding surgical morbidity and clinical benefit.[2,3] The present evidence suggests that a classification system based on aggregate numbers of lymph node metastases may also be clinically useful to estimate the risk of distant metastasis. In the present study, 972 PTC patients with complete histopathological information from a single institution aimed at evaluating a PTC patient's individual risk for (1) lung metastasis, (2) bone metastasis, and (3) other distant metastasis considering an array of clinical and pathological risk factors, including the number of lymph node metastases. As shown in Fig 1 of the original article, there is a clear correlation between the number of affected lymph nodes and distant metastases. The authors could show that in PTC, categories of 0, 1–20, and more than 20 lymph node metastases correlate better with lung metastasis than current TNMN categories N0, N1a, and N1b.

This study also has some limitations. As stated by the authors, it was not designed to estimate time to recurrence or distant metastasis, which would necessitate standardization of the initial operation and follow-up investigations as to frequency and type of imaging. Arguably, some limited lymph node dissections—leaving nodes behind in undissected areas—may have caused underestimation of the number of lymph node metastases, such that inherent differences in risk, which may exist among various brackets of lymph node metastases, may have been leveled. Some of these residual nodes may become clinically apparent later, raising the patient's risk estimate by pushing up the total number of lymph node metastases. The actual lifetime risk of lung, bone, and liver metastasis may even be higher if (1) the observation period was prolonged and (2) endoscopic procedures (thoracoscopy and laparoscopy), invasive imaging modalities (arterial hepatic angiography), and advanced imaging technologies had been employed more widely. Although the extent of disease was controlled fairly well on multivariate analysis, the predominance of patients referred for reoperation (690 of 972 patients), revealing more advanced tumors with higher rates of distant metastasis (9.9 vs 6.7%), may have raised the size effect estimates.

M. Schott, MD, PhD

References

1. Leboulleux S, Rubino C, Baudin E, et al. Prognostic factors for persistent or recurrent disease of papillary thyroid carcinoma with neck lymph node metastases

and/or tumor extension beyond the thyroid capsule at initial diagnosis. *J Clin Endocrinol Metab.* 2005;90:5723-5729.

2. Kouvaraki MA, Lee JE, Shapiro SE, et al. Preventable reoperations for persistent and recurrent papillary thyroid carcinoma. *Surgery.* 2004;136:1183-1191.

3. Famakinwa OM, Roman SA, Wang TS, et al. ATA practice guidelines for the treatment of differentiated thyroid cancer: were they followed in the United States? *Am J Surg.* 2010;199:189-198.

Role of TSH in the Spontaneous Development of Asymmetrical Thyroid Carcinoma in Mice with a Targeted Mutation in a Single Allele of the Thyroid Hormone-β Receptor

Zhao L, Zhu X, Park JW, et al (Natl Cancer Inst, Bethesda, MD; et al)
Endocrinology 153:5090-5100, 2012

Mutations of the thyroid hormone receptor-β gene (*THRB*) cause resistance to thyroid hormone (RTH). A mouse model of RTH harboring a homozygous thyroid hormone receptor (TR)-β mutation known as PV ($Thrb^{PV/PV}$ mouse) spontaneously develops follicular thyroid cancer (FTC). Similar to RTH patients with mutations of two alleles of the *THRB* gene, the $Thrb^{PV/PV}$ mouse exhibits elevated thyroid hormones accompanied by highly nonsuppressible TSH. However, the heterozygous $Thrb^{PV/+}$ mouse with mildly elevated TSH (~2-fold) does not develop FTC. The present study examined whether the mutation of a single allele of the *Thrb* gene is sufficient to induce FTC in $Thrb^{PV/+}$ mice under stimulation by high TSH. $Thrb^{PV/+}$ mice and wild-type siblings were treated with propylthiouracil (PTU) to elevate serum TSH. $Thrb^{PV/+}$ mice treated with PTU ($Thrb^{PV/+}$-PTU) spontaneously developed FTC similar to human thyroid cancer, but wild-type siblings treated with PTU did not. Interestingly, approximately 33% of $Thrb^{PV/+}$-PTU mice developed asymmetrical thyroid tumors, as is frequently observed in human thyroid cancer. Molecular analyses showed activation of the cyclin 1-cyclin-dependent kinase-4-transcription factor E2F1 pathway to increase thyroid tumor cell proliferation of $Thrb^{PV/+}$-PTU mice. Moreover, via extranuclear signaling, the PV also activated the integrin-Src-focal adhesion kinase-AKT-metalloproteinase pathway to increase migration and invasion of tumor cells. Therefore, mutation of a single allele of the *Thrb* gene is sufficient to drive the TSH-simulated hyperplastic thyroid follicular cells to undergo carcinogenesis. The present study suggests that the $Thrb^{PV/+}$-PTU mouse model potentially could be used to gain insights into the molecular basis underlying the association between thyroid cancer and RTH seen in some affected patients.

▶ The present study shows that a mutation of a single allele of the thyroid hormone receptor-β gene (*Thrb*) gene is sufficient to drive the thyroid-stimulating hormone (TSH)-simulated hyperplastic thyroid follicular cells to undergo carcinogenesis. This article describes the molecular pathway of this carcinogenesis in detail. Fig 5 in the original article, for instance, shows the increased tumor cell proliferation in these mice following treatment with propylthiouracil (PTU).

The role of TSH in thyroid carcinogenesis has been intensively studied in patients and mouse models. Increasing evidence has suggested a close association of TSH with risk of malignancy.[1] Through the use of mouse models, it has become possible to further elucidate the role of TSH in thyroid carcinogenesis at the molecular level. The *Thrb*[PV/PV] mouse, with highly elevated TSH and mutations of 2 alleles of the *Thrb* gene, spontaneously develops metastatic follicular thyroid cancer.[2] However, in *Thrb*[PV/PV] mice with the proliferation signaling of TSH blocked by knocking out the TSH receptors (*Thrb*[PV/PV] thyroid-stimulating hormone receptor[−/−] mice), thyroids show only impaired growth with no occurrence of thyroid cancer.[3] As also shown in the present studies, wild-type mice with TSH levels elevated by long-term treatment of PTU displayed only hyperplastic thyroids but no metastatic thyroid cancer.[3] Thus, growth stimulated by TSH is a prerequisite but is not sufficient for metastatic thyroid cancer to occur. Additional genetic alterations (such as PV or other oncogenic changes), destined to alter focal adhesion and migration capacities, are required to empower hyperplastic follicular cells to become metastatic cancer cells.

M. Schott, MD, PhD

References

1. Haymart MR, Glinberg SL, Liu J, Sippel RS, Jaume JC, Chen H. Higher serum TSH in thyroid cancer patients occurs independent of age and correlates with extrathyroidal extension. *Clin Endocrinol (Oxf)*. 2009;71:434-439.
2. Suzuki H, Willingham MC, Cheng SY. Mice with a mutation in the thyroid hormone receptor beta gene spontaneously develop thyroid carcinoma: a mouse model of thyroid carcinogenesis. *Thyroid*. 2002;12:963-969.
3. Lu C, Zhao L, Ying H, Willingham MC, Cheng SY. Growth activation alone is not sufficient to cause metastatic thyroid cancer in a mouse model of follicular thyroid carcinoma. *Endocrinology*. 2010;151:1929-1939.

Somatic *RAS* Mutations Occur in a Large Proportion of Sporadic *RET*-Negative Medullary Thyroid Carcinomas and Extend to a Previously Unidentified Exon

Boichard A, Croux L, Al Ghuzlan A, et al (Institut Gustave Roussy, Villejuif, France)
J Clin Endocrinol Metab 97:E2031-E2035, 2012

Context.—Medullary thyroid carcinoma (MTC) is characterized by proto-oncogene *RET* mutations in almost all hereditary cases as well as in more than 40% of sporadic cases. Recently, a high prevalence of *RAS* mutations was reported in sporadic MTC, suggesting an alternative genetic event in sporadic MTC tumorigenesis.

Objective.—This study aimed to extend this observation by screening somatic mutational status of *RET, BRAF,* and the three *RAS* proto-oncogenes in a large series of patients with MTC.

Materials and Methods.—Direct sequencing of *RET* (exons 8, 10, 11, 13, 14, 15, 16), *BRAF* (exons 11 and 15), and *KRAS, HRAS,* and *NRAS* genes (exons 2, 3, and 4) was performed on DNA prepared from 50 MTC samples, including 30 sporadic cases.

Results.—Activating *RET* mutations were detected in the 20 hereditary cases (germline mutations) and in 14 sporadic cases (somatic mutations). Among the 16 sporadic MTC without any *RET* mutation, eight *H-RAS* mutations and five *K-RAS* mutations were found. Interestingly, nine *RAS* mutations correspond to mutation hot spots in exons 2 and 3, but the other four mutations were detected in exon 4. The *RET* and *RAS* mutations were mutually exclusive. No *RAS* gene mutation was found in hereditary MTC, and no *BRAF* or *NRAS* mutation was observed in any of the 50 samples.

Conclusions.—Our study confirms that *RAS* mutations are frequent events in sporadic MTC. Moreover, we showed that *RAS* mutation analysis should not be limited to the classical mutational hot spots of *RAS* genes and should include analysis of exon 4.

▶ In this analysis, HRAS, KRAS, NRAS, and BRAF coding sequences were performed in a series of 50 tumors, including familial and sporadic forms. In this collection, mutations in RET (rearranged during transfection) and RAS genes seem to be mutually exclusive. In fact, these redundant genetic events (RAS protein signal occurs downstream of the RET receptor) do not appear to confer additional oncogenic benefit to parafollicular cells, in contrast to what has been described in other cancers such as colorectal cancer. Among the 16 RET-negative tumors, the authors observed 13 RAS mutations. Nine mutations correspond to mutation hot spots known in other types of tumors. The detection of the mutations in exon 4 could be related to the slightly higher proportion of RAS positive/RET negative sporadic medullary thyroid carcinoma (MTC) identified in this study (81%) compared with the Moura et al[1] study (78%). These mutations have been previously described only in digestive cancers and leukemias, and the authors suggest that RAS mutational status should be assessed beyond the most frequently mutated codons. To the best of my knowledge and the knowledge of the authors, these exon 4 mutations have not yet been reported in thyroid cancers. The authors confirm that an activating mutation of known oncogenes is present in 94% of our series (47 of 50 tumors). In sporadic MTC, almost half of the detected mutations are located in HRAS or KRAS genes. Moreover, the authors showed that RAS mutations are not limited to classical mutational hot spots of RAS genes and suggest that analysis should include exon 4 sequencing. To date, there are no data establishing a link between the presence of these abnormalities and efficacy of tyrosine-kinase inhibitor drugs in MTC, but this point should be considered for future drug development.

M. Schott, MD, PhD

Reference

1. Moura MM, Cavaco BM, Pinto AE, Leite V. High prevalence of RAS mutations in RET-negative sporadic medullary thyroid carcinomas. *J Clin Endocrinol Metab.* 2011;96:E863-E868.

Activation of the mTOR Pathway in Primary Medullary Thyroid Carcinoma and Lymph Node Metastases

Tamburrino A, Molinolo AA, Salerno P, et al (Natl Cancer Inst, Bethesda, MD; Natl Inst of Dental and Craniofacial Res, Bethesda, MD; et al)
Clin Cancer Res 18:3532-3540, 2012

Purpose.—Understanding the molecular pathogenesis of medullary thyroid carcinoma (MTC) is prerequisite to the design of targeted therapies for patients with advanced disease.

Experimental Design.—We studied by immunohistochemistry the phosphorylation status of proteins of the RAS/MEK/ERK and PI3K/AKT/mTOR pathways in 53 MTC tissues (18 hereditary, 35 sporadic), including 51 primary MTCs and 2 cases with only lymph node metastases (LNM). We also studied 21 autologous LNMs, matched to 21 primary MTCs. Staining was graded on a 0 to 4 scale (*S* score) based on the percentage of positive cells. We also studied the functional relevance of the mTOR pathway by measuring cell viability, motility, and tumorigenicity upon mTOR chemical blockade.

Results.—Phosphorylation of ribosomal protein S6 (pS6), a downstream target of mTOR, was evident ($S \geq 1$) in 49 (96%) of 51 primary MTC samples. This was associated with activation of AKT (phospho-Ser473, $S > 1$) in 79% of cases studied. Activation of pS6 was also observed ($S \geq 1$) in 7 (70%) of 10 hereditary C-cell hyperplasia specimens, possibly representing an early stage of C-cell transformation. It is noteworthy that 22 (96%) of 23 LNMs had a high pS6 positivity ($S \geq 3$), which was increased compared with autologous matched primary MTCs ($P = 0.024$). Chemical mTOR blockade blunted viability ($P < 0.01$), motility ($P < 0.01$), and tumorigenicity ($P < 0.01$) of human MTC cells.

Conclusion.—The AKT/mTOR pathway is activated in MTC, particularly, in LNMs. This pathway sustains malignant features of MTC cell models. These findings suggest that targeting mTOR might be efficacious in patients with advanced MTC.

▶ Medullary thyroid carcinoma (MTC), a malignancy of the parafollicular C cells of the thyroid gland, accounts for approximately 5% of all thyroid cancers and presents either sporadically (75% of patients) or in a hereditary pattern. Neither radiotherapy nor chemotherapy has demonstrated durable objective responses in patients with advanced MTC. Mutations of the RET (rearranged during transfection) gene, which codes for the transmembrane receptor for growth factors of the glial-derived neurotrophic factor family, have been consistently associated with hereditary and sporadic MTC. Germline mutations of RET are present in virtually all patients with multiple endocrine neoplasia type 2 and familial MTC, and approximately half of the patients with sporadic MTC have somatic RET mutations. MTC-associated mutations activate the RET kinase and its downstream signaling pathways. Very recently, mutations in RAS, a component of the RET signaling cascade, have been identified in RET-negative sporadic MTC samples. The aim of this study was to investigate the phosphorylation status of proteins of the RAS/MEK/ERK and PI3K/AKT/mTOR pathways in samples of primary MTC, lymph node metastases, and normal thyroid tissue. The authors evaluated the activation of these pathways as potential therapeutic targets in patients with MTC.

As shown in Fig 1 of the original article, phosphorylation of ribosomal protein S6 (pS6), a downstream target of mTOR, was evident (S > 1) in 49 of 51 (96%) primary MTC samples. Importantly, almost all lymph node metastases were also pS6 positive (Fig 3 in the original article). From the clinical point of view, mTOR blockade led to a lower viability, motility, and tumorigenicity of human MTC cells (Fig 4 in the original article). These data are of importance, as they provide the basis for future studies aimed at testing mTOR inhibitors for the treatment of metastatic MTC and may also suggest suitable biomarkers to monitor the biochemical consequences of mTOR inhibitors in MTC. Even though a new drug (vandetanib) for the treatment of growing metastatic MTC is available, mTOR inhibition might represent an alternative approach for vandetanib refractory MTC.

M. Schott, MD, PhD

Vandetanib in Patients With Locally Advanced or Metastatic Medullary Thyroid Cancer: A Randomized, Double-Blind Phase III Trial
Wells SA Jr, Robinson BG, Gagel RF, et al (Natl Insts of Health, Bethesda, MD; Univ of Sydney, Australia; Univ of Texas MD Anderson Cancer Ctr, Houston; et al)
J Clin Oncol 30:134-141, 2012

Purpose.—There is no effective therapy for patients with advanced medullary thyroid carcinoma (MTC). Vandetanib, a once-daily oral inhibitor of RET kinase, vascular endothelial growth factor receptor, and epidermal growth factor receptor signaling, has previously shown antitumor activity in a phase II study of patients with advanced hereditary MTC.

Patients and Methods.—Patients with advanced MTC were randomly assigned in a 2:1 ratio to receive vandetanib 300 mg/d or placebo. On objective disease progression, patients could elect to receive open-label vandetanib. The primary end point was progression-free survival (PFS), determined by independent central Response Evaluation Criteria in Solid Tumors (RECIST) assessments.

Results.—Between December 2006 and November 2007, 331 patients (mean age, 52 years; 90% sporadic; 95% metastatic) were randomly assigned to receive vandetanib (231) or placebo (100). At data cutoff (July 2009; median follow-up, 24 months), 37% of patients had progressed and 15% had died. The study met its primary objective of PFS prolongation with vandetanib versus placebo (hazard ratio [HR], 0.46; 95% CI, 0.31 to 0.69; $P < .001$). Statistically significant advantages for vandetanib were also seen for objective response rate ($P < .001$), disease control rate ($P = .001$), and biochemical response ($P < .001$). Overall survival data were immature at data cutoff (HR, 0.89; 95% CI, 0.48 to 1.65). A final survival analysis will take place when 50% of the patients have died. Common adverse events (any grade) occurred more frequently with vandetanib compared with placebo, including diarrhea (56% *v* 26%), rash (45% *v* 11%), nausea (33% *v* 16%), hypertension (32% *v* 5%), and headache (26% *v* 9%).

Conclusion.—Vandetanib demonstrated therapeutic efficacy in a phase III trial of patients with advanced MTC (ClinicalTrials.gov NCT00410761).

▶ Medullary thyroid carcinoma (MTC), a malignancy of the parafollicular C cells of the thyroid gland, accounts for approximately 5% of all thyroid cancers and presents either sporadically (75% of patients) or in a hereditary pattern. Neither radiotherapy nor chemotherapy has demonstrated durable objective responses in patients with advanced MTC. Germline mutations in the RET (rearranged during transfection) proto-oncogene occur in virtually all patients with hereditary MTC. Approximately 50% of patients with sporadic MTC have somatic RET mutations, and 85% of them have the M918T mutation. Evidence from preclinical studies of molecular targeted therapeutics with activity against RET demonstrate that RET kinase is a potential therapeutic target in MTC.[1] Other signaling pathways likely to contribute to the growth and invasiveness of MTC include vascular endothelial growth factor receptor (VEGFR)—dependent tumor angiogenesis and epidermal growth factor receptor (EGFR)—dependent tumor cell proliferation. Vandetanib is a once-daily oral agent that selectively targets RET, VEGFR, and EGFR signaling. The aim of the present study was to investigate the effectiveness of vandetanib in an international, randomized, placebo-controlled, double-blind, phase III trial (ZETA) to evaluate vandetanib 300 mg/d in patients with locally advanced or metastatic MTC. Between December 2006 and November 2007, 331 patients were randomly assigned to receive vandetanib or placebo. Thirty-seven percent of patients had progressed and 15% had died. The study met its primary objective of progression-free survival (PFS) prolongation with vandetanib vs placebo. This is beautifully shown in Fig 2 in the original article. Statistically significant advantages for vandetanib were also seen for objective response rate, disease control rate, and biochemical response. The benefit that was demonstrated in PFS for patients receiving vandetanib compared with placebo was observed in patients with the hereditary or the sporadic form of MTC. Because of the small number of patients with sporadic MTC who were RET-negative and the large number of patients who were RET-unknown, the subgroup analyses of PFS and objective response rate by RET mutation status are inconclusive. Unfortunately, the overall survival of both groups looks very similar (Fig 3 in the original article). However, this might be due to the crossover design of this study. Even though side effects are also seen, the drug has major implications for the treatment of metastatic (growing) MTC where no other effective therapies are available. This drug has now been approved by the Food and Drug Administration as well as by the European authorities. In Europe, this drug is, however, only approved for aggressive and symptomatic MTCs.

M. Schott, MD, PhD

Reference

1. Carlomagno F, Vitagliano D, Guida T, et al. ZD6474, an orally available inhibitor of KDR tyrosine kinase activity, efficiently blocks oncogenic RET kinases. *Cancer Res.* 2002;62:7284-7290.

Thyroid Disease in Pregnancy

Maternal Thyroid Hormone Parameters during Early Pregnancy and Birth Weight: The Generation R Study

Medici M, Timmermans S, Visser W, et al (Erasmus Med Ctr, Rotterdam, The Netherlands; et al)

J Clin Endocrinol Metab 98:59-66, 2013

Context.—Maternal hyperthyroidism during pregnancy is associated with an increased risk of low birth weight, predisposing to neonatal morbidity and mortality. However, the effects of variation in maternal serum thyroid parameters within the normal range on birth weight are largely unknown.

Objective.—The aim was to study the effects of early pregnancy maternal serum thyroid parameters within the normal range on birth weight, as well as the relation between umbilical cord thyroid parameters and birth weight.

Design, Setting, and Participants.—In early pregnancy, serum TSH, FT4 (free T_4), and thyroid peroxidase antibody levels were determined in 4464 pregnant women. Cord serum TSH and FT4 levels were determined in 2724 newborns. Small size for gestational age at birth (SGA) was defined as a gestational age-adjusted birth weight below the 2.5th percentile. The associations between normal-range maternal and cord thyroid parameters, birth weight, and SGA were studied using regression analyses.

Results.—In mothers with normal-range FT4 and TSH levels, higher maternal FT4 levels were associated with lower birth weight [$\beta = -15.4$ (3.6) g/pmol · liter, mean (SE); $P = 1.6 \times 10^{-5}$], as well as with an increased risk of SGA newborns [odds ratio (95% confidence interval) = 1.09 (1.01−1.17); $P = 0.03$]. Birth weight was positively associated with both cord TSH [$\beta = 4.1$ (1.4) g/mU · liter; $P = 0.007$] and FT4 levels [$\beta = 23.0$ (3.2) g/pmol · liter; $P = 9.2 \times 10^{-13}$].

Conclusions.—We show that maternal high-normal FT4 levels in early pregnancy are associated with lower birth weight and an increased risk of SGA new borns. Additionally, birth weightis positively associated with cord TSH and FT4 levels. These data demonstrate that even mild variation in thyroid function within the normal range can have important fetal consequences.

▶ In the present study, the authors investigated the effects of early pregnancy maternal thyroid parameters within the normal range and maternal thyroid peroxidase antibody status on birth weight as well as the relations between cord thyroid parameters and birth weight. The authors show that maternal high-normal free T_4 (FT4) levels in early pregnancy are associated with lower birth weight and an increased risk of small size for gestational age at birth newborns (Fig 1 in the original article). Additionally, birth weight is positively associated with cord thyroid-stimulating hormone and FT4 levels. Several studies have investigated the effects of maternal thyroid dysfunction during pregnancy on birth weight.[1,2] Most of these studies were performed in mothers with Graves' disease and showed a substantial increased risk of low-birth-weight (LBW) newborns.[1,2] A potential mechanism underlying this observed association is that hyperthyroid mothers have increased lipid and protein degradation, leading to a state of maternal chronic caloric deficiency, which has been shown to negatively affect birth weight.[3] Given the increased risk of LBW newborns in mothers with thyroid dysfunction during pregnancy, it is remarkable to note that limited data are available on the effects of variation in maternal thyroid parameters within the normal range on birth weight. Shields et al[4] studied the relation between thyroid function during pregnancy and birth weight in 905 mother-child pairs and found a negative association between maternal FT4 levels at 28 weeks' gestation and birth weight. This is in line with the results from the current study, in which the authors show a negative association between early pregnancy maternal FT4 levels and birth weight in 4464 mother-child pairs.

M. Schott, MD, PhD

References

1. Luewan S, Chakkabut P, Tongsong T. Outcomes of pregnancy complicated with hyperthyroidism: a cohort study. *Arch Gynecol Obstet.* 2011;283:243-247.
2. Phoojaroenchanachai M, Sriussadaporn S, Peerapatdit T, et al. Effect of maternal hyperthyroidism during late pregnancy on the risk of neonatal low birth weight. *Clin Endocrinol (Oxf).* 2001;54:365-370.
3. Belkacemi L, Nelson DM, Desai M, Ross MG. Maternal undernutrition influences placental-fetal development. *Biol Reprod.* 2010;83:325-331.
4. Shields BM, Knight BA, Hill A, Hattersley AT, Vaidya B. Fetal thyroid hormone level at birth is associated with fetal growth. *J Clin Endocrinol Metab.* 2011;96: E934-E938.

Fetal Free Thyroxine Concentrations in Pregnant Women with Autoimmune Thyroid Disease

Spremovic-Radjenovic S, Gudovic A, Lazovic G, et al (Univ of Belgrade School of Medicine, Serbia)
J Clin Endocrinol Metab 97:4014-4021, 2012

Context.—Fetuses from mothers with autoimmune thyroid disease (AITD) may be affected by antithyroid antibodies, antithyroid drugs, and iodine.

Objective.—The study correlated fetal free T$_4$ (fT4) with fetal ultrasound parameters and maternal thyroid function, thyroid antibodies, and medication dose from mothers with AITD.

Design and Setting.—The study was designed as a prospective cohort study and conducted in an academic referral center.

Patients.—Eighty-three of 85 women with AITD completed the study; 38 were treated for hyperthyroidism and 25 for hypothyroidism, and 20 were euthyroid.

Main Outcome Measures.—Outcomes were as follows: 1) fetal—fT4, TSH, ultrasound parameters (morphology, biometrics, heart rate); and 2) maternal—fT4, TSH, antithyroid drug dose, and antithyroid antibodies, thyroid peroxidase and TSH receptor (TRAK). Parameters were determined at the same time, between the 22nd and 33rd wk gestation.

Results.—A total of 48.3% of fetuses from hyperthyroid mothers, 60% of fetuses from hypothyroid mothers, and 10% of fetuses from euthyroid mothers had elevated fT4 levels ($P = 0.006$). In hypothyroid mothers, the presence of both thyroid antibodies was related to fetal hyperthyroidism, whereas absence was related to fetal euthyroidism ($P = 0.019$). Hyperthyroid mothers (TRAK-positive, thyroid peroxidase-negative) with hyperthyroid fetuses had significantly higher mean TRAK than hyperthyroid mothers with euthyroid fetuses (13.7 *vs.* 3.7 IU/liter; $P = 0.02$). Fetal fT4 correlated weakly negatively with maternal TSH within the normal range, but not with ultrasound parameters or with antithyroid drug dose.

Conclusion.—High fetal fT4 levels were unexpectedly frequent in women with AITD, including maternal autoimmune hypo- and hyperthyroidism. Further studies are needed, as well as noninvasive methods to assess fetal thyroid function.

▶ The most startling finding in this study is that treated women with autoimmune thyroid disease (AITD) had a very high incidence of abnormal fetal fT4 concentrations between 22 and 33 weeks of gestation. This is illustrated in Fig 1A of the original article. Moreover, in the group of hyperthyroid pregnant mothers, 48.3% of all fetuses had high fT4 concentrations. Previous studies have shown that neonatal hyperthyroidism was present in 9% to 10% women with Graves' disease after delivery.[1] Compared with published data referring to neonatal hyperthyroidism, this study shows that fT4 concentrations higher than normal are 5 to 10 times more frequently recorded in the fetal period than in the neonatal period. In most instances, pregnancy is associated with a progressive decrease in autoimmune activity, which leads to remission of Graves' disease and decline in thyroid antibody levels. Because fetal and maternal thyroid disease have the same pathogenesis, fetal thyroid dysfunction may also regress in the late weeks of pregnancy. As discussed by the authors, this is the first report of high fetal fT4 from hypothyroid mothers. There are no other studies on cord blood fT4 in fetuses of hypothyroid mothers for comparison. However, a 6-year study in 250 full-term newborns from hypothyroid mothers found that 44.7% of the newborns had serum fT4 levels greater than the 95th percentile of the controls. Birth weight and head circumference were significantly lower than in controls, which is a feature typically found in hyperthyroid newborns. These authors concluded that further studies to define the mechanism that might upset the fetal thyroid-pituitary axis and fetal growth were needed.

There are some limitations of the study. One important point is certainly that total T4 concentrations are strongly influenced by thyroxin-binding globulin and liver maturation. Nonetheless, this study shows that high fetal fT4 levels measured by cordocentesis are unexpectedly frequent in women with AITD, including maternal autoimmune hypo- and hyperthyroidism. Further long-term outcome studies are needed, especially those using noninvasive methods for fetal thyroid function assessment and evaluating the general health of these children in later life.

M. Schott, MD, PhD

Reference

1. Glinoer D. Management of hypo- and hyperthyroidism during pregnancy. *Growth Horm IGF Res.* 2003;13:S45-S54.

Thyroid Nodules

Preoperative Diagnosis of Benign Thyroid Nodules with Indeterminate Cytology

Alexander EK, Kennedy GC, Baloch ZW, et al (Brigham and Women's Hosp and Harvard Med School, Boston, MA; Veracyte, Inc, South San Francisco, CA; Univ of Pennsylvania, Philadelphia; et al)
N Engl J Med 367:705-715, 2012

Background.—Approximately 15 to 30% of thyroid nodules evaluated by means of fine-needle aspiration are not clearly benign or malignant. Patients with cytologically indeterminate nodules are often referred for diagnostic surgery, though most of these nodules prove to be benign. A novel diagnostic test that measures the expression of 167 genes has shown promise in improving preoperative risk assessment.

Methods.—We performed a 19-month, prospective, multicenter validation study involving 49 clinical sites, 3789 patients, and 4812 fine-needle aspirates from thyroid nodules 1 cm or larger that required evaluation. We obtained 577 cytologically indeterminate aspirates, 413 of which had corresponding histopathological specimens from excised lesions. Results of a central, blinded histopathological review served as the reference standard. After inclusion criteria were met, a gene-expression classifier was used to test 265 indeterminate nodules in this analysis, and its performance was assessed.

Results.—Of the 265 indeterminate nodules, 85 were malignant. The gene-expression classifier correctly identified 78 of the 85 nodules as suspicious (92% sensitivity; 95% confidence interval [CI], 84 to 97), with a specificity of 52% (95% CI, 44 to 59). The negative predictive values for "atypia (or follicular lesion) of undetermined clinical significance," "follicular neoplasm or lesion suspicious for follicular neoplasm," or "suspicious cytologic findings" were 95%, 94%, and 85%, respectively. Analysis of 7 aspirates with false negative results revealed that 6 had a paucity of thyroid follicular cells, suggesting insufficient sampling of the nodule.

Conclusions.—These data suggest consideration of a more conservative approach for most patients with thyroid nodules that are cytologically

TABLE 2.—Performance of Gene-Expression Classifier, According to Histopathological Subtype

Histopathological Subtype	No. of Nodules (%)	Result with Gene- Expression Classifier *No. Benign/No. Suspicious*
Benign		
Total	180 (100)	
Benign follicular nodule*	71 (39.4)	41/30
Follicular adenoma	64 (35.6)	37/27
Follicular tumor of uncertain malignant potential	11 (6.1)	5/6
Well-differentiated tumor of uncertain malignant potential	9 (5.0)	4/5
Hürthle-cell adenoma	21 (11.7)	4/17
Chronic lymphocytic thyroiditis	2 (1.1)	0/2
Hyalinizing trabecular adenoma	2 (1.1)	2/0
Malignant		
Total	85 (100)	
Papillary thyroid carcinoma[†]	42 (49.4)	4/38
Papillary thyroid carcinoma, follicular variant	19 (22.4)	2/17
Hürthle-cell carcinoma[‡]	10 (11.8)	1/9
Follicular carcinoma[§]	10 (11.8)	0/10
Medullary thyroid cancer	2 (2.4)	0/2
Malignant lymphoma	2 (2.4)	0/2

*One benign follicular nodule was a colloid nodule.
[†]One papillary thyroid carcinoma was the tall-cell variant.
[‡]Among the Hürthle-cell carcinomas, eight showed capsular invasion and two showed vascular invasion.
[§]Among the follicular carcinomas, four showed capsular invasion, one showed vascular invasion, four were well-differentiated carcinomas not otherwise specified, and one was a poorly differentiated carcinoma.

indeterminate on fine-needle aspiration and benign according to gene-expression classifier results. (Funded by Veracyte.) (Table 2).

▶ This study by Alexander et al describes the validation of a gene-expression classifier designed to identify benign, rather than malignant, nodules in a large population of fine-needle aspirates with indeterminate cytologic findings. With the use of the gene-expression classifier, the negative predictive value was 95% for aspirates classified as atypia (or follicular lesions) of undetermined significance and 94% for aspirates classified as follicular neoplasms or lesions suspicious for follicular neoplasm, implying that thyroid nodules with these cytologic abnormalities and benign gene-expression classifier results have a posttest probability of malignancy that is similar to the probability for nodules with cytologically benign features on fine-needle aspiration. Details according to the histopathologic subtype are given in Table 2. Molecular signal intensities in samples of papillary thyroid cancer are given in Fig 2 of the original article. Panels A and B show the signal intensity of markers of thyroid cancer (cytokeratin 19 and CITED1, respectively). Panels C through F show the signal intensity of follicular cell markers (cytokeratin 7, thyrotropin receptor, thyroglobulin, and thyroid transcription factor 1, respectively). Although the negative predictive value for aspirates with features suspicious for malignancy was lower, at 85%, ascertainment of a 15% risk of cancer may be useful in deciding whether to perform hemithyroidectomy or total thyroidectomy. A key strength of this investigation is the inclusion of a wide range of community and academic practice settings, geographic regions, and demographic characteristics of patients. Furthermore, the authors used local cytopathologic reports to classify nodules as having indeterminate cytologic features, and although these reports were reviewed by a central panel of expert cytopathologists to confirm the indeterminate classification, the results reflect test performance based on local cytopathologic assessment. Therefore, this approach makes the findings applicable to everyday patient care.

M. Schott, MD, PhD

Miscellaneous

Generation of functional thyroid from embryonic stem cells

Antonica F, Kasprzyk DF, Opitz R, et al (Université Libre de Bruxelles, Belgium; et al)
Nature 491:66-71, 2012

The primary function of the thyroid gland is to metabolize iodide by synthesizing thyroid hormones, which are critical regulators of growth, development and metabolism in almost all tissues. So far, research on thyroid morphogenesis has been missing an efficient stem-cell model system that allows for the *in vitro* recapitulation of the molecular and morphogenic events regulating thyroid follicular-cell differentiation and subsequent assembly into functional thyroid follicles. Here we report that a transient overexpression of the transcription factors NKX2-1 and PAX8 is sufficient to direct mouse embryonic stem-cell differentiation into thyroid follicular cells that organize into three-dimensional follicular structures when treated with thyrotropin. These *in vitro*-derived follicles showed appreciable iodide organification activity. Importantly, when grafted *in vivo* into athyroid mice, these follicles rescued thyroid hormone plasma levels and promoted subsequent symptomatic recovery. Thus, mouse embryonic stem cells can be induced to differentiate into thyroid follicular cells *in vitro* and generate functional thyroid tissue (Figs 2-4).

▶ The mammalian thyroid consists of 2 endocrine cell types, the thyroid follicular cells (TFCs) that produce the thyroid hormones T3 and T4 and the C cells that produce calcitonin. In the adult thyroid gland, TFCs are organized into follicular structures in which a monolayer of polarized TFCs enclose a luminal compartment filled with a colloidal mass containing thyroid hormone precursors bound to thyroglobulin. A follicular organization of TFCs is considered to be the prerequisite for efficient thyroid hormone biosynthesis.

It has been demonstrated that NKX2-1[1] and PAX8[2] function are vital for TFC survival, differentiation and function during thyroid organogenesis, and in mature thyroid tissue. During thyroid organogenesis, the onset of NKX2-1 and PAX8 coexpression in a small group of ventral foregut endodermal cells represents the first molecular marker of cell specification toward a TFC fate. Although NKX2-1

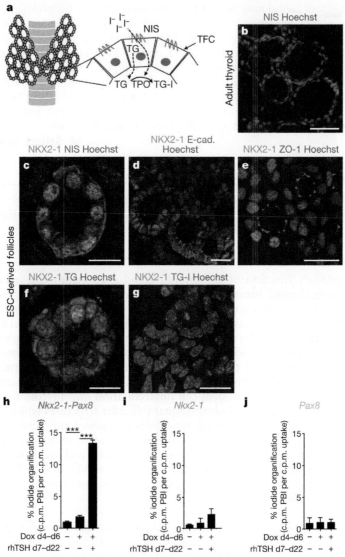

FIGURE 2.—ESC-derived thyroid cells show full morphological and functional maturation. **a**, Schematic diagram of the thyroid gland organized in follicles. **b**, Immunostaining of NIS in adult thyroid tissue. **c–f**, Immunofluorescence at day 22 of thyroid follicles derived from ESCs on ectopic expression of *Nkx2-1* and *Pax8* for NKX2-1 and NIS (**c**), NKX2-1 and E-cadherin (E-cad.) (**d**), NKX2-1 and ZO-1 (**e**) and NKX2-1 and TG (**f**). **g**, Immunodetection of TG-I in the luminal compartment of NKX2-1-positive follicles. **h–j**, Iodide-organification assay in cells differentiated after Dox induction of *Nkx2-1-Pax8* (**h**), *Nkx2-1* (**i**) and *Pax8* (**j**). Histograms show the organification percentage of iodine-125 at day 22 in cells differentiated without Dox and rhTSH (left column), in the presence of Dox only (centre column) and on Dox and rhTSH treatment (right column). Data are mean ± s.e.m. ($n = 3$). Tukey's multiple comparison test was used for statistical analysis. ***$P < 0.001$. Scale bars, 200 μm (**b**) and 20 μm (**c–g**). PBI, protein-bound [125]I. (Reprinted by permission from Macmillan Publishers Ltd: *Nature*. Antonica F, Kasprzyk DF, Opitz R, et al. Generation of functional thyroid from embryonic stem cells. *Nature*. 2012;491:66-71, Copyright 2012.)

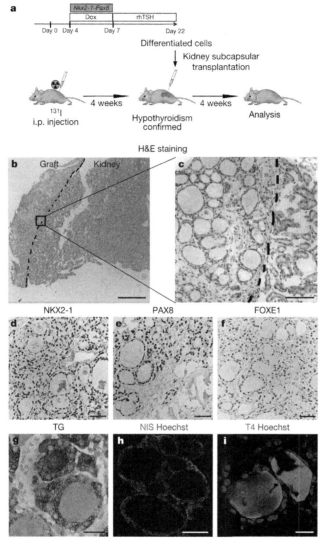

FIGURE 3.—Grafting of ESC-derived thyroid follicles in mice. a, Schematic diagram of protocol for ESC-derived thyroid follicle transplantation in the renal capsule of mice with radio-iodine-ablated thyroid (hypothyroid mice). b–i, Histological analysis of kidney sections 4 weeks after grafting. Hematoxylin and eosin staining on optimal cutting temperature embedded grafted kidney showed the localization of the transplanted tissue in the cortical area of the host organ (left side) (b) and single cuboidal epithelium organization of transplanted tissue (c), the immunohistochemistry of NKX2-1 (d), PAX8 (e), FOXE1 (f), TG (g), and the immunofluorescence of NIS (h) and T4 (i) in the grafted tissue. i.p., intraperitoneal. Scale bars, 300 μm (b), 100 μm (c), 50 μm (d, e, f, h) and 20 μm (g, i). (Reprinted by permission from Macmillan Publishers Ltd: Nature. Antonica F, Kasprzyk DF, Opitz R, et al. Generation of functional thyroid from embryonic stem cells. *Nature*. 2012;491:66-71, Copyright 2012.)

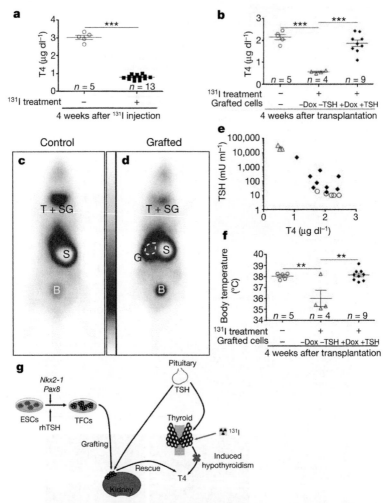

FIGURE 4.—Rescue of experimentally induced hypothyroidism by transplantation of ESC-derived thyroid follicles. **a,** Total plasma T4 levels 4 weeks after injection in untreated mice (open circles) and iodine-131-treated mice (black squares). **b,** Total plasma T4 levels 4 weeks after the transplantation of differentiated cells in iodine-131-treated mice. **c, d,** Whole-body images of mice 30 min after the injection of 99mTc-pertechnetate. Four weeks after grafting, a body scan was performed on untreated control mice (c) or iodine-131-treated mice grafted with ESC-derived follicles (d). B, bladder; G, grafted ESC-derived follicles; S, stomach; T + SG, thyroid and salivary glands. **e,** Relationship between plasma TSH and T4 levels 4 weeks after grafting. **f,** Body-temperature measurements 4 weeks after grafting. In b, e, f, open circles show iodine-131-untreated and ungrafted mice; yellow triangles show mice treated with iodine-131 and grafted with cells differentiated without Dox and rhTSH (−Dox−TSH) and black diamonds show mice treated with iodine-131 and grafted with cells differentiated with Dox and rhTSH (+Dox+TSH). The values are shown as a dot plot (a, b, f) or scatter plot (e) and data are mean ± s.e.m. Unpaired *t*-test (a) and Tukey's Multiple Comparison Test (b, f) were used for statistical analysis. *******P* < 0.01, ***P < 0.001. g, Summary diagram showing that *Nkx2-1* and *Pax8* co-expression in combination with rhTSH treatment leads to the differentiation of ESCs into fully functional thyroid follicles that promote *in vivo* hormonal and symptomatic recovery of the hypothyroid state. (Reprinted by permission from Macmillan Publishers Ltd: Nature. Antonica F, Kasprzyk DF, Opitz R, et al. Generation of functional thyroid from embryonic stem cells. *Nature.* 2012;491:66-71, Copyright 2012.)

and PAX8 are expressed individually in a variety of tissues and cell types, their coexpression is restricted to cells committed to differentiate into TFCs. It has already been shown that induced overexpression of defined transcription factors have a directing effect on the differentiation of embryonic stem cells (ESCs) into specific cell types. The aim of the present study was to show that overexpression of the transcription factors NKX2-1 and PAX8 could promote differentiation of murine ESCs into TFCs and subsequent self-formation of thyroid follicles.

Based on this protocol, the authors could demonstrate that ESC-derived thyroid cells show full morphological and functional maturation (Fig 2) and that these cells are able to form thyroid follicles in mice (under the kidney capsula where cells were injected) (Fig 3). Importantly, the generated thyroid works under the control of thyroid-stimulating hormone (secreted by the pituitary gland), resulting in an increase of T4 and the rise of body temperature (in comparison to hypothyroid mice without transplantation) (Fig 3).

In my eyes, this is the most important study published in the thyroid field in the past couple of years. The authors clearly demonstrated the generation of a completely functional thyroid from ESC. As stated in the publication, congenital hypothyroidism, resulting from either dysfunctional (15%) or dysplastic (85%) thyroid tissue, is the most common congenital endocrine disease in humans, affecting 1 in 2000 newborns. Based on that protocol, functional thyroids might be also generated sometime in the future for such patients or in patients after thyroid resection for other reasons.

M. Schott, MD, PhD

References

1. Kimura S, Hara Y, Pineau T, et al. The T/ebp null mouse: thyroid-specific enhancer-binding protein is essential for the organogenesis of the thyroid, lung, ventral forebrain, and pituitary. *Genes Dev.* 1996;10:60-69.
2. Mansouri A, Chowdhury K, Gruss P. Follicular cells of the thyroid gland require Pax8 gene function. *Nat Genet.* 1998;19:87-90.

Genome-wide analysis of thyroid hormone receptors shared and specific functions in neural cells

Chatonnet F, Guyot R, Benoît G, et al (Université de Lyon, France; Centre de Génétique et de Physiologie Moléculaire et Cellulaire, Villeurbanne, France)
Proc Natl Acad Sci U S A 110:E766-E775, 2013

TRα1 and TRβ1, the two main thyroid hormone receptors in mammals, are transcription factors that share similar properties. However, their respective functions are very different. This functional divergence might be explained in two ways: it can reflect different expression patterns or result from different intrinsic properties of the receptors. We tested this second hypothesis by comparing the repertoires of 3,3',5-triiodo-L-thyronine (T3)-responsive genes of two neural cell lines, expressing either TRα1 or TRβ1. Using transcriptome analysis, we found that a substantial fraction of the T3 target genes display a marked preference for one of the two

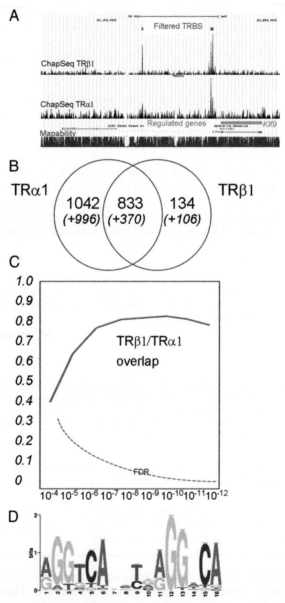

FIGURE 5.—TRα1 and TRβ1 cistromes. (*A*) representative view of the UCSC mouse genome browser (http://genome.ucsc.edu/cgi-bin/hgGateway) around the *Klf9* locus. (*Bottom*) *Klf9* position and exon/intron composition are indicated by boxes (exons) and bars (introns). Mapability for 36-mer tags is indicated as a red line ranging from 0 (not mapable) to 1 (fully mapable) for every position. Each ChAP-Seq experiment is represented as a signal track, providing the number of tags sequenced on 10-bp sliding windows (scale on the right-hand side is the number of counted tags). Two shared TRBS and one binding site detected only for TRα1 are located upstream of *Klf9*. Note that for *Klf9*, the TRBS are not at the previously reported position (57). (*B*) Venn diagrams representing the number of binding sites for each ChAP/ChIP-Seq experiment and the number of shared TRBS. The threshold *P* value is 10^{-7} for the sites identified

receptors. So when placed alone in identical situations, the two receptors have different repertoires of target genes. Chromatin occupancy analysis, performed at a genome-wide scale, revealed that TRα1 and TRβ1 cistromes were also different. However, receptor-selective regulation of T3 target genes did not result from receptor-selective chromatin occupancy of their promoter regions. We conclude that modification of TRα1 and TRβ1 intrinsic properties contributes in a large part to the divergent evolution of the receptors' function, at least during neurodevelopment (Fig 5).

▶ Thyroid hormone 3,3′,5-triiodo-L-thyronine (T3) exerts a broad influence on vertebrate development and maintains adult homeostasis. The aim of this study was to investigate the functional divergence of TRα1 and TRβ1, which might be explained by different intrinsic properties of the receptors. Using transcriptome analysis, the authors found that a substantial fraction of the T3 target genes display a marked preference for 1 of the 2 receptors. The authors found that when placed alone in identical situations, the 2 receptors have different repertoires of target genes. Chromatin occupancy analysis, performed on a genome-wide scale, revealed that TRα1 and TRβ1 cistromes were also different (Fig 5). However, receptor-selective regulation of T3 target genes did not result from receptor-selective chromatin occupancy of their promoter regions.

The authors' observation that T3 can act in a receptor-selective manner suggests that ancestral gene duplication allowed each receptor to gain specific intrinsic properties and functions during vertebrate evolution. Further work is required to transpose these data from the C17.2 neural cell line to the developing brain and possibly to the other organs where both receptors are present. The authors believe, however, that the receptor-selective response is a major factor defining the respective developmental and physiological functions of TRα1 and TRβ1, which may have general consequences for our understanding of T3 signaling. Notably, it should clarify the links between the *Thra* or *Thrb* germline and somatic mutations and their phenotypical or clinical manifestations. Another significant consequence is for the development of T3 analogs tested to treat dyslipidemia.[1] The possibility for these drugs to regulate only a subset of the T3 target might raise other putative indications.

M. Schott, MD, PhD

in a single experiment. Additional sites (in parentheses and italics) are the ones observed in more than one experiment, using a 10^{-4} threshold for peak calling, taking into account the data of the RXR ChIP-Seq experiment (Fig. S3). (C) Limited overlap between TRα1 and TRβ1 cistromes. Depending on the *P* value used for peak calling, the fraction of TRβ1-binding sites overlapping with TRα1-binding site varies. However, unlike what is observed between TRα1 and RXR (Fig. S3), overlap never exceeds 0.8 even for *P* value $<10^{-7}$. The false discovery rate was calculated by assuming that all TRα1-binding sites should be also identified in the RXR ChIP-Seq experiment performed on C17.2α cells. (D) Consensus sequence defined by the CHIP-MEME algorithm using all of the TRBS is close to a direct repeat with a 4-nt spacer (DR4). According to structure analysis, RXR recognizes the 5′ half-site (5′AGGTCA) and TR recognizes the 3′ half-site (5′AGGNCA). (Reprinted from Chatonnet F, Guyot R, Benoît G, et al. Genome-wide analysis of thyroid hormone receptors shared and specific functions in neural cells. Proc Natl Acad Sci U S A. 2013;110:E766-E775, Copyright 2013, National Academy of Sciences, U.S.A.)

Reference

1. Baxter JD, Webb P. Thyroid hormone mimetics: potential applications in athero-sclerosis, obesity and type 2 diabetes. *Nat Rev Drug Discov.* 2009;8:308-320.

Thyroid hormone triggers the developmental loss of axonal regenerative capacity via thyroid hormone receptor $\alpha1$ and krüppel-like factor 9 in Purkinje cells

Avci HX, Lebrun C, Wehrlé R, et al (Université Pierre et Marie Curie (UPMC) Paris 06, France; et al)
Proc Natl Acad Sci U S A 109:14206-14211, 2012

Neurons in the CNS of higher vertebrates lose their ability to regenerate their axons at a stage of development that coincides with peak circulating thyroid hormone (T_3) levels. Here, we examined whether this peak in T_3 is involved in the loss of axonal regenerative capacity in Purkinje cells (PCs). This event occurs at the end of the first postnatal week in mice. Using organotypic culture, we found that the loss of axon regenerative capacity was triggered prematurely by early exposure of mouse PCs to T_3, whereas it was delayed in the absence of T_3. Analysis of mutant mice showed that this effect was mainly mediated by the T_3 receptor $\alpha1$. Using gain- and loss-of-function approaches, we also showed that Krüppel-like factor 9 was a key mediator of this effect of T_3. These results indicate that the sudden physiological increase in T_3 during development is involved in the onset of the loss of axon regenerative capacity in PCs. This loss of regenerative capacity might be part of the general program triggered by T_3 throughout the body, which adapts the animal to its postnatal environment (Figs 1 and 2).

▶ In higher vertebrates, there is a period of development during which central nervous system (CNS) neurons can regenerate their axons after injury. The molecular mechanisms underlying the subsequent loss of this ability are not fully understood, but the onset of an inhibitory environment in the developing CNS is known to prevent axon regeneration,[1] together with intrinsic neuronal maturation.[2] The aim of this article was to investigate whether the (coincidental) peak in T_3 is involved in the loss of axonal regenerative capacity in Purkinje cells

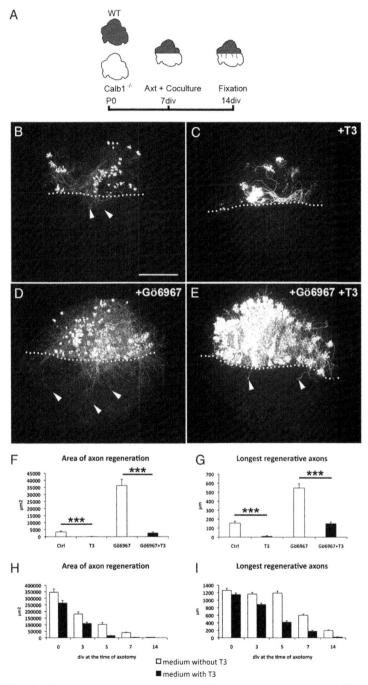

FIGURE 1.—T_3 accelerates the developmental loss of PC axon regenerative capacity. (*A*) Slice culture regeneration assay. Cerebellar slices from newborn mice (P0) were cultured, thus preserving PCs and their

(PCs). Fig 1 shows that T_3 accelerates the developmental loss of PC axon regenerative capacity. Fig 2 shows that T_3 depletion prolongs the period of developmental plasticity of PC axons. This study shows that T_3 is a key factor to determine the time at which PCs lose their ability to regenerate their axons in organotypic cultures. This function of T_3 is mainly mediated by thyroid hormone receptor-$\alpha 1$ and involves its downstream target Krüppel-like factor-9. This effect of T_3 on developing mammalian CNS neurons is a unique finding, because T_3 has previously been shown to promote axon regeneration in sectioned adult mammal nerves in the peripheral nervous system.[3]

M. Schott, MD, PhD

References

1. He Z, Koprivica V. The Nogo signaling pathway for regeneration block. *Annu Rev Neurosci*. 2004;27:341-368.
2. Liu K, Tedeschi A, Park KK, He Z. Neuronal intrinsic mechanisms of axon regeneration. *Annu Rev Neurosci*. 2011;34:131-152.
3. Panaite PA, Barakat-Walter I. Thyroid hormone enhances transected axonal regeneration and muscle reinnervation following rat sciatic nerve injury. *J Neurosci Res*. 2010;88:1751-1763.

targets (deep cerebellar nuclei neurons) in the same slice. Axotomy (axt) was performed in vitro. After 7 div, the ventral halves containing the deep cerebellar nuclei neurons were amputated and replaced by the ventral half of a cerebellar slice taken from age-matched (P0 + 7 div) Calb1$^{-/-}$ mice. Hence, all Calb1-immunoreactive axons in the ventral half of the slice were regenerative axons. These slice cocultures were kept for another 7 div to allow regeneration to proceed. Photomicrographs of cocultured slices immunostained with Calb1 antibodies are shown: untreated coculture (*B*), T_3-treated cocultures (*C* and *E*), and Gö6976-treated cocultures (*D* and *E*). The dotted lines indicate the sites of axotomy, and arrowheads show regenerating axons. Note that the axons are thicker in T_3-treated cultures than in untreated cultures. (Scale bar: 475 μm.) (*F* and *G*) Quantitative analysis of regeneration in the presence and absence of T_3 and Gö6976. Axotomy was always performed after 7 div. (*H* and *I*) Quantitative analysis of regeneration to determine the time dependency of the T_3 effect. Axotomy was performed at various time points (0, 3, 5, 7, and 14 div). All cultures were grown in the presence of Gö6976, with (black bars) or without (white bars) T_3. The area covered by Calb1$^+$ regenerating axons (*F* and *H*) and mean length of the three longest regenerating axons in the Calb1$^{-/-}$ slice (*G* and *I*) are shown. Values are means ± SEM [***$P < 0.001$, nonparametric Kruskal−Wallis one-way ANOVA with the Mann−Whitney post hoc test (*F* and *G*) and two-way ANOVA (T_3 effect and age) with post hoc protected least significant difference (PLSD) of the Fisher exact test (*H* and *I*)]. In F and G, n = 27, 27, 34, and 46 for Ctrl, T_3, Gö6976, and Gö6976 + T_3, respectively. In *H* and *I*, n = 24, 32, 24, 22, and 23 in the absence of T_3 and n = 23, 36, 20, 21, and 22 in the presence of T_3 for axotomy at 0, 3, 5, 7, and 14 div, respectively. (Reprinted from Avci HX, Lebrun C, Wehrlé R, et al. Thyroid hormone triggers the developmental loss of axonal regenerative capacity via thyroid hormone receptor α1 and krüppel-like factor 9 in Purkinje cells. *Proc Natl Acad Sci U S A*. 2012;109:14206-14211, Copyright 2012, National Academy of Sciences, U.S.A.)

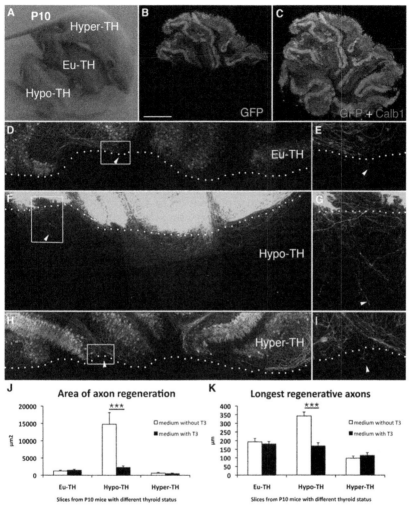

FIGURE 2.—T3 depletion prolongs the period of developmental plasticity of PC axons. (*A*) To study PC regenerative capacity in P10 animals in T₃-depleted conditions, we generated euthyroid (Eu-TH), hypothyroid (Hypo-TH), and hyperthyroid (Hyper-TH) pups of the L7-GFP-BAC line. Thyroid status can be detected visually: Euthyroid pups are bigger than hypothyroid pups but smaller than hyperthyroid pups. (*B* and *C*) Only half of the litter expressed GFP in all PCs when Swiss females were crossed with transgenic L7-GFP-BAC heterozygous males. The dorsal half of cerebellar slices from L7-GFP-BAC mice were cultured and apposed to the ventral half from their GFP-negative littermates. Thus, all the GFP-immunoreactive axons present in the ventral half were regenerative PC axons. The ventral half was visualized by immunostaining with anti-Calb1 antibodies (*C*). Photomicrographs of euthyroid (*D* and *E*), hypothyroid (*F* and *G*), and hyperthyroid (*H* and *I*) cocultures. *E*, *G*, and *I* are magnified views of *D*, *F*, and *H*, respectively. The arrowheads indicate regenerating axons, and the dotted lines indicate the sites of axotomy. Quantitative analysis of the area of axon regeneration (*J*) and the longest regenerative axons (*K*) is shown. The cocultures were grown in the presence (black bars) or absence (white bars) of T₃. Values are means ± SEM (***P < 0.001, Kruskal—Wallis test with Mann—Whitney post hoc test). (Scale bar: *B* and *C*, 450 μm; *D*, *F*, and *H*, 240 μm; *E*, *G*, and *I*, 80 μm.) *n* = 17, 18, and 17 for Eu- TH, Hypo-TH, and Hyper-TH, and *n* = 15, 18, and 17 in the presence of T₃ for Eu-TH, Hypo-TH, and Hyper-TH, respectively. (Reprinted from Avci HX, Lebrun C, Wehrlé R, et al. Thyroid hormone triggers the developmental loss of axonal regenerative capacity via thyroid hormone receptor α1 and krüppel-like factor 9 in Purkinje cells. *Proc Natl Acad Sci U S A*. 2012;109:14206-14211, Copyright 2012, National Academy of Sciences, U.S.A.)

Thyroid hormone is required for hypothalamic neurons regulating cardiovascular functions

Mittag J, Lyons DJ, Sällström J, et al (Karolinska Institutet, Stockholm, Sweden; et al)
J Clin Invest 123:509-516, 2013

Thyroid hormone is well known for its profound direct effects on cardiovascular function and metabolism. Recent evidence, however, suggests that the hormone also regulates these systems indirectly through the central nervous system. While some of the molecular mechanisms underlying the hormone's central control of metabolism have been identified, its actions in the central cardiovascular control have remained enigmatic. Here, we describe a previously unknown population of parvalbuminergic neurons in the anterior hypothalamus that requires thyroid hormone receptor

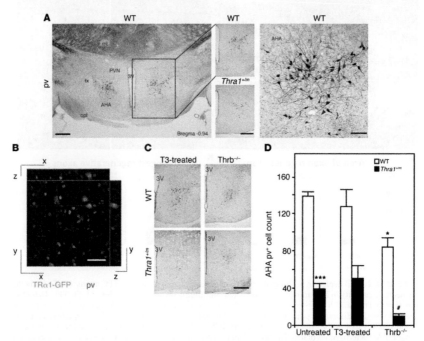

FIGURE 2.—Reduced number of pv cells in the anterior hypothalamus of $Thra1^{+/m}$ mice. (A) Immunohistochemistry for pv in the anterior hypothalamus, as overview (left; scale bar: 250 μm) and high magnification (right; scale bar: 50 μm) in wild-type and $Thra1^{+/m}$ mice (middle; scale bar: 250 μm). fx, fornix; mt, mamillothalamic tract; PVN, paraventricular nucleus of the hypothalamus; 3V, 3rd ventricle; opt, optic tract. (B) Double immunohistochemistry for GFP (green) and pv (red) in the AHA of a mouse strain expressing a chimeric TRα1-GFP protein. Yellow indicates overlapping staining. Scale bar: 25 μm. (C) pv neurons in T3-treated wild-type and $Thra1^{+/m}$ mice or crossings with hyperthyroid $Thrb^{-/-}$ mice. Scale bar: 250 μm. (D) Quantification of pv neurons in the AHA of the different animal models. All values are mean ± SEM; $n = 4-9$. *$P < 0.05$ to untreated wild type; ***$P < 0.001$ to untreated wild type; #$P < 0.05$ to untreated $Thra1^{+/m}$. For Interpretation of the references to color in this figure legend, the reader is referred to web version of this article. (Reprinted from Mittag J, Lyons DJ, Sällström J, et al. Thyroid hormone is required for hypothalamic neurons regulating cardiovascular functions. *J Clin Invest.* 2013;123:509-516, © 2013, American Society of Clinical Investigation.)

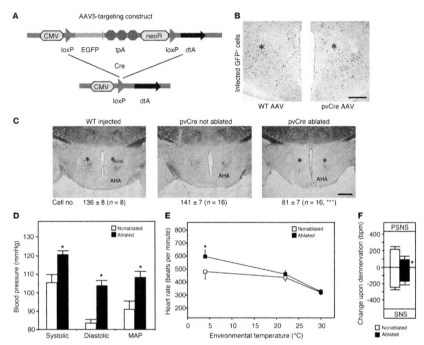

FIGURE 4.—Effect of the in vivo ablation of AHA pv cells in pvCre mice. (A) AAV construct before and after Cre recombination. CMV, cytomegalovirus promotor; loxP, Cre recombination site; tpA, triple polyadenylation site; neoR, neomycin resistance gene; dtA, diphtheria toxin A. (B) Immunohistochemistry for EGFP at the site of the injection (indicated by asterisks) showing AAV-infected cells (scale bar: 250 μm). (C) Immunohistochemistry for pv in AAV-injected wild-type, nonablated pvCre, or AAV-injected ablated pvCre mice (the overall ablation efficiency is shown in the cell count at the bottom; ***$P < 0.001$ to nonablated, unpaired 2-tailed Student's t test; the respective groups for the subsequent cardiac and metabolic analyses had cell counts of 81 ± 13 in the ablated animals vs. 142 ± 10 in the non-ablated animals; $n = 6$, $P = 0.002$; scale bar: 500 μm). Asterisks indicate the site of injection. (D) Systolic, diastolic, and mean arterial blood pressure in mice with reduced numbers of pv$^+$ cells in the AHA (black bars) and controls (white bars; *$P < 0.05$ for ablated vs. nonablated, unpaired 2-tailed Student's t test). (E) Heart rates in these mice (*$P < 0.05$ for ablated vs. nonablated at 4°C, 2-way ANOVA). (F) Change in heart rate upon pharmacological deinnervation of the parasympathetic nervous system (PSNS) (scopolamine methyl bromide) or the sympathetic nervous system (SNS) (timolol) in mice with reduced numbers of pv$^+$ cells in the AHA (black bars) and controls (white bars; *$P < 0.05$ for ablation, 2-way ANOVA). All values are mean ± SEM. (Reprinted from Mittag J, Lyons DJ, Sällström J, et al. Thyroid hormone is required for hypothalamic neurons regulating cardiovascular functions. *J Clin Invest*. 2013; 123:509-516, © 2013, American Society of Clinical Investigation.)

signaling for proper development. Specific stereotaxic ablation of these cells in the mouse resulted in hypertension and temperature-dependent tachycardia, indicating a role in the central autonomic control of blood pressure and heart rate. Moreover, the neurons exhibited intrinsic temperature sensitivity in patch-clamping experiments, providing a new connection between cardiovascular function and core temperature. Thus, the data identify what we believe to be a novel hypothalamic cell population potentially important for understanding hypertension and indicate developmental hypothyroidism as an epigenetic risk factor for cardiovascular disorders. Furthermore, the findings may be beneficial for treatment of the recently identified patients that have a mutation in thyroid hormone receptor α1 (Figs 2 and 4).

▶ Thyroid hormone is a well-known regulator of cardiovascular function and metabolic rate. Hyperthyroid patients display increased metabolic rate and weight loss, despite increased food intake, as well as a profound tachycardia. Conversely, hypothyroid patients often suffer from weight gain and bradycardia. Although most of the cardiovascular and metabolic effects of thyroid hormone have been attributed to direct actions in the corresponding peripheral tissues, such as heart or skeletal muscle and fat, recent studies have found that the hormone modulates these processes also through the brain.[1] In this study, the authors show that both thyroid hormone receptors are required for the development of a previously unknown population of parvalbuminergic cells in the anterior hypothalamus in a mouse model with heterozygous mutations in the thyroid hormone receptor α1 (TRα1) (Figs 2 and 4). These data link, for the first time to our knowledge, defects in thyroid hormone signaling during development to a permanent cellular alteration in the hypothalamus. Moreover, as the cells are associated with the control of cardiovascular function, this study shows that developmental hypothyroidism may represent a previously unknown risk factor for cardiovascular disorders.

What are the consequences for patients? Several types of patients with genetic defects in thyroid hormone signaling have been identified during the last decade, including those with mutations in thyroid hormone transporters and receptors. In mice and humans, these defects often result in strongly impaired brain function. Thus, it would not be surprising if the central autonomic control was also affected in these patients. However, the first patient with a mutant TRα1 exhibited low blood pressure and did not present hypertension when treated with thyroxine[2]—a difference that is likely explained by the fact that her particular TRα1 mutation cannot be reactivated. Further analyses of the angiotensin system and the cardiovascular responses to temperature will be required in patients with thyroid hormone receptor mutations or defective thyroid hormone transporters to fully elucidate whether thyroid hormone exerts a similar role in the central control of cardiovascular function in humans.

M. Schott, MD, PhD

References

1. Fliers E, Klieverik LP, Kalsbeek A. Novel neural pathways for metabolic effects of thyroid hormone. *Trends Endocrinol Metab.* 2010;21:230-236.
2. Bochukova E, Schoenmakers N, Agostini M, et al. A mutation in the thyroid hormone receptor alpha gene. *N Engl J Med.* 2012;366:243-249.

Tetrac Can Replace Thyroid Hormone During Brain Development in Mouse Mutants Deficient in the Thyroid Hormone Transporter Mct8

Horn S, Kersseboom S, Mayerl S, et al (Leibniz Inst for Age Res/Fritz Lipmann Inst, Jena, Germany; Erasmus Med Ctr, Rotterdam, The Netherlands)
Endocrinology 154:968-979, 2013

The monocarboxylate transporter 8 (MCT8) plays a critical role in mediating the uptake of thyroid hormones (THs) into the brain. In patients, inactivating mutations in the *MCT8* gene are associated with a severe form of psychomotor retardation and abnormal serum TH levels. Here, we evaluate the therapeutic potential of the TH analog 3,5,3′,5′-tetraiodothyroacetic acid (tetrac) as a replacement for T_4 in brain development. Using COS1 cells transfected with TH transporter and deiodinase constructs, we could show that tetrac, albeit not being transported by MCT8, can be metabolized to the TH receptor active compound 3,3′,5-triiodothyroacetic acid (triac) by type 2 deiodinase and inactivated by type 3 deiodinase. Triac in turn is capable of replacing T_3 in primary murine cerebellar cultures where it potently stimulates Purkinje cell development. In vivo effects of tetrac were assessed in congenital hypothyroid *Pax8*-knockout (KO) and *Mct8/Pax8* double-KO mice as well as in *Mct8*-KO and wild-type animals after daily injection of tetrac (400 ng/g body weight) during the first postnatal weeks. This treatment was sufficient to promote TH-dependent neuronal differentiation in the cerebellum, cerebral cortex, and striatum but was ineffective in suppressing hypothalamic TRH expression. In contrast, TSH transcript levels in the pituitary were strongly down-regulated in response to tetrac. Based on our findings we propose that tetrac administration offers the opportunity to provide neurons during the postnatal stage with a potent TH receptor agonist, thereby eventually reducing the neurological damage in patients with MCT8 mutations without deteriorating the thyrotoxic situation in peripheral tissues.

▶ Because patients with inactivating monocarboxylate transporter 8 (MCT8) mutations suffer from severe neurological impairments, it seems of utmost importance to develop a therapeutic strategy that could improve the situation of these patients. Unfortunately, the exact mechanisms that result in the development of the neurological symptoms are still not known. Parameters such as decreased thyroid hormone (TH) concentrations in the cerebrospinal fluid and delayed myelination as found in several patients support the hypothesis that a strongly diminished TH supply during critical stages of brain development is substantially linked to the phenotype. In the present study by Horn et al, it has been shown that the TH analog Triac is capable of replacing T3 in primary murine cerebellar cultures where it potently stimulates Purkinje cell development. In vivo effects of tetrac were assessed in congenital hypothyroid Pax8-knockout (KO) and Mct8/Pax8 double-KO mice as well as in Mct8-KO and wild-type animals after daily injection of tetrac during the first postnatal weeks. This treatment was sufficient to promote TH-dependent neuronal differentiation in the cerebellum, cerebral cortex, and striatum but was ineffective in suppressing hypothalamic thyroid-releasing hormone expression (Fig 5 in the original article). In contrast, thyroid-stimulating hormone transcript levels in the pituitary were strongly downregulated in response to tetrac (Fig 6 in the original article). A major disadvantage for the clinical application of TA3 is its short half-life of 6 hours in humans. Consequently, TA3 has to be administered at least 3 to 4 times daily or as a continuous-release formulation, which has not been tested in clinical studies. Therefore, the authors considered TA4 as an alternative because TA4 does not only have a longer half-life of 3 to 4 days, but it can also act as a prohormone for TA3, which, much like T4, is a prohormone for T3. In summary, this article demonstrates the potency of TA4 in replacing TH during brain development, even in the absence of MCT8. Thus, TA4 may be considered as a therapeutic option for patients with MCT8 mutations, particularly when these patients are diagnosed very early in life and irreversible brain damage as a consequence of insufficient TH supply can still be prevented. For normalizing serum TH parameters later in life, application of lower TA4 doses may be suited due to the strong suppressive effects of TA4 on endogenous TH production.

M. Schott, MD, PhD

Higher Free Thyroxine Levels Predict Increased Incidence of Dementia in Older Men: The Health In Men Study

Yeap BB, Alfonso H, Chubb SAP, et al (Univ of Western Australia, Australia; et al)
J Clin Endocrinol Metab 97:E2230-E2237, 2012

Context.—Both hypothyroidism and subclinical hyperthyroidism hinder cognitive function.

Objective.—We aimed to determine whether more subtle alterations of thyroid hormone levels predict increased incidence of dementia in aging men.

Participants and Design.—Community-dwelling men aged 70–89 yr participated in this prospective longitudinal study.

Main Outcome Measures.—The Standardized Mini-Mental State Examination was performed at baseline (2001–2004), and circulating TSH and free T_4 (FT_4) were assayed. Men with known thyroid disease or dementia, or Standardized Mini-Mental State Examination scores below 24 were excluded from follow-up. New-onset dementia, defined by International Classification of Disease (ICD) codes, was ascertained using data linkage (2001–2009).

Results.—During follow-up, 145 of 3401 men (4.3%) were diagnosed for the first time with dementia. Men who developed dementia had higher baseline FT_4 (16.5 ± 2.2 *vs.* 15.9 ± 2.2 pmol/liter, $P = 0.004$) but similar TSH (2.2 ± 1.4 *vs.* 2.3 ± 1.6 mU/liter, $P = 0.23$) compared with men who did not receive this diagnosis. After adjusting for covariates, higher FT_4 predicted new-onset dementia (11%increased risk per 1 pmol/liter increase in FT_4, $P = 0.005$; quartiles Q2–4 *vs.* Q1: adjusted hazard ratio = 1.76, 95% confidence interval = 1.03–3.00, $P = 0.04$). There was no association between TSH quartiles and incident dementia. When the analysis was restricted to euthyroid men (excluding those with subclinical hyper- or hypothyroidism), higher FT_4 remained associated with incident dementia (11% increase per unit increment, $P = 0.03$; Q2—4 *vs.* Q1: adjusted hazard ratio $= 2.02$, 95% confidence interval $= 1.10$—3.71, $P = 0.024$).

Conclusions.—Higher FT_4 levels predict new-onset dementia in older men, independently of conventional risk factors for cognitive decline. Additional studies are needed to explore potential underlying mechanisms and to clarify the utility of thyroid function testing in older men at risk of dementia.

▶ Dementia is a syndrome that leads to progressive cognitive decline and functional impairment, the prevalence of which increases with age. The aim of this study was to investigate the possible correlation of free thyroxine levels and the incidence of dementia. Subclinical hyperthyroidism has already been reported to be associated with lower scores on cognitive testing and with prevalent dementia in cross-sectional studies.[1] An association between subclinical hyperthyroidism and dementia has been suggested by previous epidemiologic studies,[2] but the association in the elderly has not been established, and the effect of treating subclinical hyperthyroidism on cognitive function has not been studied in large, randomized trials. Furthermore, it is also uncertain whether there is a differential cognitive effect of thyroid function among euthyroid subjects, as has been shown for other clinical parameters, including metabolic syndrome, atrial fibrillation, bone density, and the risk of fracture. This study now shows that there is a clear correlation between free thyroxine levels and the incidence of dementia (Fig 1 in the original article). This correlation might be explained by the reduced brain glucose metabolism, which has been shown in positron emission tomography (PET) and which could be corrected by T4 therapy.[3] Of note, PET studies show that hyperthyroid patients exhibit lower glucose metabolism in the limbic system and frontal and temporal lobes and that cerebral glucose metabolism is increased after treatment. Therefore, both deficiency and excess of thyroid hormone acting via dysregulation of cerebral glucose metabolism could mediate increased risk of dementia. Higher free thyroxine is associated with hippocampal and amygdalar atrophy on magnetic resonance imaging scans of the brain. An alternative explanation is that subtle brain changes associated with early neurodegeneration led to minor dysregulation of thyroid function and represent a marker of early brain pathology rather than a true cause of dementia. The authors, therefore, hypothesize that exposure to high-normal thyroid hormone levels over a long period leads to cumulative effects that predispose to dementia, becoming apparent in older men. This may differ from the actions of exogenous thyroxine on cognition measured over a shorter time frame.

M. Schott, MD, PhD

References

1. Ceresini G, Lauretani F, Maggio M, et al. Thyroid function abnormalities and cognitive impairment in elderly people: results of the Invecchiare in Chianti study. *J Am Geriatr Soc.* 2009;57:89-93.

2. Vadiveloo T, Donnan PT, Cochrane L, Leese GP. The Thyroid Epidemiology, Audit, and Research Study (TEARS): morbidity in patients with endogenous subclinical hyperthyroidism. *J Clin Endocrinol Metab.* 2011;96:1344-1351.
3. Bauer M, Silverman DH, Schlagenhauf F, et al. Brain glucose metabolism in hypothyroidism: a positron emission tomography study before and after thyroid hormone replacement therapy. *J Clin Endocrinol Metab.* 2009;94:2922-2929.

Hyperthyroid-associated osteoporosis is exacerbated by the loss of TSH signaling

Baliram R, Sun L, Cao J, et al (Mount Sinai School of Medicine, NY; Human Nutrition Res Ctr, Grand Forks, ND; et al)
J Clin Invest 122:3737-3741, 2012

The osteoporosis associated with human hyperthyroidism has traditionally been attributed to elevated thyroid hormone levels. There is evidence, however, that thyroid-stimulating hormone (TSH), which is low in most hyperthyroid states, directly affects the skeleton. Importantly, *Tshr*-knockout mice are osteopenic. In order to determine whether low TSH levels contribute to bone loss in hyperthyroidism, we compared the skeletal phenotypes of wild-type and *Tshr*-knockout mice that were rendered hyperthyroid. We found that hyperthyroid mice lacking TSHR had greater bone

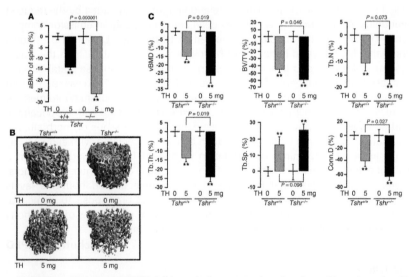

FIGURE 1.—Hyperthyroid TSHR-deficient mice have greater bone loss than wild-type hyperthyroid mice with intact TSH signaling. aBMD (A), micro-CT images (B), and individual parameters from vertebral bodies (C) of wild-type (*Tshr*[+/+]) and *Tshr*[−/−] mice implanted with 0-mg (placebo) or 5-mg T_4 pellets (TH) for 21 days. Mean percent changes (± SEM) in vBMD, BV/TV, Tb.N, Tb.Th, Tb.Sp, and Conn.D are shown. **$P < 0.01$; $n = 6-8$ mice/group. (Reprinted from Baliram R, Sun L, Cao J, et al. Hyperthyroid-associated osteoporosis is exacerbated by the loss of TSH signaling. *J Clin Invest.* 2012;122:3737-3741, © 2012, American Society of Clinical Investigation.)

loss and resorption than hyperthyroid wild-type mice, thereby demonstrating that the absence of TSH signaling contributes to bone loss. Further, we identified a TSH-like factor that may confer osteoprotection. These studies suggest that therapeutic suppression of TSH to very low levels may contribute to bone loss in people (Fig 1).

▶ The present mouse study by Baliram et al shows that hyperthyroid-associated osteoporosis is exacerbated by the loss of thyroid-stimulating hormone (TSH) signaling. This has been shown in a thyroid-stimulating hormone receptor$^{-/-}$ knockout mouse model. These mice have a greater bone loss compared with wild-type mice (Fig 1). This observation is relevant both clinically and biologically. There is growing evidence for an association between low TSH, low bone mineral density (BMD), and increased bone turnover in hyperthyroidism. The risk of vertebral and nonvertebral fractures increases 4.5- and 3.2-fold, respectively, with serum TSH levels of 0.1 IU/L or less.[1] Likewise, euthyroid women with serum TSH levels in the lowest tertile of the normal range have a higher incidence of vertebral fractures, independent of thyroid hormone levels.[2] Analysis of the National Health and Nutrition Examination Survey data show that the odds ratio for correlations between TSH and bone mass range between 2 and 3.4.[3] Moreover, in the Tromso study, participants with serum TSH levels below 2 SD had significantly lower BMDs.[4] In patients taking suppressive doses of T4 for thyroid cancer, serum cathepsin K levels were grossly elevated.[5] Importantly, and of clinical relevance, greater bone loss occurs in T4-treated patients with suppressed TSH levels than in those without suppression. The present mouse study attempts to reinforce the idea that these clinical observations may not simply be correlative; instead, low TSH may facilitate the excessive bone loss in human hyperthyroidism. There is, therefore, a need for caution when T4 supplementation is initiated so as not to unnecessarily lower serum TSH to undetectable levels.

M. Schott, MD, PhD

References

1. Martini G, Gennari L, De P, et al. The effects of recombinant TSH on bone turnover markers and serum osteoprotegerin and RANKL levels. *Thyroid.* 2008;18:455-460.
2. Mazziotti G, Porcelli T, Patelli I, Vescovi PP, Giustina A. Serum TSH values and risk of vertebral fractures in euthyroid post-menopausal women with low bone mineral density. *Bone.* 2010;46:747-751.
3. Morris MS. The association between serum thyroid-stimulating hormone in its reference range and bone status in postmenopausal American women. *Bone.* 2007;40: 1128-1134.
4. Grimnes G, Emaus N, Joakimsen RM, Figenschau Y, Jorde R. The relationship between serum TSH and bone mineral density in men and postmenopausal women: the Tromsø study. *Thyroid.* 2008;18:1147-1155.
5. Mikosch P, Kerschan-Schindl K, Woloszczuk W, et al. High cathepsin K levels in men with differentiated thyroid cancer on suppressive L-thyroxine therapy. *Thyroid.* 2008;18:27-33.

5 Calcium and Bone Metabolism

Introduction

Many significant clinical studies were published in the area of calcium and bone disorders during the last year. Due to revived interest and controversy regarding calcium and vitamin D metabolism, the first section of this chapter focuses on a number of important papers evaluating effects of calcium and/ or vitamin D on long-term outcomes regarding health or mortality. The second longest section focuses on a variety of studies describing results of pathophysiology studies or major clinical trials published in the clinically important area of osteoporosis. The third section describes several papers reporting advances in treatment or understanding of the pathophysiology of metabolic bone disease.

These studies collectively focus attention on major advances in our understanding of calcium and bone disorders reported during the past year. These studies have already impacted clinical practice of endocrinology significantly. As with any review of selected publications from the literature, there were many other significant studies published this past year that could not be included in this short chapter.

The first section contains 7 studies focusing on the effect of calcium and vitamin D on long-term outcomes regarding health or mortality. The first study (5-1; selection 1) provides evidence that serum 25-hydroxyvitamin D levels of 20 ng/mL may minimize the composite risk of hip fracture, myocardial infarction, cancer, or death in older adults. This level corresponds to the recommended target serum 25-hydroxyvitamin D level given in the 2011 Institute of Medicine recommendations for maintenance of skeletal health. Whether this target level will prove to be appropriate for prevention of skeletal or other disease outcomes remains to be seen. The second study (5-2; selection 2) is a large, multi-year cohort study that raises concern that excessive calcium intake through diet and/or supplements might increase the risk of myocardial infarction and overall cardiovascular mortality in men and women. No benefit was seen for stroke risk. Subjects taking calcium supplements had an increased risk of myocardial infarction, and this risk was increased further if subjects took only calcium supplements. The third study (5-3; selection 3) showed that all-cause mortality, cardiovascular disease, and ischemic heart disease were increased in women taking 1400 mg or greater dietary calcium each day. Only 6% of subjects took calcium supplements, and they were not associated with all-cause or cause-specific mortality. However, all-cause mortality was increased significantly in subjects taking calcium supplements with dietary calcium intake of greater than 1400 mg. The study concluded that high calcium intake in women was associated with increased all-cause mortality and mortality from cardiovascular disease, but not mortality from stroke. The fourth study (5-4; selection 4) is a large meta-analysis that reported that, while vitamin D supplementation alone did not reduce death, combination calcium and vitamin D supplementation reduced mortality. These findings suggest that calcium and vitamin D supplementation should be taken in combination, and that the adverse effects of calcium supplementation alone reported in other studies may be mitigated by taking calcium in combination with vitamin D. The fifth study (5-5; selection 5) reported that treatment with paricalcitol, an active form of vitamin D, did not improve left ventricular mass index or left ventricular diastolic function in subjects with late stage chronic kidney disease (CKD) and mild-to-moderate left ventricular hypertrophy over 48 weeks. However, paricalcitol did reduce hospitalizations for cardiovascular disease during the study, and it also limited increases in B-natriuretic peptide in subjects with prominent left ventricular hypertrophy at baseline. These findings imply that reduction in cardiovascular events caused by vitamin D in other treatment trials is not due simply to changes in cardiac structure or function. The sixth study (5-6; selection 6) evaluated pooled, participant-level vitamin D intake data from 11 double-blind, randomized, controlled trials of oral vitamin D supplementation with or without calcium, compared to placebo or calcium alone, in subjects 65 years or older. A total of 31 022 subjects of mean age 72 years, with 91% women, had 1111 incident hip fractures and 3770 nonvertebral fractures. Those randomized to receive vitamin D had a nonsignificant reduction in hip fractures of 10%, and a significant 7% reduction in nonvertebral fractures, compared to placebo or calcium alone. Reduction in risk of fractures was seen only in the highest quartile of vitamin D intake, with median intake above 800 International Units (IU) daily, with 30% reduction in risk of hip fracture, and 14% reduction in risk of nonvertebral fracture. This study suggests that vitamin D supplementation of at least 800 IU each day may reduce hip and nonvertebral fracture risk in older adults. The seventh study (5-7; selection 7) is the first randomized, controlled, dose-response study of supplemental vitamin D in vitamin D-deficient white postmenopausal women. Interindividual variation in serum 25-hydroxyvitamin D levels achieved with varying doses of vitamin D3 from 400 to 4800 IU each day for 1 year was broad, but on average, vitamin D 800 IU each day achieved a mean serum 25-hydroxyvitamin D level of 20 ng/mL, and 1600 IU each day achieved a mean serum level of 30 ng/mL. The 20 ng/mL value corresponds to the 2011 Institute of Medicine recommendation for maintenance of skeletal health.

The second section describes 15 studies reporting results of pathophysiology studies or major clinical trials published in the clinically important area of osteoporosis. The first study (5-8; selection 8) suggests that atypical subtrochanteric femoral fractures are associated with long-term bisphosphonate use. However, these fractures were quite rare, but their incidence had increased over the preceding 10 years. The risk of atypical femoral fractures increased with longer-term bisphosphonate use without evidence of a threshold or plateau in risk. The study concluded that the risk to benefit ratio for bisphosphonate treatment of osteoporosis appeared favorable, given the very rare risk of atypical fractures. The second study (5-9; selection 9) is a very important study that quantified the risk of atypical nontraumatic diaphyseal femoral fracture stratified by years of bisphosphonate use. The age-adjusted incidence rates for atypical femoral fracture were 1.78/ 100 000/year with exposure from 0.1 to 1.9 years, 16.1/100 000/year after 4.0-5.9 years, and 113.1/100 000/year after 8.0 to 9.9 years. No relation was seen between the atypical fractures and duration of bisphosphonate use, age, or bone mineral density (BMD). The findings of this study support the current Food and Drug Administration (FDA) recommendation to consider stopping bisphosphonate therapy after 5 years of continuous therapy. The third study (5-10; selection 19) demonstrated that the FRAX fracture risk algorithm predicted fractures in obese women almost as well as in nonobese women. The findings indicate that fracture risk estimates obtained in obese women using clinical risk factors plus BMD are better than fracture risk estimates obtained with clinical risk factors alone, and that it is not necessary to apply a correction factor to the risk estimate obtained because obese women have higher hip BMD and body mass index than nonobese women. The fourth study (5-11; selection 11) demonstrated that there was not a significant interaction between alendronate and FRAX scores for nonvertebral fractures, clinical fractures, major osteoporotic fractures, or radiographic vertebral fractures. The study concluded that the effect of alendronate on fracture risk reduction did not depend on baseline FRAX score. The fifth study (5-12; selection 12) is a significant observational study that demonstrated that fracture reduction in a large cohort of patients treated with glucocorticoid therapy with weekly alendronate or risedronate was similar to that seen in previous randomized, controlled clinical trials in postmenopausal women and men. The efficacies of these 2 bisphosphonates on surrogate markers, including BMD and bone turnover markers, was also similar to that seen in previous trials. This is the first large study to demonstrate fracture efficacy of weekly alendronate and risedronate in glucocorticoid-induced osteoporosis, with the study showing reduction not just in vertebral fractures, but also nonvertebral fractures. The sixth study (5-13; selection 13) confirms and extends previous observations regarding bisphosphonate-associated osteonecrosis of the jaw in cancer patients. Unlike most previous studies, this study reports findings from a large cohort not restricted to multiple myeloma or breast cancer patients. The overall risk of jaw osteonecrosis was low at 3.1%, but the prevalence was higher at 7.2% in patients with multiple myeloma, and 4.2% in patients with breast cancer. Risk factors for jaw osteonecrosis included type of bisphosphonate used, diabetes, hypothyroidism, smoking, corticosteroid therapy, alcohol, prior dental extractions, and higher number of bisphosph-onate infusions. The study concluded that increased cumulative bisphosph-onate dose and prolonged bisphosphonate therapy were the most important risk factors associated with jaw osteonecrosis in cancer patients. The seventh study (5-14; selection 14) gives reassurance that the risk of eye inflammatory reactions is very low in patients treated with bisphosphonate therapies. The study concluded that subsets of the population of osteopo-rosis patients may be at increased risk, especially those with rheumatic or pulmonary disorders. Patients at highest risk appeared to be those with sero-negative rheumatoid arthritis, necrotizing vascular disorders, and Sjogren syndrome, implying that underlying inflammatory disease was the most likely cause for the eye reactions. The eighth study (5-15; selection 24) demonstrated that 2 infusions of zoledronic acid over 2 years reduced the relative risk of new vertebral morphometric fractures in osteoporotic men by 67%. These results are similar to the findings with zoledronic acid in postmenopausal women with osteoporosis, indicating that the antifracture effect of zoledronic acid is similar in men and women. The study was not powered to show an effect on nonvertebral fractures.

The next 4 studies demonstrate the effects of teriparatide on the skeleton. The ninth study (5-16; selection 16) demonstrated that combination anabolic and antiresorptive therapy had significant benefit in treatment of postmenopausal osteoporosis. The timing and sequence of parathyroid hormone (PTH) 1-84 in combination with a bisphosphonate appeared to determine skeletal outcomes. Combination therapy with concurrent or sequential PTH 1-84 and monthly ibandronate resulted in significantly increased lumbar spine areal and volumetric BMD, and increased markers of bone formation. These findings suggested that combination therapy with anabolic and antiresorptive agents may significantly improve BMD, depending on the sequence of administration. The 10th study (5-17; selec-tion 17) showed unexpected variance in treatment results on bone micro-architecture and strength using 2 different forms of PTH, compared to findings with zoledronic acid, when assessed by high resolution peripheral quantitative computed tomography scanning. Both PTH 1-34 and PTH 1-84 caused an increase in cortical porosity and decrease in cortical bone density at the radius and tibia. Trabecular number in the tibia increased with both agents, as did cortical thickness in both the radius and tibia with PTH 1-34. Zoledronic acid did not change cortical porosity at the radius or tibia, while trabecular bone volume increased. Bone strength esti-mated by finite element analysis remained stable with PTH 1-34 and zole-dronic acid, while PTH 1-84 caused bone strength to decrease at both the radius and tibia. Further study will be required to establish whether PTH 1-34 and PTH 1-84 differ in terms of their treatment effect on bone strength. The 11th study (5-18; selection 18) emphasizes the importance of reporting full histomorphometric indices when distinguishing the mechanism of action of new osteoporosis drugs, particularly in conditions of low bone turnover. There was very little overlap in the effect of teriparatide and zoledronic acid on dynamic histomorphometric indices, with the clearest separation occurring in mineralizing surface/bone surface, bone formation rate/bone surface, and total formation period. Both drugs caused similar changes in mineral apposition rate, indicating that this was not a good parameter to distinguish antiresorptive from anabolic agents. Static histomorphometric indices for these 2 drugs differed only in magnitude rather than direction of change. These considerations will be important when analyzing new drugs under development, especially as some drugs may be formation-sparing or mixed antiresorptive/anabolic agents. The 12th study (5-19; selection 20) provides good evidence that teriparatide treatment for up to 18 months reduced clinical fractures by 30-36 months compared to the first 6 months in elderly postmenopausal women 75 years of age or older. The study also showed an improvement in health-related quality of life and early reduction in back pain symptoms that persisted for 18 months after discontinuation of teriparatide and initiation of other osteoporosis medication. These findings indicate that teriparatide prevents fractures in elderly women at high risk of fracture when treated as part of a sequential regimen.

The next 2 studies describe effects of denosumab on BMD and fracture healing. The 13th study (5-20; selection 15) showed that denosumab continued to stimulate increases in lumbar spine and total hip BMD over 8 years of continued therapy, distinctly different from most other antiresorptive agents that demonstrate a plateauing effect after 3 to 4 years. This study was not powered to demonstrate fracture reduction, however, so it was not clear than the continued increase in BMD resulted in reduced vertebral and hip fractures. The 14th study (5-21; selection 25) provides reassuring findings of additional evidence that current FDA-approved treatments for osteoporosis have no apparent adverse effects on fracture healing or postsurgical fracture repair. Because these agents potently suppress both bone resorption and bone formation required for fracture repair, they could potentially cause prolonged fracture healing or nonunion of fracture, especially if given closely around the time of fracture. This study showed that denosumab caused very rapid suppression of bone resorption and bone formation, but no evidence of complications related to fracture or surgical repair of fracture when given within 6 weeks of fracture.

The last study (5-22; selection 22) in this section demonstrated that daily low-frequency vibration treatment for 1 year in healthy osteopenic postmenopausal women did not result in an improvement in BMD or bone structure. Previous studies showing benefit from vibrating platforms had smaller sample sizes, greater loss to follow-up, and did not provide calcium or vitamin D supplementation to participants. It is possible that daily high-magnitude whole body vibration treatment might have a different effect on skeletal outcomes, but this remains controversial.

The third section describes several papers reporting advances in treatment or understanding of the pathophysiology of metabolic bone disease. The first study (5-23; selection 10) is the largest longitudinal study assessing BMD and body composition changes that occurred in a group of healthy women from before pregnancy to 9 months postpartum. The study demonstrated that pregnancy and breastfeeding caused reversible bone loss at all sites, but that bone loss returned to baseline by 19 months postpartum regardless of the length of breastfeeding. The second study (5-24; selection 21) showed that cinacalcet, a calcimimetic agent that acts as an allosteric regulator of the calcium-sensing receptor, did not reduce death or cardiovascular mortality in patients with stage V CKD receiving hemodialysis. In spite of reducing the rate of parathyroidectomy by more than 50%, cinacalcet was not able to reduce death or cardiovascular endpoints in this high-risk population over almost 2 years of follow-up. Further studies in the late-stage CKD population will be necessary to demonstrate therapies able to reduce mortality and cardiovascular death. The third study (5-25; selection 22) is a long-term clinical trial showing that 4 years of continuous treatment with PTH 1-84 is effective therapy for patients with chronic hypoparathyroidism. PTH 1-84 was able to maintain mineral metabolism parameters in the desired goal ranges in spite of significantly reduced calcium and calcitriol supplementation, and returned markedly decreased markers of bone turnover to more normal levels after a short period of increased levels.

In conclusion, these selected papers reflect a sampling of the wide variety of excellent clinical studies published in the area of calcium and bone disorders over the last year. It is evident that many other significant papers could not be included in this perspective due to space constraints. Most of the studies reviewed here add incrementally to current concepts regarding calcium and bone disorders based on previous knowledge and clinical experience, whereas others demonstrate significant advances or clarification of understanding of physiological functions of the skeleton. Future clinical investigation will continue to advance our knowledge regarding skeletal function in health and disease.

Bart L. Clarke, MD

Mineral and Vitamin D Metabolism

Serum 25-Hydroxyvitamin D Concentration and Risk for Major Clinical Disease Events in a Community-Based Population of Older Adults: A Cohort Study

de Boer IH, Levin G, Robinson-Cohen C, et al (Univ of Washington, Seattle)
Ann Intern Med 156:627-634, 2012

Background.—Circulating concentrations of 25-hydroxyvitamin D [25-(OH)D] are used to define vitamin D deficiency. Current clinical 25-(OH) D targets based on associations with intermediate markers of bone metabolism may not reflect optimal levels for other chronic diseases and do not account for known seasonal variation in 25-(OH)D concentration.

Objective.—To evaluate the relationship of 25-(OH)D concentration with the incidence of major clinical disease events that are pathophysiologically relevant to vitamin D.

Design.—Cohort study.

Setting.—The Cardiovascular Health Study conducted in 4 U.S. communities. Data from 1992 to 2006 were included in this analysis.

Participants.—1621 white older adults.

Measurements.—Serum 25-(OH)D concentration (using a high-performance liquid chromatography—tandem mass spectrometry assay that conforms to National Institute of Standards and Technology reference standards) and associations with time to a composite outcome of incident hip fracture, myocardial infarction, cancer, or death.

Results.—Over a median 11-year follow-up, the composite outcome occurred in 1018 participants (63%). Defining events included 137 hip fractures, 186 myocardial infarctions, 335 incidences of cancer, and 360 deaths. The association of low 25-(OH)D concentration with risk for the composite outcome varied by season ($P = 0.057$). A concentration lower than a season-specific Z score of -0.54 best discriminated risk for the composite outcome and was associated with a 24% higher risk in adjusted analyses (95% CI, 9% to 42%). Corresponding season-specific 25-(OH)D concentrations were 43, 50, 61, and 55 nmol/L (17, 20, 24, and 22 ng/mL) in winter, spring, summer, and autumn, respectively.

Limitation.—The observational study was restricted to white participants.

Conclusion.—Threshold concentrations of 25-(OH)D associated with increased risk for relevant clinical disease events center near 50 nmol/L (20 ng/mL). Season-specific targets for 25-(OH)D concentration may be more appropriate than static targets when evaluating health risk.

▶ The optimal level of serum 25-hydroxyvitamin D to prevent disease remains controversial. Serum 1,25-dihydroxyvitamin D has been shown to suppress the renin-angiotensin-aldosterone system, regulate immune system function, and reduce abnormal cell proliferation.[1] Several studies have shown an association between vitamin D deficiency and all-cause mortality, coronary heart disease, and cancer,[2-4] but there is no consensus yet on the serum 25-hydroxyvitamin D level required to prevent or treat these diseases. That vitamin D could exert effects on diseases other than calcium and bone disorders depends on the fact that vitamin D has well-recognized pleiotropic effects on other tissues and biologic processes. The few randomized trials with vitamin D treatment that have been published have shown generally disappointing results.

This observational study evaluated a composite outcome involving incident hip fracture, myocardial infarction, cancer, or death in the Cardiovascular Health Study, a cohort study of 1621 white adults in 4 U.S. communities, analyzing data from 1992 to 2006. Over a median of 11 years of follow-up, 1018 (63%) subjects had a composite outcome event. The association of serum 25-hydroxyvitamin D with risk of composite outcome varied by season, with a serum concentration Z-score of -0.54 best discriminating risk of composite outcome (Fig 1 in the original article). This Z-score was associated with 24% higher risk of outcome in adjusted analyses. Corresponding season-specific serum 25-hydroxyvitamin D levels were 17, 20, 24, and 22 ng/mL in winter, spring, summer, and autumn, respectively. Risk of hip fracture at this Z-score was increased by 34%. The study concluded that threshold concentrations of serum 25-hydroxyvitamin D center on 20 ng/mL and suggested that season-specific targets for 25-hydroxy-vitamin D may be more appropriate than a fixed target when evaluating health risk.

This study provides evidence that a target serum 25-hydroxyvitamin D level centering around 20 ng/mL may be reasonable for minimizing the composite risk of hip fracture, myocardial infarction, cancer, or death. This level matches the recommended target serum 25-hydroxyvitamin D level given by the Institute of Medicine recommendations for maintenance of skeletal health, as published in November 2011.[5] Whether this target level will prove to be appropriate for prevention of individual or other disease outcomes remains to be seen. Nevertheless, it appears that a serum 25-hydroxyvitamin D level close to 20 ng/mL may reduce risk of hip fracture, myocardial infarction, cancer, and death.

B. L. Clarke, MD

References

1. Dusso AS, Brown AJ, Slatopolsky E. Vitamin D. *Am J Physiol Renal Physiol.* 2005;289:F8-F28.
2. Cauley JA, Lacroix AZ, Wu L, et al. Serum 25-hydroxyvitamin D concentrations and risk for hip fractures. *Ann Intern Med.* 2008;149:242-250.
3. Robinson-Cohen C, Katz R, Hoofnagle AN, et al. Mineral metabolism markers and the long-term risk of hip fracture: the Cardiovascular Health Study. *J Clin Endocrinol Metab.* 2011;96:2186-2193.
4. Kestenbaum B, Katz R, de Boer I, et al. Vitamin D, parathyroid hormone, and cardiovascular events among older adults. *J Am Coll Cardiol.* 2011;58:1433-1441.
5. Ross AC, Taylor CL, Yaktine AL, Del Valle HB, Committee to Review Dietary Reference Intakes for Vitamin D and Calcium, Institute of Medicine, eds. Dietary Reference Intakes for Calcium and Vitamin D. Washington, DC: The National Academies Press; 2011.

Associations of dietary calcium intake and calcium supplementation with myocardial infarction and stroke risk and overall cardiovascular mortality in the Heidelberg cohort of the European Prospective Investigation into Cancer and Nutrition study (EPIC-Heidelberg)

Li K, Kaaks R, Linseisen J, et al (German Cancer Res Centre, Heidelberg, Germany)

Heart 98:920-925, 2012

Background.—It has been suggested that a higher calcium intake might favourably modify cardiovascular risk factors. However, findings of an ultimately decreased risk of cardiovascular disease (CVD) are limited. Instead, recent evidence warns that taking calcium supplements might increase myocardial infarction (MI) risk.

Objective.—To prospectively evaluate the associations of dietary calcium intake and calcium supplementation with MI and stroke risk and overall CVD mortality.

Methods.—Data from 23 980 Heidelberg cohort participants of the European Prospective Investigation into Cancer and Nutrition study, aged 35—64 years and free of major CVD events at recruitment, were analysed.

Multivariate Cox regression models were used to estimate HRs and 95% CIs.

Results.—After an average follow-up time of 11 years, 354 MI and 260 stroke cases and 267 CVD deaths were documented. Compared with the lowest quartile, the third quartile of total dietary and dairy calcium intake had a significantly reduced MI risk, with a HR of 0.69 (95% CI 0.50 to 0.94) and 0.68 (95% CI 0.50 to 0.93), respectively. Associations for stroke risk and CVD mortality were overall null. In comparison with non-users of any supplements, users of calcium supplements had a statistically significantly increased MI risk (HR = 1.86; 95% CI 1.17 to 2.96), which was more pronounced for calcium supplement only users (HR = 2.39; 95% CI 1.12 to 5.12).

Conclusions.—Increasing calcium intake from diet might not confer significant cardiovascular benefits, while calcium supplements, which might raise MI risk, should be taken with caution.

▶ A variety of epidemiological studies have shown reduction in risk of hypertension, obesity, and type 2 diabetes in individuals taking calcium supplementation.[1-3] These studies suggest that calcium supplementation might reduce the risk of cardiovascular events. Three studies showed that dietary calcium intake decreased risk of ischemic stroke,[4,5] and another study showed that dietary calcium reduced risk of ischemic heart disease mortality.[6] Other studies have shown no cardiovascular benefit, and 2 recent meta-analyses showed increased risk of myocardial infarction (MI).[7,8]

This study prospectively evaluated the association of dietary calcium intake and supplementation with the risk of MI, stroke, and overall cardiovascular disease mortality in a cohort of 23 980 adults aged 35 to 64 years and free of major cardiovascular disease events at recruitment in Heidelberg, Germany. The subjects were participants in the European Prospective investigation into Cancer and Nutrition study. After average follow-up of 11 years, subjects with total dietary and dairy calcium intake in the third quartile had reduced MI risk by 31% and 32%, respectively. No benefit was seen for stroke risk and cardiovascular disease mortality. Subjects taking calcium supplements had an increased risk of MI, and this risk was increased further if subjects took only calcium supplements. The study concluded that increased dietary calcium intake might not reduce cardiovascular disease outcomes, and that calcium supplements might increase the risk of MI.

This study has several important limitations. Dietary calcium intake within 1 year of recruitment was reported by self-administered food frequency questionnaire, but it was not followed over the multiple years of the study, so the study was unable to capture long-term variation in the diet or calcium supplements. Supplement intake within 4 weeks of recruitment was assessed by interview and questionnaire, but supplement names and doses were not recorded, so it was impossible to assess risk of cardiovascular disease by calcium supplement dose. Finally, subjects were excluded if they had preexisting MI, stroke, and/or transient ischemic attack, but not other forms of preexisting cardiovascular disease. This study raises concern that calcium intake might increase the risk of cardiovascular outcomes, but the limitations compromise the ability of this study to clearly show increased risk based on dietary or supplemental calcium intake.

B. L. Clarke, MD

References

1. Bucher HC, Cook RJ, Guyatt GH, et al. Effects of dietary calcium supplementation on blood pressure. A meta-analysis of randomized controlled trials. *JAMA.* 1996;275:1016-1022.
2. Villegas R, Gao YT, Dai Q, et al. Dietary calcium and magnesium intakes and the risk of type 2 diabetes: the Shanghai Women's Health Study. *Am J Clin Nutr.* 2009; 89:1059-1067.
3. Teegarden D. Calcium intake and reduction in weight or fat mass. *J Nutr.* 2003; 133:249S-251S.
4. Iso H, Stampfer MJ, Manson JE, et al. Prospective study of calcium, potassium, and magnesium intake and risk of stroke in women. *Stroke.* 1999;30:1772-1779.
5. Abbott RD, Curb JD, Rodriguez BL, et al. Effect of dietary calcium and milk consumption on risk of thromboembolic stroke in older middle-aged men. The Honolulu Heart Program. *Stroke.* 1996;27:813-818.
6. Bostick RM, Kuishi LH, Wu Y, et al. Relation of calcium, vitamin D, and dairy food intake to ischemic heart disease mortality among postmenopausal women. *Am J Epidemiol.* 1999;149:151-161.
7. Bolland MJ, Grey A, Gamble GD, Reid IR. Calcium and vitamin D supplements and health outcomes: a reanalysis of the Women's Health Initiative (WHI) limited-access data set. *Am J Clin Nutr.* 2011;94:1144-1149.
8. Bolland MJ, Avenell A, Baron JA, et al. Effect of calcium supplements on risk of myocardial infarction and cardiovascular events: meta-analysis. *BMJ.* 2010;341: c3691.

Long term calcium intake and rates of all cause and cardiovascular mortality: community based prospective longitudinal cohort study
Michaëlsson K, Melhus H, Warensjö Lemming E, et al (Uppsala Univ, Sweden; et al)
BMJ 346:f228, 2013

Objective.—To investigate the association between long term intake of dietary and supplemental calcium and death from all causes and cardiovascular disease.

Design.—Prospective longitudinal cohort study.

Setting.—Swedish mammography cohort, a population based cohort established in 1987-90.

Participants.—61 433 women (born between 1914 and 1948) followed-up for a median of 19 years.

Main Outcome Measures.—Primary outcome measures, identified from registry data, were time to death from all causes (n = 11 944) and cause specific cardiovascular disease (n = 3862), ischaemic heart disease (n = 1932), and stroke (n = 1100). Diet was assessed by food frequency questionnaires at baseline and in 1997 for 38 984 women, and intakes of calcium were estimated. Total calcium intake was the sum of dietary and supplemental calcium.

Results.—The risk patterns with dietary calcium intake were non-linear, with higher rates concentrated around the highest intakes ($\geq$1400 mg/day). Compared with intakes between 600 and 1000 mg/day, intakes above 1400 mg/day were associated with higher death rates from all causes (hazard ratio 1.40, 95% confidence interval 1.17 to 1.67), cardiovascular disease (1 49, 1.09 to 2.02), and ischaemic heart disease (2.14, 1.48 to 3.09) but not from stroke (0.73, 0.33 to 1.65). After sensitivity analysis including marginal structural models, the higher death rate with low dietary calcium intake (<600 mg/day) or with low and high total calcium intake was no longer apparent. Use of calcium tablets (6% users; 500 mg calcium per tablet) was not on average associated with all cause or cause specific mortality but among calcium tablet users with a dietary calcium intake above 1400 mg/day the hazard ratio for all cause mortality was 2.57 (95% confidence interval 1.19 to 5.55).

Conclusion.—High intakes of calcium in women are associated with higher death rates from all causes and cardiovascular disease but not from stroke.

▶ Postmenopausal women in Western countries commonly take supplemental calcium to prevent osteoporotic fractures. More than 60% of middle-aged and older women in the United States are regular users of calcium supplements.[1] Three recent reanalyses of randomized trials showed an increased risk of ischemic heart disease and stroke in women taking calcium supplements.[2-4] Reanalysis of another randomized trial, however, did not show the same findings.[5] Most cohort studies of women have evaluated the risk of stroke with dietary and/or supplemental calcium, rather than cardiovascular disease and mortality, with variable findings.

This Swedish mammography prospective, longitudinal, cohort study of 61 433 women initially evaluated self-reported food frequency questionnaire dietary and supplemental calcium intake between 1987 and 1990, with reassessment in 1997. All-cause mortality, cause-specific cardiovascular disease, ischemic heart disease, and stroke were assessed by registry data over a median follow-up of 19 years. The study showed that all-cause mortality, cardiovascular disease, and ischemic heart disease were increased in subjects taking less than 600 mg or 1400 mg or greater dietary calcium each day at baseline. Model adjustment resulted in loss of significance of the higher death rate with dietary calcium less than 600 mg and total calcium intake less than 600 mg or greater than 1400 mg. Only 6% of subjects took calcium supplements, and this was not associated with all-cause or cause-specific mortality, but all-cause mortality was increased significantly in subjects taking calcium supplements with dietary calcium intake of greater than 1400 mg. The study concluded that high calcium intake in women was associated with increased all-cause mortality and mortality from cardiovascular disease, but not mortality from stroke.

This study has similar limitations to the previous study, including assessment of baseline dietary calcium intake using a self-reported food frequency questionnaire. Food frequency questionnaires tend to overestimate calcium intake, and this study used age-standardized portion sizes rather than actual individual portion sizes. Dietary and supplemental calcium intake tends to vary over time, and the study did not reassess self-reported intakes over time. Vitamin D intake was not reported, and it is known that vitamin D intake minimizes cardiovascular outcomes in this age population. The findings are concerning, however, and suggest that high calcium dietary intake may be associated with increased death rates from all causes and cardiovascular disease.

B. L. Clarke, MD

References

1. Mangano KM, Walsh SJ, Insogna KL, Kenny AM, Kerstetter JE. Calcium intake in the United States from dietary and supplemental sources across adult age groups: new estimates from the National Health and Nutrition Examination Survey 2003-2006. *J Am Diet Assoc.* 2011;111:687-695.
2. Bolland MJ, Avenell A, Baron JA, et al. Effect of calcium supplements on risk of myocardial infarction and cardiovascular events: meta-analysis. *BMJ.* 2010;341: c3691.
3. Bolland MJ, Grey A, Avenell A, Gamble GD, Reid IR. Calcium supplements with or without vitamin D and risk of cardiovascular events: reanalysis of the Women's Health Initiative (WHI) limited access dataset and meta-analysis. *BMJ.* 2010;342: d2040.
4. Bolland MJ, Barber PA, Doughtly RN, et al. Vascular events in healthy older women receiving calcium supplementation: randomised controlled trial. *BMJ.* 2008;336:262-266.
5. Lewis JR, Calver J, Zhu K, Flicker L, Prince RL. Calcium supplementation and the risks of atherosclerotic vascular disease in older women: results of a 5-year RCT and a 4.5-year follow-up. *J Bone Miner Res.* 2011;26:35-41.

Vitamin D with Calcium Reduces Mortality: Patient Level Pooled Analysis of 70,528 Patients from Eight Major Vitamin D Trials

Rejnmark L, Avenell A, Masud T, et al (Aarhus Univ Hosp, Denmark; Univ of Aberdeen, UK; Nottingham Univ Hosps, Nottingham, UK; et al)
J Clin Endocrinol Metab 97:2670-2681, 2012

Introduction.—Vitamin D may affect multiple health outcomes. If so, an effect on mortality is to be expected. Using pooled data from randomized controlled trials, we performed individual patient data (IPD) and trial level meta-analyses to assess mortality among participants randomized to either vitamin D alone or vitamin D with calcium.

Subjects and Methods.—Through a systematic literature search, we identified 24 randomized controlled trials reporting data on mortality in which vitamin D was given either alone or with calcium. From a total of 13 trials with more than 1000 participants each, eight trials were included in our IPD analysis. Using a stratified Cox regression model, we calculated risk of death during 3 yr of treatment in an intention-to-treat analysis. Also, we performed a trial level meta-analysis including data from all studies.

Results.—The IPD analysis yielded data on 70,528 randomized participants (86.8% females) with a median age of 70 (interquartile range, 62–77) yr. Vitamin D with or without calcium reduced mortality by 7%

[hazard ratio, 0.93; 95% confidence interval (CI), 0.88—0.99]. However, vitamin D alone did not affect mortality, but risk of death was reduced if vitamin D was given with calcium (hazard ratio, 0.91; 95% CI, 0.84—0.98). The number needed to treat with vitamin D plus calcium for 3 yr to prevent one death was 151. Trial level meta-analysis (24 trials with 88,097 participants) showed similar results, *i.e.* mortality was reduced with vitamin D plus calcium (odds ratio, 0.94; 95% CI, 0.88—0.99), but not with vitamin D alone (odds ratio, 0.98; 95% CI, 0.91—1.06).

Conclusion.—Vitamin D with calcium reduces mortality in the elderly, whereas available data do not support an effect of vitamin D alone.

▶ A meta-analysis of randomized controlled trials published in 2007 showed that vitamin D supplementation reduced all-cause mortality rate by 7%.[1] Three subsequent meta-analyses using updated literature searches and different study inclusion criteria did not show that vitamin D alone reduced mortality.[2-4] Two of these studies, however, showed that vitamin D reduced mortality if it was combined with calcium supplementation.[3,4] These study level meta-analyses may give biased assessments and are limited in their ability to explain heterogeneity. Individual patient data meta-analyses have greater statistical power than study-level meta-analyses.

This individual patient data meta-analysis evaluated 24 randomized controlled trials that reported mortality in subjects receiving vitamin D alone or in combination with calcium. Of these 24 trials, 13 included more than 1000 subjects each, and 8 had individual data available for inclusion in this analysis. The 8 trials included a total of 70 528 subjects, with 86.8% female, of median age 70 years. Vitamin D with or without calcium reduced mortality rate by 7%, whereas vitamin D alone did not affect mortality. Risk of death was decreased if vitamin D was given with calcium, with 151 subjects needing to be treated for 3 years to prevent 1 death. Trial-level data meta-analysis of the 24 trials with 88 097 subjects showed similar results with vitamin D and calcium, but not with vitamin D alone. The study concluded that vitamin D with calcium reduces mortality in elderly patients, whereas vitamin D alone does not.

This large meta-analysis further clarifies the relative risks of calcium and vitamin D supplementation. Whereas calcium intake alone may increase mortality or cardiovascular disease,[5] vitamin D alone does not appear to reduce death, but the combination of calcium and vitamin D supplementation seems to reduce mortality. These findings may be interpreted as suggesting that calcium and vitamin D supplementation should not be taken separately but, rather, in combination. The adverse effects of calcium alone may be mitigated by taking this in combination with vitamin D. Given that most patients taking these supplements for osteoporosis or skeletal health take both, concerns regarding the adverse effects of each alone may be overstated.

B. L. Clarke, MD

References

1. Autier P, Gandini S. Vitamin D supplementation and total mortality: a meta-analysis of randomized controlled trials. *Arch Intern Med.* 2007;167:1730-1737.

2. Chung M, Balk EM, Brendel M, et al. Vitamin D and calcium: a systematic review of health outcomes. *Evid Rep Technol Assess (Full Rep)*. 2009;183:1-420.
3. Avenell A, Gillespie WJ, Gillespie LD, O'Connell D. Vitamin D and vitamin D analogues for preventing fractures associated with involutional and post-menopausal osteoporosis. *Cochrane Database Syst Rev*. 2009;2:CD000227.
4. Bjelakovic G, Gluud LL, Nikalova D, et al. Vitamin D supplementation for prevention of mortality in adults. *Cochrane Database Syst Rev*. 2011;7:CD007470.
5. Michaëlsson K, Melhus H, Warensjö Lemming E, et al. Long term calcium intake and rates of all cause and cardiovascular mortality: community based prospective longitudinal cohort study. *BMJ*. 2013;346:f228.

Vitamin D Therapy and Cardiac Structure and Function in Patients With Chronic Kidney Disease: The PRIMO Randomized Controlled Trial

Thadhani R, Appelbaum E, Pritchett Y, et al (Massachusetts General Hosp, Boston; Beth Israel Deaconess Med Ctr, Boston, MA; Brigham and Women's Hosp, Boston, MA; et al)
JAMA 307:674-684, 2012

Context.—Vitamin D is associated with decreased cardiovascular-related morbidity and mortality, possibly by modifying cardiac structure and function, yet firm evidence for either remains lacking.

Objective.—To determine the effects of an active vitamin D compound, paricalcitol, on left ventricular mass over 48 weeks in patients with an estimated glomerular filtration rate of 15 to 60 mL/min/1.73 m^2.

Design, Setting, and Participants.—Multinational, double-blind, randomized placebocontrolled trial among 227 patients with chronic kidney disease, mild to moderate left ventricular hypertrophy, and preserved left ventricular ejection fraction, conducted in 11 countries from July 2008 through September 2010.

Intervention.—Participants were randomly assigned to receive oral paricalcitol, 2 μg/d (n = 115), or matching placebo (n = 112).

Main Outcome Measures.—Change in left ventricular mass index over 48 weeks by cardiovascular magnetic resonance imaging. Secondary end points included echocardiographic changes in left ventricular diastolic function.

Results.—Treatment with paricalcitol reduced parathyroid hormone levels within 4 weeks and maintained levels within the normal range throughout the study duration. At 48 weeks, the change in left ventricular mass index did not differ between treatment groups (paricalcitol group, 0.34 g/m$^{2.7}$ [95% CI, −0.14 to 0.83 g/m$^{2.7}$] vs placebo group, −0.07 g/m$^{2.7}$ [95% CI, −0.55 to 0.42 g/m$^{2.7}$]). Doppler measures of diastolic function including peak early diastolic lateral mitral annular tissue velocity (paricalcitol group, −0.01 cm/s [95% CI, −0.63 to 0.60 cm/s] vs placebo group, −0.30 cm/s [95% CI, −0.93 to 0.34 cm/s]) also did not differ. Episodes of hypercalcemia were more frequent in the paricalcitol group compared with the placebo group.

Conclusion.—Forty-eight week therapy with paricalcitol did not alter left ventricular mass index or improve certain measures of diastolic dysfunction in patients with chronic kidney disease.

Trial Registration.—clinicaltrials.gov Identifier: NCT00497146.

▶ Serum 25-hydroxyvitamin D levels are associated with decreased cardiovascular-related morbidity and mortality. Possible mechanisms for these associations remain elusive, but vitamin D receptors have been identified in vascular smooth muscle, endothelial cells, and possibly cardiac tissue.[1,2] A variety of observational studies, small clinical trials, and meta-analyses have demonstrated that vitamin D therapy reduces cardiovascular events in healthy older men and women.[3,4]

Patients with chronic kidney disease (CKD) frequently develop low serum 1,25-dihydroxyvitamin D levels because of low serum 25-hydroxyvitamin D levels and reduced renal 1α-hydroxylase activity. Vitamin D deficiency contributes to secondary hyperparathyroidism, which results in metabolic bone disease. Observational studies in patients with CKD have shown that vitamin D deficiency is associated with increased risk of cardiovascular events.[5,6] Other observational studies showed that therapy with calcitriol or related analogs resulted in reduced risk of cardiovascular events.[7,8] It has been proposed that vitamin D treatment reduces left ventricular hypertrophy, improves left ventricular diastolic dysfunction, and reduces episodes of congestive heart failure.

This multinational, prospective, double-blind, randomized clinical trial evaluated the effects of paricalcitol, an active vitamin D analogue, 2 mcg each day or placebo on left ventricular mass over 48 weeks in 227 patients with estimated glomerular filtration rate of 15 to 60 mL/min/1.73 m^2. These subjects had stage III-IV CKD, with mild-to-moderate left ventricular hypertrophy and preserved left ventricular ejection fraction. Treatment with paricalcitol reduced parathyroid hormone levels to within the normal range within 4 weeks and maintained them in the normal range for the remainder of the study. The change in left ventricular mass index at 48 weeks by cardiovascular magnetic resonance imaging did not differ between the paricalcitol or placebo treatment groups. Doppler assessment of left ventricular diastolic function also did not change between treatment groups over this interval, and hypercalcemia was more frequent in the paricalcitol group.

This study demonstrated that an active form of vitamin D was unable to improve left ventricular mass index or left ventricular diastolic function in subjects with stage III-IV CKD and mild-to-moderate left ventricular hypertrophy. However, paricalcitol reduced hospitalizations for cardiovascular disease during the study and limited increases in B-natriuretic peptide in subjects with prominent left ventricular hypertrophy at baseline. These findings suggest that the reduction in cardiovascular events by vitamin D seen in other treatment trials is not due simply to changes in cardiac structure or function. These findings apply strictly to patients with stage III-IV CKD, but they may also apply to others in the general population.

B. L. Clarke, MD

References

1. Holick MF. Vitamin D deficiency. *N Engl J Med.* 2007;357:266-281.
2. Levin A, Djurdev O, Thompson C, et al. Canadian randomized trial of hemo-globin maintenance to prevent or delay left ventricular mass growth in patients with CKD. *Am J Kidney Dis.* 2005;46:799-811.
3. Autier P, Gandini S. Vitamin D supplementation and total mortality: a meta-analysis of randomized controlled trials. *Arch Intern Med.* 2007;167:173-1737.
4. Wang TJ, Pencina MJ, Booth SL, et al. Vitamin D deficiency and cardiovascular disease. *Circulation.* 2008;117:502-511.
5. Drechsler C, Pilz S, Obermayer-Pitsch B, et al. Vitamin D deficiency is associated with sudden cardiac death, combined cardiovascular events, and mortality in hemodialysis patients. *Eur Heart J.* 2010;31:2253-2261.
6. Kalantar-Zadeh K, Kuwae N, Regidor DL, et al. Survival predictability of time-varying indicators of bone disease in maintenance hemodialysis patients. *Kidney Int.* 2006;70:771-780.
7. Teng M, Wolf M, Lowrie E, Ofsthun N, Lazarus JM, Thadhani R. Survival of patients undergoing hemodialysis with paricalcitol or calcitriol therapy. *N Engl J Med.* 2003;349:446-456.
8. Teng M, Wolf M, Ofsthun MN, et al. Activated injectable vitamin D and hemodi-alysis survival: a historical cohort study. *J Am Soc Nephrol.* 2005;16:1115-1125.

A Pooled Analysis of Vitamin D Dose Requirements for Fracture Prevention

Bischoff-Ferrari HA, Willett WC, Orav EJ, et al (Univ Hosp Zurich, Switzerland; Harvard School of Public Health, Boston, MA; et al)
N Engl J Med 367:40-49, 2012

Background.—The results of meta-analyses examining the relationship between vitamin D supplementation and fracture reduction have been inconsistent.

Methods.—We pooled participant-level data from 11 double-blind, randomized, controlled trials of oral vitamin D supplementation (daily, weekly, or every 4 months), with or without calcium, as compared with placebo or calcium alone in persons 65 years of age or older. Primary end points were the incidence of hip and any nonvertebral fractures according to Cox regression analyses, with adjustment for age group, sex, type of dwelling, and study. Our primary aim was to compare data from quartiles of actual intake of vitamin D (including each individual participant's adher-ence to the treatment and supplement use outside the study protocol) in the treatment groups of all trials with data from the control groups.

Results.—We included 31,022 persons (mean age, 76 years; 91% women) with 1111 incident hip fractures and 3770 nonvertebral fractures. Participants who were randomly assigned to receive vitamin D, as compared with those assigned to control groups, had a nonsignificant 10% reduction in the risk of hip fracture (hazard ratio, 0.90; 95% confidence interval [CI], 0.80 to 1.01) and a 7% reduction in the risk of nonvertebral fracture (hazard ratio, 0.93; 95% CI, 0.87 to 0.99). By quartiles of actual intake, reduction in the risk of fracture was shown only at the highest intake level (median, 800 IU daily; range, 792 to 2000), with a 30% reduction in the risk of hip fracture (hazard ratio, 0.70; 95% CI, 0.58 to 0.86) and a 14% reduction in the risk of any nonvertebral fracture (hazard ratio, 0.86; 95% CI, 0.76 to 0.96). Benefits at the highest level of vitamin D intake were fairly consistent across subgroups defined by age group, type of dwelling, baseline 25-hydroxyvitamin D level, and additional calcium intake.

Conclusions.—High-dose vitamin D supplementation (≥800 IU daily) was somewhat favorable in the prevention of hip fracture and any nonvertebral fracture in persons 65 years of age or older. (Funded by the Swiss National Foundations and others.)

▶ Although the majority of studies of calcium supplementation alone have not shown evidence of fracture reduction, study-level meta-analyses of the relationship between vitamin D supplementation and fracture reduction have given variable results. One trial-level meta-analysis of double-blind, randomized, controlled trials reported an 18% reduction in hip fractures and a 20% reduction in nonvertebral fractures at doses of at least 482 International Units (IU) of vitamin D each day.[1] Three other study-level meta-analyses[2-4] and 1 pooled analysis of participant-level data from open-design and blinded trials[5] showed that vitamin D supplementation had no effect on total fractures, or a reduction of hip fractures by 7% to 16% if combined with calcium supplementation, regardless of the dose of vitamin D given. These variable results have been attributed to differences in inclusion criteria for the analyses with respect to blinding, oral vs injectable vitamin D formulation used, or accommodation for nonadherence to therapy.

To minimize these confounders, this study pooled participant-level actual vitamin D intake data from 11 double-blind, randomized, controlled trials of oral vitamin D supplementation with or without calcium, compared with placebo or calcium alone, in subjects 65 years of age or older. A total of 31 022 subjects of mean age 72 years, 91% of whom were women, had 1111 incident hip fractures and 3770 nonvertebral fractures. Those randomized to receive vitamin D had a nonsignificant reduction in hip fractures of 10%, and a significant 7% reduction in nonvertebral fractures, compared with placebo or calcium alone (Fig 1 in the original article). Reduction in risk of fractures was seen only in the highest quartile of vitamin D intake, with median intake above 800 IU daily, with 30% reduction in risk of hip fracture and 14% reduction in risk of nonvertebral fracture. Reduction in fracture in the highest quartile of vitamin D supplement was consistent across subgroups by age, type of dwelling, baseline 25-hydroxy vitamin D level, or additional calcium intake. The study concluded that high-dose vitamin D intake of more than 800 IU each day helped prevent hip and nonvertebral fractures in adults 65 years of age or older.

This study suggests that high-dose, but not lower-dose, vitamin D supplementation alone may help reduce hip and nonvertebral fracture risk in older adults. Previous studies of vitamin D supplementation and fracture reduction have not always achieved actual intake of the assigned doses, as this study did. This study reported benefit even for community-dwelling adults not living in institutions, unlike in previous studies. This study demonstrated that vitamin D dose still mattered even when vitamin D was given with calcium supplementation, and that calcium supplementation of less than 1000 mg each day was optimal for fracture reduction. The findings in this study support the recommendations in the 2011 Institute of Medicine report.[6]

B. L. Clarke, MD

References

1. Bischoff-Ferrari HA, Willett WC, Wong JB, et al. Prevention of nonvertebral fractures with oral vitamin D and dose dependency: a meta-analysis of randomized controlled trials. *Arch Intern Med.* 2009;169:551-561.
2. Cranney A, Horsley T, O'Donnell S, et al. Effectiveness and safety of vitamin D in relation to bone health. *Evid Rep Technol Assess (Full Rep).* 2007:1-235.
3. Boonen S, Lips P, Bouillon R, et al. Need for additional calcium to reduce the risk of hip fracture with vitamin D supplementation: evidence from a comparative metaanalysis of randomized controlled trials. *J Clin Endocrinol Metab.* 2007;92: 1415-1423.
4. Avenell A, Gillespie WJ, Gillespie LD, O'Connell D. Vitamin D and vitamin D analogues for preventing fractures associated with involutional and postmenopausal osteoporosis. *Cochrane Database Syst Rev.* 2009;2:CD000227.
5. DIPART (Vitamin D Individual Patient Analysis of Randomized Trials) Group. Patient level pooled analysis of 68 500 patients from seven major vitamin D fracture trials in US and Europe. *BMJ.* 2010;340:b5463.
6. Ross AC, Manson JE, Abrams SA, et al. The 2011 Dietary Reference Intakes for Calcium and Vitamin D: what dietetics practitioners need to know. *J Am Diet Assoc.* 2011;111:524-527.

Epidemiology and Pathophysiology of Osteoporosis

Dose Response to Vitamin D Supplementation in Postmenopausal Women: A Randomized Trial

Gallagher JC, Sai A, Templin T II, et al (Univ of Nebraska Med Ctr, Omaha)
Ann Intern Med 156:425-437, 2012

Background.—Serum 25-hydroxyvitamin D (25-[OH]D) is considered the best biomarker of clinical vitamin D status.

Objective.—To determine the effect of increasing oral doses of vitamin D3 on serum 25-(OH)D and serum parathyroid hormone (PTH) levels in postmenopausal white women with vitamin D insufficiency (defined as a 25-[OH]D level ≤50 nmol/L) in the presence of adequate calcium intake. These results can be used as a guide to estimate the Recommended Dietary Allowance (RDA) (defined as meeting the needs of 97.5% of the population) for vitamin D_3.

Design.—Randomized, placebo-controlled trial. (ClinicalTrials.gov registration number: NCT00472823)

Setting.—Creighton University Medical Center, Omaha, Nebraska.

Participants.—163 healthy postmenopausal white women with vitamin D insufficiency enrolled in the winter or spring of 2007 to 2008 and followed for 1 year.

Intervention.—Participants were randomly assigned to receive placebo or vitamin D_3, 400, 800, 1600, 2400, 3200, 4000, or 4800 IU once daily. Daily calcium supplements were provided to increase the total daily calcium intake to 1200 to 1400 mg.

Measurements.—The primary outcomes were 25-(OH)D and PTH levels at 6 and 12 months.

Results.—The mean baseline 25-(OH)D level was 39 nmol/L. The dose response was curvilinear and tended to plateau at approximately 112 nmol/L in patients receiving more than 3200 IU/d of vitamin D_3. The RDA of vitamin D_3 to achieve a 25-(OH)D level greater than 50 nmol/L was 800 IU/d. A mixed-effects model predicted that 600 IU of vitamin D_3 daily could also meet this goal. Compared with participants with a normal body mass index (<25 kg/m^2), obese women (≥30 kg/m^2) had a 25-(OH)D level that was 17.8 nmol/L lower. Parathyroid hormone levels at 12 months decreased with an increasing dose of vitamin D_3 ($P = 0.012$). Depending on the criteria used, hypercalcemia occurred in 2.8% to 9.0% and hypercalciuria in 12.0% to 33.0% of participants; events were unrelated to dose.

Limitation.—Findings may not be generalizable to other age groups or persons with substantial comorbid conditions.

Conclusion.—A vitamin D_3 dosage of 800 IU/d increased serum 25-(OH)D levels to greater than 50 nmol/L in 97.5% of women; however, a model predicted the same response with a vitamin D3 dosage of 600 IU/d. These results can be used as a guide for the RDA of vitamin D_3, but prospective trials are needed to confirm the clinical significance of these results.

▶ Vitamin D plays a critical role in bone metabolism and calcium homeostasis. To quantify the requirements for dietary intake of vitamin D and other nutrients, the Institute of Medicine and US National Academy of Sciences have developed Dietary Reference Intakes.[1] Dietary Reference Intakes include both Estimated Average Requirements, which meet the need of 50% of the population, and Recommended Dietary Allowances, which meet the need of 97.5% of the population. Tolerable Upper Intake Levels refer to the highest average daily intake that is likely to pose no risk for adverse health effects for nearly all individuals in the population.

Prior to this study, there were no comprehensive studies on the relationship between vitamin D dose and serum 25-hydroxyvitamin D levels on which to base a recommended daily allowance for vitamin D. In addition, there were no treatment trials that could establish a level of serum 25-hydroxyvitamin D linked to clinical outcomes. Most studies evaluating calcium and vitamin D treatment reported combined, and not separate, levels or effects.[2] Serum 25-hydroxyvitamin D levels also depend on sunlight exposure,[3] body mass index (BMI),[4] and skin color.[5,6]

This study reports the effect of increasing oral doses of vitamin D3 on serum 25-hydroxyvitamin D and parathyroid hormone levels in 163 postmenopausal white women with vitamin D insufficiency, defined as baseline serum 25-hydroxyvitamin D levels of ≤20 ng/mL (≤50 nmol/L), and adequate calcium intake. Subjects were recruited in the winter to minimize the effect of sunlight on baseline vitamin D levels and were followed for 1 year after randomization to vitamin D3 ranging from 400 to 4800 International Units (IU) each day. Daily calcium intake was supplemented to maintain intake at 1200 to 1400 mg elemental calcium. Subjects had a mean baseline 25-hydroxyvitamin D level of 15.6 ng/mL

(39 mmol/L), with a curvilinear response to supplementation that plateaued at around 45 ng/mL when given more than 3200 IU each day (Fig 2 in the original article). To achieve a serum 25-hydroxyvitamin D level of 20 ng/mL (50 nmol/L), the Recommended Dietary Allowance for vitamin D3 was 800 IU each day. Mixed-effects modeling showed that this level could be achieved with 600 IU each day.

This is the first randomized, controlled, dose-response study of supplemental vitamin D in vitamin D–deficient white postmenopausal women. Interindividual variation in serum 25-hydroxyvitamin D levels achieved with varying doses of vitamin D3 was broad, but on average, vitamin D 800 IU each day achieved a mean serum 25-hydroxyvitamin D level of 20 ng/mL and 1600 IU each day achieved 30 ng/mL. Obese subjects with BMI $\geq$30 kg/m^2 achieved serum 25-hydroxymitan D levels 7 ng/mL (17.8 nmol/L) lower than subjects with BMI < 25 kg/m^2. Hypercalcemia occurred in 2.8% to 9.0% of subjects while hypercalciuria occurred in 12.0% to 33.0% of subjects during the trial.

B. L. Clarke, MD

References

1. Institute of Medicine, Standing Committee on the Scientific Evaluation of Dietary Reference Intakes. Food, and Nutrition Board. Vitamin D. In: Dietary Reference Intakes for Calcium, Phosphorus, Magnesium, Vitamin D, and Fluoride. Washington, DC: National Academies Press; 1997. www.nap.edu/openbook. php?record_id=5776. Accessed February 16, 2013.
2. Ross AC, Taylor CL, Yaktine AL, Del Valle HB, Institute of Medicine Committee to Review Dietary Reference Intakes for Vitamin D and Calcium, eds. Dietary Reference Intakes for Calcium and Vitamin D. Washington, DC: National Academies Press; 2011.
3. Holick MF, Matsuoka LY, Wortsman J. Age, vitamin D, and solar ultraviolet [letter]. *Lancet*. 1989;2:1104-1105.
4. Wortsman J, Matsuoka LY, Chen TC, Lu Z, Holick MF. Decreased bioavailability of vitamin D in obesity. *Am J Clin Nutr*. 2000;72:690-693.
5. Looker AC. Body fat and vitamin D status in black versus white women. *J Clin Endocrinol Metab*. 2005;90:635-640.
6. Aloia JF, Patel M, Dimaano R, et al. Vitamin D intake to attain a desired serum 25-hydroxyvitamin D concentration. *Am J Clin Nutr*. 2008;87:1952-1958.

Increasing Occurrence of Atypical Femoral Fractures Associated With Bisphosphonate Use
Meier RPH, Perneger TV, Stern R, et al (Univ Hosps of Geneva and Faculty of Medicine, Switzerland)
Arch Intern Med 172:930-936, 2012

Background.—Current evidence suggests that there is an association between bisphosphonate therapy and atypical femoral fractures, but the extent of this risk remains unclear.

Methods.—Between 1999 and 2010, a total of 477 patients 50 years and older were hospitalized with a subtrochanteric or femoral shaft fracture at a single university medical center. Admission radiographs and medical and

Incidence of Atypical Nontraumatic Diaphyseal Fractures of the Femur

Dell RM, Adams AL, Greene DF, et al (Kaiser Permanente Southern California, Gardena; et al)
J Bone Miner Res 27:2544-2550, 2012

Bisphosphonates reduce the rate of osteoporotic fractures in clinical trials and community practice. "Atypical" nontraumatic fractures of the diaphyseal (subtrochanteric or shaft) part of the femur have been observed in patients taking bisphosphonates. We calculated the incidence of these fractures within a defined population and examined the incidence rates according to duration of bisphosphonate use. We identified all femur fractures from January 1, 2007 until December 31, 2011 in 1,835,116 patients older than 45 years who were enrolled in the Healthy Bones Program at Kaiser Southern California, an integrated health care provider. Potential atypical fractures were identified by diagnostic or procedure codes and adjudicated by examination of radiographs. Bisphosphonate exposure was derived from internal pharmacy records. The results showed that 142 patients had atypical fractures; of these, 128 had bisphosphonate exposure. There was no significant correlation between duration of use (5.5 ± 3.4 years) and age (69.3 ± 8.6 years) or bone density (*T*-score −2.1 ± 1.0). There were 188,814 patients who had used bisphosphonates. The age-adjusted incidence rates for an atypical fracture were 1.78/100,000/year (95% confidence interval [CI], 1.5−2.0) with exposure from 0.1 to 1.9 years, and increased to 113.1/100,000/year (95% CI, 69.3−156.8) with exposure from 8 to 9.9 years. We conclude that the incidence of atypical fractures of the femur increases with longer duration of bisphosphonate use. The rate is much lower than the expected rate of devastating hip fractures in elderly osteoporotic patients. Patients at risk for osteoporotic fractures should not be discouraged from initiating bisphosphonates, because clinical trials have documented that these medicines can substantially reduce the incidence of typical hip fractures. The increased risk of atypical fractures should be taken into consideration when continuing bisphosphonates beyond 5 years.

▶ Previous studies have demonstrated that bisphosphonates reduce the risk of osteoporotic fractures in clinical trials[1] and in community practice.[2,3] Atypical subtrochanteric and femoral shaft fractures have been rarely reported in patients who have taken bisphosphonates for prolonged periods.[4-6] These fractures are different for typical osteoporotic fractures in their radiographic appearance and circumstances in which they occur. These fractures are typically transverse, associated with thickening or beaking of the lateral cortex, resemble stress fractures, and occur with no or minimal preceding trauma. Typical osteoporotic fractures, on the other hand, occur in a spiral or comminuted pattern, are associated with thin cortices, and occur with minimal-to-moderate preceding trauma. Atypical fractures were rarely reported prior to the introduction of bisphosphonate therapies.

This study estimates the overall incidence and incidence by duration of exposure of atypical femur fractures within a very large US managed care organization from 2007–2011. The study population included 1 835 116 patients older than 45 years of age who were enrolled in an osteoporosis prevention program. All atypical fractures were initially identified by diagnostic and procedure billing codes and confirmed by x-ray review. Duration of bisphosphonate exposure was determined from internal pharmacy records. The study identified 142 atypical nontraumatic diaphyseal femoral fractures, with 128 of these occurring after treatment with bisphosphonate therapy. No correlation was seen between these atypical fractures and duration of bisphosphonate use, age, or bone mineral density. The database contained 188 814 patients who had received bisphosphonates. The age-adjusted incidence rates for atypical diaphyseal femoral fracture were 1.78/100 000/year with exposure from 0.1 to 1.9 years. The age-adjusted incidence rate increased to 16.1/100 000/year after 4.0 to 5.9 years, and 113.1/100 000/year after 8.0 to 9.9 years. The study concluded that atypical femur fractures are rare, but that they increase with increasing duration of bisphosphonate exposure. The authors recommended that patients at high risk of osteoporotic fracture not be discouraged from considering bisphosphonate therapy because the rate of atypical femur fractures is much lower than the risk of typical femoral osteoporotic fractures.

This important study provides quantification of the risk of atypical nontraumatic diaphyseal femoral fracture stratified by years of bisphosphonate use. Strengths of the study include the large size, duration of follow-up for detection of atypical fractures, and x-ray adjudication of all atypical fractures included. As in other studies, a small percentage (10%) of patients with atypical femur fractures did not have prior exposure to bisphosphonate therapy. Compared with the risks of atypical femur fracture reported in this study, the risk of typical osteoporotic hip fractures in subjects without prior vertebral fracture who were receiving placebo during clinical trials has been reported as 750/100 000/year,[7] or 833/100 000/year in those with vertebral fracture.[8] In osteoporotic subjects 70–79 years of age, the rate was reported to increase to 1390/100 000/year,[9] and in osteoporotic subjects older than 80 the rate was 4200/100 000/year.[9] The findings of this study support current US Food and Drug Administration recommendations to consider stopping bisphosphonate therapy after 5 years of continuous therapy.

B. L. Clarke, MD

References

1. Bilezikian JP. Efficacy of bisphosphonates in reducing fracture risk in postmenopausal osteoporosis. *Am J Med.* 2009;122:S14-S21.
2. Dell RM, Greene D, Anderson D, Williams K. Osteoporosis disease management: what every orthopaedic surgeon should know. *J Bone Joint Surg Am.* 2009;91:79-86.
3. Adams AL, Shi J, Takayanagi M, Dell RM, Funahashi TT, Jacobsen SJ. Ten-year hip fracture incidence rate trends in a large California population, 1997–2006. *Osteoporos Int.* 2013;24:373-376.
4. Goh SK, Yang KY, Koh JS, et al. Subtrochanteric insufficiency fractures in patients on alendronate therapy: a caution. *J Bone Joint Surg Br.* 2007;89:349-353.
5. Lenart BA, Lorich DG, Lane JM. Atypical fractures of the femoral diaphysis in postmenopausal women taking alendronate. *N Engl J Med.* 2008;358:1304-1306.

6. Giusti A, Hamdy NA, Papapoulos SE. Atypical fractures of the femur and bisphosphonate therapy: a systematic review of case/case series studies. *Bone.* 2010;47:169-180.

7. Black DM, Cummings SR, Karpf DB, et al. Randomised trial of effect of alendronate on risk of fracture in women with existing vertebral fractures. Fracture Intervention Trial Research Group. *Lancet.* 1996;348:1535-1541.

8. Black DM, Delmas PD, Eastell R, et al. Once-yearly zoledronic acid for treatment of postmenopausal osteoporosis. *N Engl J Med.* 2007;356:1809-1822.

9. McClung MR, Geusens P, Miller PD, et al; Hip Intervention Program Study Group. Effect of risedronate on the risk of hip fracture in elderly women. Hip Intervention Program Study Group. *N Engl J Med.* 2001;344:333-340.

Changes in bone mineral density and body composition during pregnancy and postpartum. A controlled cohort study

Møller UK, vi Streym S, Mosekilde L, et al (Aarhus Univ Hosp, Aarhus C, Denmark)

Osteoporos Int 23:1213-1223, 2012

In a controlled cohort study, bone mineral density (BMD) was measured in 153 women prepregnancy; during pregnancy; and 0.5, 4, 9, and 19 months postpartum. Seventy-five age-matched controls, without pregnancy plans, were followed in parallel. Pregnancy and breastfeeding cause a reversible bone loss, which, initially, is most pronounced at trabecular sites but also involves cortical sites during prolonged breastfeeding.

Introduction.—Conflicting results have been reported on effects of pregnancy and breastfeeding on BMD and body composition (BC). In a controlled cohort study, we elucidate changes in BMD and BC during and following a pregnancy.

Methods.—We measured BMD and BC in 153 women planning pregnancy (n = 92 conceived), once in each trimester during pregnancy and 15, 129, and 280 days postpartum. Moreover, BMD was measured 19 months postpartum (n = 31). Seventy-five age-matched controls, without pregnancy plans, were followed in parallel.

Results.—Compared with controls, BMD decreased significantly during pregnancy by $1.8 \pm 0.5\%$ at the lumbar spine, $3.2 \pm 0.5\%$ at the total hip, $2.4 \pm 0.3\%$ at the whole body, and $4.2 \pm 0.7\%$ at the ultra distal forearm. Postpartum, BMD decreased further with an effect of breastfeeding. At 9 months postpartum, women who had breastfed for <9 months had a BMD similar to that of the controls, whereas BMD at the lumbar spine and hip was decreased in women who were still breastfeeding. During prolonged breastfeeding, BMD at sites which consist of mostly trabecular bone started to be regained, whereas BMD at sites rich in cortical bone decreased further. At 19 months postpartum, BMD did not differ from baseline at any site. During pregnancy, fat- and lean-tissue mass increased by $19 \pm 22\%$ and $5 \pm 6\%$ ($p < 0.001$), respectively. Postpartum, changes in fat mass differed according to breastfeeding status with a slower decline in women who continued breastfeeding. Calcium and vitamin D intake was not associated with BMD changes.

Conclusion.—Pregnancy and breastfeeding cause a reversible bone loss. At 19 months postpartum, BMD has returned to pre-pregnancy level independently of breastfeeding length. Reversal of changes in fat mass depends on breastfeeding status.

▶ It has been known for many years that pregnancy and breastfeeding result in major changes in maternal calcium homeostasis and bone metabolism to provide calcium to the fetus and newborn infant. Some studies have reported that pregnancy causes bone loss in the mother because of transfer of calcium to the fetus and increased urinary calcium loss.[1,2] Other studies have shown no change or increased bone density and attributed this to the increased levels of estradiol and increased intestinal calcium absorption during pregnancy.[3,4] Postpartum studies show that most new mothers lose bone density, but the effect of breastfeeding at different sites in the skeleton remains controversial.[5,6] Moreover, pregnancy and breastfeeding result in large changes in body weight and body composition, and this may affect bone density also.[7,8]

This important study was designed to improve understanding of the simultaneous physiological changes that occur in bone density and bone composition during pregnancy and breastfeeding. A cohort of 153 women 25 to 35 years of age planning conception was followed from before pregnancy until a mean of 9 months postpartum. Compared with 75 healthy age-matched controls without plans for pregnancy, the 92 women who conceived lost significant bone density at the lumbar spine (1.8 ± 0.5%), total hip (3.2 ± 0.5%), whole body (2.4 ± 0.3%), and ultradistal forearm (4.2 ± 0.7%). Eight women had miscarriages during pregnancy. After parturition, women continued to lose bone density. Women who breastfed for less than 9 months had bone density similar to controls at 9 months, whereas women who continued breastfeeding had further bone loss at their lumbar spine and hip. With continued breastfeeding, sites rich in trabecular bone tended to increase in bone density, whereas cortical sites continued to lose bone density. At 19 months, bone density was the same in all subjects as at baseline. Although the pregnant women had higher daily calcium and vitamin D intakes compared with controls, calcium and vitamin D intake was not associated with changes in bone density. Fat and lean mass increased during pregnancy by 19 ± 22% and 5 ± 6%, respectively. Changes in lean mass quickly returned to baseline after parturition, whereas changes in fat mass differed according to whether women continued breastfeeding or not, with a slower decrease in women who continued breastfeeding. However, the changes in body composition did not explain the changes in bone density seen. The study concluded that pregnancy and breastfeeding caused reversible bone loss at all sites, but that bone loss returned to baseline by 19 months postpartum regardless of the length of breastfeeding.

This is the largest longitudinal study assessing bone density and body composition changes that occur in a group of healthy women from prepregnancy to 9 months postpartum. The findings confirm that a small amount of bone loss occurs during pregnancy at all skeletal sites, and that bone loss continues postpartum as long as breastfeeding continues. Women who breastfed for less than 9 months recovered their baseline bone density by 9 months, whereas women who breastfed for longer had continued bone loss at their lumbar spine and hip. Long-term breastfeeding seemed to cause continued bone loss at cortical sites and regain of bone density at trabecular sites. Regardless of the duration of breast-feeding, women regained their baseline bone density at all sites by 19 months. During pregnancy, body composition changes included increased fat and lean mass, with slower loss of fat mass with continued breastfeeding.

B. L. Clarke, MD

References

1. Black AJ, Topping J, Durham B, Farquharson RG, Fraser WD. A detailed assessment of alterations in bone turnover, calcium homeostasis, and bone density in normal pregnancy. *J Bone Miner Res.* 2000;15:557-563.
2. Gallacher SJ, Fraser WD, Owens OJ, et al. Changes in calciotrophic hormones and biochemical markers of bone turnover in normal human pregnancy. *Eur J Endocrinol.* 1994;131:369-374.
3. Cross NA, Hillman LS, Allen SH, Krause GF, Vieira NE. Calcium homeostasis and bone metabolism during pregnancy, lactation, and postweaning: a longitudinal study. *Am J Clin Nutr.* 1995;61:514-523.
4. Ritchie LD, Fung EB, Halloran BP, et al. A longitudinal study of calcium homeostasis during human pregnancy and lactation and after resumption of menses. *Am J Clin Nutr.* 1998;67:693-701.
5. López JM, González G, Reyes V, Campino C, Díaz S. Bone turnover and density in healthy women during breastfeeding and after weaning. *Osteoporos Int.* 1996;6:153-159.
6. Karlsson C, Obrant KJ, Karlsson M. Pregnancy and lactation confer reversible bone loss in humans. *Osteoporos Int.* 2001;12:828-834.
7. Sohlström A, Forsum E. Changes in adipose tissue volume and distribution during reproduction in Swedish women as assessed by magnetic resonance imaging. *Am J Clin Nutr.* 1995;61:287-295.
8. Butte NF, Hopkinson JM. Body composition changes during lactation are highly variable among women. *J Nutr.* 1998;128:381S-385S.

Current Issues in Osteoporosis Therapy

Effect of Alendronate for Reducing Fracture by FRAX Score and Femoral Neck Bone Mineral Density: The Fracture Intervention Trial

Donaldson MG, Palermo L, Ensrud KE, et al (California Pacific Med Res Inst, San Francisco; Univ of California, San Francisco; Univ of Minnesota, Minneapolis; et al)

J Bone Miner Res 27:1804-1810, 2012

The WHO Fracture Risk Assessment Tool (FRAX; http://www.shef.ac.uk/FRAX) estimates the 10-year probability of major osteoporotic fracture. Clodronate and bazedoxifene reduced nonvertebral and clinical fracture more effectively on a relative scale in women with higher FRAX scores. We used data from the Fracture Intervention Trial (FIT) to evaluate the interaction between FRAX score and treatment with alendronate. We combined the Clinical Fracture (CF) arm and Vertebral Fracture (VF) arm of FIT. The CF and VF arm of FIT randomized 4432 and 2027 women, respectively, to placebo or alendronate for 4 and 3 years, respectively. FRAX risk factors were assessed at baseline. FRAX scores were calculated by WHO. We used Poisson regression models to assess the interaction between alendronate and FRAX score on the risk of nonvertebral, clinical, major osteoporotic, and radiographic vertebral fractures. Overall, alendronate significantly reduced the risk of nonvertebral fracture (incidence rate ratio [IRR] 0.86; 95% confidence interval [CI], 0.75–0.99), but the effect was greater for femoral neck (FN) bone mineral density (BMD) T-score $\leq$−2.5 (IRR 0.76; 95% CI, 0.62–0.93) than for FN T-score >−2.5 (IRR 0.96; 95% CI, 0.80–1.16) ($p = 0.02$, interaction between alendronate and FN BMD). However, there was no evidence of an interaction between alendronate and FRAX score with FN BMD for risk of nonvertebral fracture (interaction $p = 0.61$). The absolute benefit of alendronate was greatest among women with highest FRAX scores. Results were similar for clinical fractures, major osteoporotic fractures, and radiographic vertebral fractures and whether or not FRAX scores included FN BMD. Among this cohort of women with low bone mass there was no significant interaction between FRAX score and alendronate for nonvertebral, clinical or major osteoporotic fractures, or radiographic vertebral fractures. These results suggest that the effect of alendronate on a relative scale does not vary by FRAX score. A randomized controlled trial testing the effect of antifracture agents among women with high FRAX score but without osteoporosis is warranted.

▶ Four recent studies have performed post hoc analyses of placebo-controlled, randomized clinical trials to evaluate for an interaction between 10-year probability of fracture by Fracture Risk Assessment Tool (FRAX) and hip fracture reduction resulting from treatment with the pharmacological agent.[1,2] For clodronate[3] and bazedoxifene,[4] the studies demonstrated that higher baseline fracture risk was associated with greater reduction in clinical fractures. However, for raloxifene[5] and strontium ranelate,[6] the studies did not show an interaction. Alendronate has been reported to reduce fractures in women with postmenopausal osteoporosis but not in women with femoral neck bone mineral density (BMD) T scores between −1.6 and −2.5 who have not had a previous spine or hip fracture.[7]

This study evaluated the interaction between the FRAX score and treatment with alendronate, combining the data from the Clinical Fracture and Vertebral Fracture arms of FRAX. These studies randomized 4432 and 2027 women to placebo or alendronate for 4 or 3 years, respectively. This study showed that alendronate significantly reduced the risk of nonvertebral fractures, with the effect greater if femoral neck BMD was less than or equal to −2.5 than if femoral neck BMD was greater than −2.5. However, no interaction between alendronate and FRAX score with femoral neck BMD was seen for risk of nonvertebral fracture. The absolute benefit of alendronate was greatest among women with the highest T scores. Similar results were seen with clinical fractures, major osteoporotic fractures, radiographic fractures, and whether or not FRAX scores included femoral neck BMD. There was no significant interaction between alendronate and FRAX scores for nonvertebral fractures, clinical fractures, major osteoporotic fractures, or radiographic vertebral fractures. The study concluded that the effect of alendronate on a relative scale does not vary by FRAX score. In light of these findings, a randomized, controlled trial evaluating the effect of antifracture agents in postmenopausal women with high FRAX scores but without osteoporosis was recommended.

It is widely acknowledged that the World Health Organization FRAX algorithm predicts hip or major osteoporotic fractures in patients with osteopenia. One of the main purposes of FRAX is to identify those at highest risk of fracture. The clodronate and bazedoxifene analyses mentioned earlier showed that FRAX was able to identify subgroups of patients that had the greatest reduction in relative risk of fracture with treatment. However, this study did not find similar results, indicating that benefit from alendronate did not depend on baseline FRAX scores. The reasons for this lack of association are unclear, and a randomized, controlled trial evaluating alendronate in postmenopausal women with high FRAX scores but not osteoporosis will be required to sort these issues out.

B. L. Clarke, MD

References

1. Kanis JA, Oden A, Johnell O, et al. The use of clinical risk factors enhances the performance of BMD in the prediction of hip and osteoporotic fractures in men and women. *Osteoporos Int.* 2007;18:1033-1046.
2. Kanis JA, Johnell O, Oden A, Johansson H, McCloskey E. FRAX and the assessment of fracture probability in men and women from the UK. *Osteoporos Int.* 2008;19:385-397.
3. McCloskey EV, Johansson H, Oden A, et al. Ten-year fracture probability identifies women who will benefit from clodronate therapy — additional results from a double-blind, placebo controlled randomized study. *Osteoporos Int.* 2009;20: 811-817.
4. Kanis JA, Johansson H, Oden A, McCloskey EV. A meta-analysis of the efficacy of raloxifene on all clinical and vertebral fractures and its dependency on FRAX. *Bone.* 2010;47:729-735.
5. Kanis JA, Johansson H, Oden A, McCloskey EV. Bazedoxifene reduces vertebral and clinical fractures in postmenopausal women at high risk assessed with FRAX. *Bone.* 2009;44:1049-1054.
6. Kanis JA, Johansson H, Oden A, McCloskey EV. A meta-analysis of the effect of strontium ranelate on the risk of vertebral and non-vertebral fracture in postmenopausal osteoporosis and the interaction with FRAX. *Osteoporos Int.* 2011;22: 2347-2355.
7. Cummings SR, Black DM, Thompson DE, et al. Effect of alendronate on risk of fracture in women with low bone density but without vertebral fractures: results from the Fracture Intervention Trial. *JAMA.* 1998;280:2077-2082.

Oral bisphosphonates reduce the risk of clinical fractures in glucocorticoid-induced osteoporosis in clinical practice
Thomas T, Horlait S, Ringe JD, et al (Univ Hosp of Saint-Etienne, Cedex 2, France; Warner Chilcott, Paris, France; Univ of Cologne, Germany)
Osteoporos Int 24:263-269, 2013

This study aims to estimate bisphosphonate effectiveness by comparing fracture incidence over time on therapy in glucocorticoid-induced osteoporosis (GIO). From this observational study, alendronate and risedronate decreased clinical vertebral and nonvertebral fractures over time. The effectiveness of each bisphosphonate is consistent with their efficacies demonstrated on surrogate markers in randomized controlled trials (RCTs).

Introduction.—This study aims to estimate bisphosphonate effectiveness by comparing fracture incidence over time on therapy with fracture incidence during a short period after starting a therapy.

Methods.—The study population was a subgroup of a larger cohort study comprising two cohorts of women aged ≥ 65 years, prescribed with alendronate or risedronate. Within the two study cohorts, 11,007 women were identified as having received glucocorticoids. Within each cohort, the baseline incidence of clinical fractures at nonvertebral and vertebral sites was defined by the initial 3-month period after starting therapy. Relative to these baseline data, we then compared the fracture incidence during the subsequent 12 months on therapy.

Results.—The baseline incidence of clinical nonvertebral and vertebral fractures was similar in the alendronate cohort (5.22 and 5.79/100 person-years, respectively) and in the risedronate cohort (5.51 and 5.68/100 person-years, respectively). Relative to the baseline incidence, fracture incidence was significantly lower in the subsequent 12 months in both cohorts of alendronate (33% lower at nonvertebral sites and 59% at vertebral sites) and risedronate (28% lower at nonvertebral sites and 54% at vertebral sites).

Conclusion.—From this observational study not designed to compare drugs, both alendronate and risedronate decreased clinical vertebral and nonvertebral fractures over time. The reductions observed in fracture incidence, within each cohort, suggest that the effectiveness of each bisphosphonate in clinical practice is consistent with their efficacies demonstrated on surrogate markers in randomized controlled trials.

▶ It has been estimated that 1% of the general population is prescribed long-term glucocorticoid therapy to treat different disease states[1] and that up to 2.5% of adults 70 to 79 years of age require chronic glucocorticoid therapy.[2] Therefore, it is not surprising that glucocorticoid-induced osteoporosis is the most common secondary cause of osteoporosis. Initiation of glucocorticoid therapy for inflammatory disorders causes rapid suppression of bone formation and increased bone resorption as well as alterations in bone and muscle tissues that contribute to increased risk of vertebral and nonvertebral fractures within months of starting therapy. Stopping glucocorticoid therapy leads to gradual partial reversal of increased fracture risk.[2] Cohort studies have not been able to show a safe threshold below which glucocorticoid therapy does not cause increased fracture risk—even doses less than 7.5 mg/day are associated with increased risk.[3] Randomized, controlled trials have shown that bisphosphonates and teriparatide are able to prevent bone loss and reduce markers of bone turnover.[4] Because of low baseline fracture risk and short duration of therapy, none of these trials has shown fracture risk reduction. Post-hoc analysis combining data from 2 risedronate trials in patients taking glucocorticoid therapy for less than 3 months[5] or longer than 6 months[6] demonstrated 70% reduction in fractures.

This observational study evaluated fracture risk in a large administrative database of older women treated clinically with weekly alendronate or risedronate. The study was not designed to compare efficacy or safety of these drugs. Within the study cohort, 11 007 women were identified as having taken glucocorticoid therapy. Baseline clinical vertebral and nonvertebral fractures occurring in these women within the first 3 months of bisphosphonate therapy were identified and compared with fractures occurring over the next 12 months. Baseline clinical vertebral and nonvertebral fractures in the alendronate-treated women occurred at incidence rates of 5.79/100 person-years and 5.22/100 person-years, respectively. For risedronate, the incidence rates were 5.68/100 person-years and 5.51/100 person-years, respectively. Over the next 12 months, alendronate-treated subjects had 59% fewer clinical vertebral fractures and 33% fewer nonvertebral fractures, whereas risedronate-treated subjects had 54% fewer clinical vertebral fractures and 28% fewer nonvertebral fractures. The study concluded that fracture reduction with alendronate and risedronate in clinical practice was similar to fracture reduction seen with these drugs in randomized, controlled trials.

This significant observational study demonstrated that fracture reduction in a large cohort with 2 different weekly bisphosphonates was similar to their efficacies on surrogate markers, including bone mineral density and bone turnover markers, in previous randomized, controlled trials. This is the first large study to demonstrate fracture efficacy of weekly bisphosphonates in glucocorticoid-induced osteoporosis. The study showed reduction not just in vertebral fractures, but also in nonvertebral fractures. Previous randomized, controlled trials had shown nonsignificant reduction in vertebral fractures only. Weaknesses of this study include possible misclassification of fractures from billing code diagnoses without x-ray adjudication to verify occurrence of fractures. It is reassuring that fracture efficacy of alendronate and risedronate appears to be similar in this observational cohort of glucocorticoid-treated women to the efficacy seen in randomized, controlled trials.

B. L. Clarke, MD

References

1. Walsh LJ, Wong CA, Pringle M, Tattersfield AE. Use of oral corticosteroids in the community and the prevention of secondary osteoporosis: a cross sectional study. *BMJ.* 1996;313:344-346.
2. van Staa TP, Leufkens HG, Abenhaim L, Begaud B, Zhang B, Cooper C. Use of oral corticosteroids in the United Kingdom. *QJM.* 2000;93:105-111.
3. Van Staa TP, Leufkens HG, Abenhaim L, Zhang B, Cooper C. Use of oral corticosteroids and risk of fractures. *J Bone Miner Res.* 2000;15:993-1000.
4. Curtis JR, Westfall AO, Allison JJ, et al. Longitudinal patterns in the prevention of osteoporosis in glucocorticoid-treated patients. *Arthritis Rheum.* 2005;52:2485-2494.
5. Cohen S, Levy RM, Keller M, et al. Risedronate therapy prevents corticosteroid-induced bone loss: a twelve-month, multicenter, randomized, double-blind, placebo-controlled, parallel-group study. *Arthritis Rheum.* 1999;42:2309-2318.
6. Reid DM, Hughes RA, Laan RF, et al. Efficacy and safety of daily risedronate in the treatment of corticosteroid-induced osteoporosis in men and women: a randomized trial. European Corticosteroid-Induced Osteoporosis Treatment Study. *J Bone Miner Res.* 2000;15:1006-1013.

A Retrospective Study Evaluating Frequency and Risk Factors of Osteonecrosis of the Jaw in 576 Cancer Patients Receiving Intravenous Bisphosphonates

Thumbigere-Math V, Tu L, Huckabay S, et al (Univ of Minnesota School of Dentistry, Minneapolis)

Am J Clin Oncol 35:386-392, 2012

Objective.—To evaluate the frequency, risk factors, and clinical presentation of bisphosphonate (BP)-related osteonecrosis of the jaw (BRONJ).

Study Design.—We performed a retrospective analysis of 576 patients with cancer treated with intravenous pamidronate and/or zoledronate between January, 2003 and December, 2007 at the University of Minnesota Masonic Cancer Center and Park Nicollet Institute.

Results.—Eighteen of 576 identified patients (3.1%) developed BRONJ including 8 of 190 patients (4.2%) with breast cancer, 6 of 83 patients (7.2%) with multiple myeloma, 2 of 84 patients (2.4%) with prostate cancer, 1 of 76 patients (1.3%) with lung cancer, 1 of 52 patients (1.9%) with renal cell carcinoma, and in none of the 73 patients with other malignancies. Ten patients (59%) developed BRONJ after tooth extraction, whereas 7 (41%) developed it spontaneously (missing data for 1 patient). The mean number of BP infusions (38.1 ± 19.06 infusions vs. 10.5 ± 12.81 infusions; $P < 0.001$) and duration of BP treatment (44.3 ± 24.34 mo vs. 14.6 ± 18.09 mo; $P < 0.001$) were significantly higher in patients with BRONJ compared with patients without BRONJ. Multivariate Cox proportional hazards regression analysis showed that diabetes [hazard ratio (HR) = 3.40; 95% confidence interval (CI), 1.14-10.11; $P = 0.028$], hypothyroidism (HR = 3.59; 95% CI, 1.31-9.83; $P = 0.013$), smoking (HR = 3.44; 95% CI, 1.28-9.26; $P = 0.015$), and higher number of zoledronate infusions (HR = 1.07; 95% CI, 1.03-1.11; $P = 0.001$) significantly increased the risk of developing BRONJ.

Conclusions.—Increased cumulative doses and long-term BP treatment are the most important risk factors for BRONJ development. Type of BP, diabetes, hypothyroidism, smoking, and prior dental extractions may play a role in BRONJ development.

▶ The risk of osteonecrosis of the jaw is very low in patients with osteoporosis, but it is much higher in cancer patients treated with intravenous bisphosphonates. Besides their benefit for reducing osteoporotic fractures because of their antiresorptive effects on osteoclasts,[1] bisphosphonates are used to treat metastatic cancer in the skeleton because of their direct antiproliferative and proapoptotic activities on cancer cells.[2] Bisphosphonates also have been shown to have anti-angiogenesis effects that reduce tumor cell growth.[3] As a consequence of these effects, bisphosphonates have been shown to reduce pathological fractures, bone pain, and skeletal events due to skeletal metastases.[4,5] Most patients who develop osteonecrosis of the jaw in association with bisphosphonate therapy have cancer and have been treated with intravenous bisphosphonates.[6,7]

This retrospective study evaluated 576 cancer patients treated with intravenous pamidronate or zoledronic acid for jaw osteonecrosis at 2 institutions between 2003 and 2007. Most patients (72%) had been treated with zoledronic acid, with 15% having received pamidronate and 13% having received both drugs sequentially. A total of 18 patients (3.1%) developed jaw osteonecrosis, with 8 having breast cancer and 6 having multiple myeloma. Of the others, 2 patients had prostate cancer, 1 had lung cancer, and 1 had renal cell carcinoma. Jaw osteonecrosis developed after tooth extraction in 10 patients, whereas it was spontaneous in the others. Patients with jaw osteonecrosis had received intravenous bisphosphonate therapy for 44.3 ± 24.3 months, whereas the 558 patients not developing jaw osteonecrosis had received intravenous bisphosphonate therapy for 14.6 ± 18.1 months. Patients with jaw osteonecrosis had received 38.1 ± 19.1 infusions, whereas those not developing jaw osteonecrosis had received 10.5 ± 12.8 infusions. Risk factors for jaw osteonecrosis in this cohort included type of bisphosphonate, diabetes, hypothyroidism, smoking, corticosteroid therapy, alcohol, prior dental extractions, and higher number of bisphosphonate infusions. The study concluded that increased cumulative bisphosphonate doses and prolonged bisphosphonate therapy were the most important risk factors associated with jaw osteonecrosis.

This study confirms and extends previous observations regarding osteonecrosis of the jaw in cancer patients. Because the true incidence, etiology, and risk factors that contribute to the pathogenesis of jaw osteonecrosis remain unknown, this study adds significant information. Unlike most previous studies, this study reports findings from a large cohort not restricted to multiple myeloma or breast cancer patients. Overall risk of jaw osteonecrosis was low at 3.1%, but the prevalence was higher at 7.2% in patients with multiple myeloma, and 4.2% in patients with breast cancer. The risk of jaw osteonecrosis was higher in patients receiving zoledronic acid than in those receiving pamidronate. This study identified hypothyroidism as a new risk factor for jaw osteonecrosis. In summary, osteonecrosis of the jaw remains infrequent in cancer patients, but cumulative dose and duration of intravenous bisphosphonate therapy, dental extraction, and corticosteroid therapy continue to be strong risk factors for this condition.

B. L. Clarke, MD

References

1. Fleisch H. Bisphosphonates: mechanisms of action. *Endocr Rev.* 1998;19:80-100.
2. Diel IJ, Solomayer EF, Bastert G. Bisphosphonates and the prevention of metastasis: first evidences from preclinical and clinical studies. *Cancer.* 2000;88:3080-3088.
3. Fournier P, Boissier S, Filleur S, et al. Bisphosphonates inhibit angiogenesis in vitro and testosterone-stimulated vascular regrowth in the ventral prostate in castrated rats. *Cancer Res.* 2002;62:6538-6544.
4. Berenson JR, Lichtenstein A, Porter L, et al. Efficacy of pamidronate in reducing skeletal events in patients with advanced multiple myeloma. Myeloma Aredia Study Group. *N Engl J Med.* 1996;334:488-493.
5. Hillner BE, Ingle JN, Chlebowski RT, et al. American Society of Clinical Oncology 2003 update on the role of bisphosphonates and bone health issues in women with breast cancer. *J Clin Oncol.* 2003;21:4042-4057.
6. Woo SB, Hellstein JW, Kalmar JR. Narrative [corrected] review: bisphosphonates and osteonecrosis of the jaws. *Ann Intern Med.* 2006;144:753-761.

7. Hoff AO, Toth BB, Altundag K, et al. Frequency and risk factors associated with osteonecrosis of the jaw in cancer patients treated with intravenous bisphosphonates. *J Bone Miner Res.* 2008;23:826-836.

Inflammatory Eye Reactions in Patients Treated With Bisphosphonates and Other Osteoporosis Medications: Cohort Analysis Using a National Prescription Database

Pazianas M, Clark EM, Eiken PA, et al (Oxford Univ Inst of Musculoskeletal Sciences, UK; Univ of Bristol, UK; Hillerød Hosp, Denmark; et al)
J Bone Miner Res 28:455-463, 2013

Ocular inflammatory reactions have been described in patients on bisphosphonate treatment. We estimated the incidence rate of ocular inflammation at 3 and 12 months in patients treated for osteoporosis using a register-based cohort linked to prescription data (hospitals and private practice) and hospital data. From January 1, 1997 to December 31, 2007, a total of 88,202 patients beginning osteoporosis therapy were identified. Of those patients, 82,404 (93%) began oral bisphosphonates and 5798 (7%) nonbisphosphonates. Within the first year of treatment, 4769 (5.4%) of patients on osteoporosis therapy filled one or more prescriptions for topical eye steroids (TES). TES treatment rates (per 1000 patient-years) in the first year of osteoporosis treatment were 44 (95% confidence interval [CI] 42 to 46) for alendronate, 40 (95% CI 38 to 43) for etidronate, 45 (95% CI 35 to 57) for risedronate, 32 (95% CI 27 to 37) for raloxifene, and 64 (95% CI 49 to 83) for strontium ranelate. After adjustment for age, Charlson index, and the number of comedications, pulmonary disease in men was associated with an increased use of TES (odds ratio [OR] = 1.48; 95% CI 1.17 to 1.86; $p = 0.001$). In women, malignant disease (OR = 1.27; 95% CI 1.02 to 1.60; $p = 0.04$) and pulmonary disease (OR = 1.32; 95% CI 1.07 to 1.62; $p = 0.01$) were significant predictors at 3 months and rheumatic diseases at 12 months (OR = 1.20; 95% CI 1.10 to 1.31; $p < 0.001$). There was no significant difference between the different drug classes (bisphosphonates versus nonbisphosphonates, alendronate versus nonalendronate-bisphosphonates) for risk of ocular inflammation, with age and the number of comedications being the only significant predictors. Hospital-treated uveitis (48 patients, or 0.05%) showed a similar trend. In conclusion, after initiation of treatment for osteoporosis, the risk of inflammatory eye reactions requiring TES is relatively low and not significantly different between bisphosphonate and nonbisphosphonate users. Patients with a rheumatic or pulmonary disease are at increased risk.

▶ Rare case reports, small case series, and the major randomized placebo-controlled trials have reported inflammatory eye reactions, including conjunctivitis, scleritis, episcleritis, uveitis, and keratitis, associated with oral or intravenous bisphosphonate use.[1-4] The first case reports of conjunctivitis occurred with etidronate, and later clodronate, both non–nitrogen-containing bisphosphonates. The majority of reports have linked these rare reactions to nitrogen-containing bisphosphonates, including alendronate, risedronate, ibandronate, pamidronate, and zoledronic acid. Inflammatory eye reactions may also occur because of the underlying disease in patients with rheumatoid arthritis, inflammatory bowel disease, or sarcoidosis. It is not yet clear whether these reactions occur because of the bisphosphonate therapy, or underlying disease, or an interaction between the two, when patients have inflammatory disorders. In other cases without evidence of systemic inflammation, bisphosphonates may be causally associated.

Two very large cohort studies have shown conflicting results regarding the association of bisphosphonates with eye inflammatory disorders. The US Veterans Cohort Study included 5.7 million persons, including 35 252 new bisphosphonate users, 85% of whom were taking alendronate, and 3736 cases of uveitis or scleritis.[5] The prevalence of inflammatory eye reactions was low, and similar rates of uveitis and scleritis were seen in users and nonusers of bisphosphonates. The rate of inflammatory eye reactions in new users at 6 months of therapy was 7.9 new cases per 10 000 persons, with a relative risk of 1.23 (95% CI, 0.85-1.79) compared with veterans not exposed. Nearly half of the veterans with inflammatory eye reactions had systemic disorders associated with inflammation of the uveal tract or sclera. The Canadian Pharmaco-Epidemiological Cohort Study evaluated 934 147 patients, including 10 827 first-time users of bisphosphonates.[6] First-time users had an increased relative risk of uveitis of 1.45 (95% CI, 1.25-1.68) and relative risk of scleritis of 1.51 (95% CI, 1.34-1.68). Adjustment for age, sex, and medical conditions, including inflammatory disorders, did not change the associations found. The number needed to harm was 1100 for uveitis and 370 for scleritis.

This study evaluated 88 202 patients beginning osteoporosis therapy in 2007 in a Danish national register—based cohort linked to prescription and hospital data for ocular inflammation 3 and 12 months after starting therapy. Of these patients, 82 404 (93%) began oral bisphosphonates and 5798 (7%) started non-bisphosphonate therapy. Within the first year of treatment, 4769 (5.4%) also filled 1 or more prescriptions of topical eye steroids, which were used as a surrogate for eye inflammation. Treatment rates with topical eye steroids for alendronate users were 44/1000 person-years, 40/1000 for etidronate, 45 for risedronate, 32 for raloxifene, and 64 for strontium ranelate. Predictors of eye inflammation included pulmonary disease in both men and women, and cancer in women. There was no significant difference between the different drug classes for risk of eye inflammation, with age and number of concomitant medications being the only significant predictors of inflammatory eye reactions. Hospital-treated uveitis in 48 patients (0.05%) showed similar findings. The study concluded that risk of inflammatory eye reactions requiring topical eye steroid treatment is low and not significantly different between patients treated with bisphosphonate or nonbisphosphonates and that patients with underlying rheumatic or pulmonary disease are at increased risk.

These findings are reassuring that the risk of eye inflammatory reactions is low in patients treated with bisphosphonate therapies. In addition, the risk of severe uveitis is very low, at least in Denmark. Nevertheless, subsets of the population of osteoporotic patients may be at increased risk, especially those with rheumatic or pulmonary disorders. Patients at highest risk included those with seronegative rheumatoid arthritis, necrotizing vascular disorders, and Sjogren syndrome, suggesting that underlying inflammatory disease is the most likely cause for the eye reactions. These findings support those of the US Veterans Cohort Study but differ from the findings of the Canadian Pharmaco-Epidemiological Cohort Study. Limitations of this observational study include the relatively short study duration of one year and a lack of information regarding patients with uveitis or other eye inflammatory reactions managed in general practice or by office-based ophthalmologists. Most eye inflammatory reactions have been reported to occur within 1 year of starting bisphosphonate therapy, and a lack of long-term persistence with therapy makes longer-term studies of this issue difficult.

B. L. Clarke, MD

References

1. Siris ES. Bisphosphonates and iritis. *Lancet.* 1993;341:436-437.
2. Ghose K, Waterworth R, Trolove P, Highton J. Uveitis associated with pamidronate. *Aust N Z J Med.* 1994;24:320.
3. Mbekeani JN, Slamovits TL, Schwartz BH, Sauer HL. Ocular inflammation associated with alendronate therapy. *Arch Ophthalmol.* 1999;117:837-838.
4. Black DM, Delmas PD, Eastell R, et al; HORIZON Pivotal Fracture Trial. Once-yearly zoledronic acid for treatment of postmenopausal osteoporosis. *N Engl J Med.* 2007;356:1809-1822.
5. French DD, Margo CE. Postmarketing surveillance rates of uveitis and scleritis with bisphosphonates among a national veteran cohort. *Retina.* 2008;28:889-893.
6. Etminan M, Forooghian F, Maberley D. Inflammatory ocular adverse events with the use of oral bisphosphonates: a retrospective cohort study. *CMAJ.* 2012;184: E431-434.

Effect of denosumab on bone mineral density and biochemical markers of bone turnover: 8-year results of a phase 2 clinical trial
McClung MR, Lewiecki EM, Geller ML, et al (Oregon Osteoporosis Ctr, Portland; New Mexico Clinical Res & Osteoporosis Ctr, Albuquerque; Amgen Inc, Thousand Oaks, CA; et al)
Osteoporos Int 24:227-235, 2013

In a phase 2 study, continued denosumab treatment for up to 8 years was associated with continued gains in bone mineral density and persistent reductions in bone turnover markers. Denosumab treatment was well tolerated throughout the 8-year study.

Introduction.—The purpose of this study is to present the effects of 8 years of continued denosumab treatment on bone mineral density (BMD) and bone turnover markers (BTM) from a phase 2 study.

Methods.—In the 4-year parent study, postmenopausal women with low BMD were randomized to receive placebo, alendronate, or denosumab. After 2 years, subjects were reallocated to continue, discontinue, or discontinue and reinitiate denosumab; discontinue alendronate; or maintain placebo for two more years. The parent study was then extended for 4 years where all subjects received denosumab.

Results.—Of the 262 subjects who completed the parent study, 200 enrolled in the extension, and of these, 138 completed the extension. For the subjects who received 8 years of continued denosumab treatment, BMD at the lumbar spine ($N = 88$) and total hip ($N = 87$) increased by 16.5 and 6.8 %, respectively, compared with their parent study baseline, and by 5.7 and 1.8 %, respectively, compared with their extension study baseline. For the 12 subjects in the original placebo group, 4 years of denosumab resulted in BMD gains comparable with those observed during the 4 years of denosumab in the parent study. Reductions in BTM were sustained over the course of continued denosumab treatment. Reductions also were observed when the placebo group transitioned to denosumab. Adverse event profile was consistent with previous reports and an aging cohort.

Conclusion.—Continued denosumab treatment for 8 years was associated with progressive gains in BMD, persistent reductions in BTM, and was well tolerated.

▶ The RANK/RANK ligand pathway is the major modulator of osteoclast activity.[1-3] Increased production of RANK ligand leads to upregulation of osteoclast recruitment and activation, resulting in increased bone remodeling and bone loss in postmenopausal women.[4,5] Denosumab is a fully human immunoglobulin G2 monoclonal antibody that binds to RANK ligand with very high specificity.[6] Denosumab, thereby, functions as a very potent antiresorptive agent, reducing the formation, activity, and survival of osteoclasts.[7,8] Denosumab has previously been shown to reduce bone loss[9] and prevent fractures.[10]

This study presents the 4-year extension data of the 4-year phase 2 dose-ranging study for denosumab in postmenopausal women. Denosumab treatment over 8 years resulted in continued gains in bone mineral density and persistent decreases in markers of bone turnover and was well tolerated. Of 262 subjects who enrolled in the initial phase 2 study, 200 enrolled in the extension study and 138 completed the extension study. In those completing the extension study, lumbar spine bone density increased by 16.5% and total hip bone density by 6.8% from baseline, and they increased by 5.7% and 1.8%, respectively, from the beginning of the extension study. Markers of bone turnover continued to be reduced over continued denosumab treatment. Adverse events were consistent with previous reports and an aging cohort, without increased risk of rare infections. The study concluded that denosumab treatment continued for 8 years was associated with continued increases in bone mineral density and reductions in markers of bone turnover and was well tolerated.

These findings indicate that denosumab continues to stimulate increases in lumbar spine and total hip bone mineral density over prolonged use, different in magnitude from most other antiresorptive agents that result in plateauing of effect after 3 to 4 years. Bone density at the 1/3 distal radius did not continue to increase, however. This study was not powered to demonstrate fracture reduction, however, so it is not yet clear that the continued increases in bone mineral density seen result in reduced vertebral and hip fractures. Findings from the long-term extension of the FREEDOM Trial over 7 and 10 years are anticipated to help clarify this issue.[11] Although this small trial is unable to fully assess the safety of denosumab in postmenopausal women, the fact that adverse events, serious adverse events, and deaths were similar in years 5 to 8 of treatment to what was seen in years 1 to 4 of treatment suggests that longer-term treatment does not increase the risk of rare infections, skin disorders, or other side effects. The study found no increased risk of jaw osteonecrosis, atypical femur fractures, or impaired fracture healing, and no evidence of immune system impairment. This study supports the continued efficacy and safety of long-term denosumab use.

B. L. Clarke, MD

References

1. Lacey DL, Timms E, Tan HL, et al. Osteoprotegerin ligand is a cytokine that regulates osteoclast differentiation and activation. *Cell.* 1998;93:165-176.
2. Yasuda H, Shima N, Nakagawa N, et al. Osteoclast differentiation factor is a ligand for osteoprotegerin/osteoclastogenesis-inhibitory factor and is identical to TRANCE/RANKL. *Proc Natl Acad Sci U S A.* 1998;95:3597-3602.
3. Boyle WJ, Simonet WS, Lacey DL. Osteoclast differentiation and activation. *Nature.* 2003;423:337-342.
4. D'Amelio P, Grimaldi A, Di Bella S, et al. Estrogen deficiency increases osteoclastogenesis up-regulating T cells activity: a key mechanism in osteoporosis. *Bone.* 2008;43:92-100.
5. Eghbali-Fatourechi G, Khosla S, Sanyal A, et al. Role of RANK ligand in mediating increased bone resorption in early postmenopausal women. *J Clin Invest.* 2003;111:1221-1230.
6. Kosteniuk PJ, Nguyen HQ, McCabe, et al. Denosumab, a fully human monoclonal antibody to RANKL, inhibits bone resorption and increases BMD in knock-in mice that express chimeric (murine/human) RANKL. *J Bone Miner Res.* 2009;24:182-195.
7. Lacey DL, Tan HL, Lu J, et al. Osteoprotegerin ligand modulates murine osteoclast survival in vitro and in vivo. *Am J Pathol.* 2000;157:435-448.
8. Udagawa N, Takahashi N, Yasuda H, et al. Osteoprotegerin produced by osteoblasts is an important regulator in osteoclast development and function. *Endocrinology.* 2000;141:3478-3484.
9. McClung MR, Lewiecki EM, Cohen SB, et al. Denosumab in postmenopausal women with low bone mineral density. *N Engl J Med.* 2006;354:821-831.
10. Cummings SR, San Martin J, McClung MR, et al. Denosumab for the prevention of fractures in postmenopausal women with osteoporosis. *N Engl J Med.* 2009; 361:756-765.
11. Papapoulos S, Chapurlat R, Libanati C, et al. Five years of denosumab exposure i women with postmenopausal osteoporosis: results from the first two years of the FREEDOM extension. *J Bone Miner Res.* 2011;27:694-701.

Skeletal Histomorphometry in Subjects on Teriparatide or Zoledronic Acid Therapy (SHOTZ) Study: A Randomized Controlled Trial
Dempster DW, Zhou H, Recker RR, et al (Helen Hayes Hosp, West Haverstraw, NY; Creighton Univ, Omaha, Nebraska; et al)
J Clin Endocrinol Metab 97:2799-2808, 2012

Context.—Recent studies on the mechanism of action (MOA) of bone-active drugs have rekindled interest in how to present and interpret dynamic histomorphometric parameters of bone remodeling.

Objective.—We compared the effects of an established anabolic agent, teriparatide (TPTD), with those of a prototypical antiresorptive agent, zoledronic acid (ZOL).

Design.—This was a 12-month, randomized, double-blind, active-comparator controlled, cross-sectional biopsy study.

Setting.—The study was conducted at 12 U.S. and Canadian centers.

Subjects.—Healthy postmenopausal women with osteoporosis participated in the study.

Interventions.—Subjects received TPTD 20 µg once daily by sc injection (n = 34) or ZOL 5 mg by iv infusion at baseline (n = 35).

Main Outcome Measures.—The primary end point was mineralizing surface/bone surface (MS/BS), a dynamic measure of bone formation, at month 6. A standard panel of dynamic and static histomorphometric indices was also assessed. When specimens with missing labels were encountered, several methods were used to calculate mineral apposition rate (MAR). Serum markers of bone turnover were also measured.

Results.—Among 58 subjects with evaluable biopsies (TPTD = 28; ZOL = 30), MS/BS was significantly higher in the TPTD group (median: 5.60 vs. 0.16%, $P < 0.001$). Other bone formation indices, including MAR, were also higher in the TPTD group ($P < 0.05$). TPTD significantly increased procollagen type 1 N-terminal propeptide (PINP) at months 1, 3, 6, and 12 and carboxyterminal cross-linking telopeptide of collagen type 1 (CTX) from months 3 to 12. ZOL significantly decreased PINP and CTX below baseline at all time points.

Conclusions.—TPTD and ZOL possess fundamentally different mechanisms of action with opposite effects on bone formation based on this analysis of both histomorphometric data and serum markers of bone formation and resorption. An important mechanistic difference was a substantially higher MS/BS in the TPTD group. Overall, these results define the dynamic histomorphometric characteristics of anabolic activity relative to antiresorptive activity after treatment with these two drugs.

▶ Tetracycline-labeled bone histomorphometry allows assessment of bone remodeling at the tissue level.[1,2] This technique permits drugs used to treat osteoporosis to be classified as antiresorptive (anticatabolic) or anabolic. Antiresorptive medications primarily prevent osteoclast-mediated bone resorption, slowing bone loss, filling in the remodeling space, and permitting more complete secondary mineralization.[3] Anabolic agents primarily stimulate osteoblast-mediated new bone formation, leading to positive bone balance within each bone remodeling unit and to increased bone mineral density.[4] The mechanism of action of osteoporosis drugs is characterized by several dynamic parameters of bone formation, including mineralizing surface/bone surface, mineral apposition rate, and bone formation rate.[5] Determination of mineral apposition rate has been challenging in studies of potent antiresorptive drugs that reduce bone turnover, such as bisphosphonates[6,7] or denosumab.[8]

This study compared the histomorphometric profile of teriparatide and zoledronic acid using a standard panel of static and dynamic parameters in 34 patients randomized to treatment with teriparatide 20 mcg subcutaneously each day for 1 year, and 35 patients treated with zoledronic acid 5 mg intravenously once a year. Among 58 patients with evaluable biopsies, mineralizing surface/bone surface was significantly increased in the teriparatide group, with other bone formation indices, including mineral apposition rate, also increased, compared with the zoledronic acid group. Markers of bone turnover were significantly increased by teriparatide and decreased by zoledronic acid. The study concluded that teriparatide and zoledronic acid prevent bone loss and fractures by very different mechanisms, with opposite effects on bone formation, and significantly increased mineralizing surface with teriparatide.

These findings confirm previously published studies comparing the effect of the 2 study drugs to placebo. There is very little overlap in the effect of these drugs on dynamic histomorphometric indices, with the clearest separation in mineralizing surface/bone surface, bone formation rate/bone surface, and total formation period. However, both drugs caused similar changes in mineral apposition rate, indicating that this is not a good parameter to distinguish antiresorptive from anabolic agents. Static histomorphometric indices for the 2 drugs differed only in magnitude rather than direction of change. The study emphasizes the importance of reporting full histomorphometric indices when distinguishing the mechanism of action of new osteoporosis drugs as well as number of samples with double, single, or no labels, and the method used to calculate the mineral apposition rate, particularly in conditions of low bone turnover. These requirements will be important when analyzing new drugs under development, especially because some drugs may be formation-sparing or mixed antiresorptive/anabolic agents.

B. L. Clarke, MD

References

1. Parfitt AM, Drezner MK, Glorieux FH, et al. Bone histomorphometry: standardization of nomenclature, symbols, and units. Report of the ASBMR Histomorphometry Nomenclature Committee. *J Bone Miner Res.* 1987;2:595-610.
2. Dempster DW, Compston JE, Drezner MK, et al. Standardized nomenclature, symbols, and units for bone histomorphometry: a 2012 update of the report of the ASBMR Histomorphometry Nomenclature Committee. *J Bone Miner Res.* 2013;28:2-17.
3. Hernandez CJ, Beaupré GS, Marcus R, Carter DR. A theoretical analysis of the contributions of remodeling space, mineralization, and bone balance to changes in bone mineral density during alendronate treatment. *Bone.* 2001;29:511-516.
4. Riggs BL, Parfitt AM. Drugs used to treat osteoporosis: the critical need for a uniform nomenclature based on their action on bone remodeling. *J Bone Miner Res.* 2005;20:177-184.

5. Recker RR, Kimmel DB, Dempster D, Weinstein RS, Wronski TJ, Burr DB. Issues in modern bone histomorphometry. *Bone*. 2011;49:955-964.
6. Eriksen EF, Melsen F, Sod E, Barton I, Chines A. Effects of long-term risedronate on bone quality and bone turnover in women with postmenopausal osteoporosis. *Bone*. 2002;31:620-625.
7. Recker RR, Delmas PD, Halse J, et al. Effects of intravenous zoledronic acid once yearly on bone remodeling and bone structure. *J Bone Miner Res*. 2008;23:6-16.
8. Reid IR, Miller PD, Brown JP, et al. Effects of denosumab on bone histomorphometry: the FREEDOM and STAND studies. *J Bone Miner Res*. 2010;25:2256-2265.

Predictive Value of FRAX for Fracture in Obese Older Women

Premaor M, for the Study of Osteoporotic Fractures (SOF) Research Group (Federal Univ of Santa Maria, Brazil; et al)

J Bone Miner Res 28:188-195, 2013

Recent studies indicate that obesity is not protective against fracture in postmenopausal women and increases the risk of fracture at some sites. Risk factors for fracture in obese women may differ from those in the nonobese. We aimed to compare the ability of FRAX with and without bone mineral density (BMD) to predict fractures in obese and nonobese older postmenopausal women who were participants in the Study of Osteoporotic Fractures. Data for FRAX clinical risk factors and femoral neck BMD were available in 6049 women, of whom 18.5% were obese. Hip fractures, major osteoporotic fractures, and any clinical fractures were ascertained during a mean follow-up period of 9.03 years. Receiving operator curve (ROC) analysis, model calibration, and decision curve analysis were used to compare fracture prediction in obese and nonobese women. ROC analysis revealed no significant differences between obese and nonobese women in fracture prediction by FRAX, with or without BMD. Predicted hip fracture risk was lower than observed risk in both groups of women, particularly when FRAX+BMD was used, but there was good calibration for FRAX+BMD in prediction of major osteoporotic fracture in both groups. Decision curve analysis demonstrated that both FRAX models were useful for hip fracture prediction in obese and nonobese women for threshold 10-year fracture probabilities in the range of 4% to 10%, although in obese women FRAX+BMD was superior to FRAX alone. For major osteoporotic fracture, both FRAX models were useful in both groups of women for threshold probabilities in the range of 10% to 30%. For all clinical fractures, the FRAX models were not useful at threshold probabilities below 30%. We conclude that FRAX is of value in predicting hip and major osteoporotic fractures in obese postmenopausal women, particularly when used with BMD.

▶ Obesity was previously presumed to be protective against bone loss and fractures. More recent studies have shown that obesity may not reduce the risk of fractures.[1,2] Risk factors for fracture may differ between obese and nonobese women.

Fractures in obese women are more common in the leg, ankle, and humerus, and less common in the hip, wrist, and pelvis.[3,4]

The World Health Organization fracture risk assessment tool (FRAX) is a web-based computer algorithm used to predict 10-year absolute risk of hip fracture and major osteoporotic fractures, including hip, clinical vertebral, wrist, and humerus fractures.[5,6] FRAX uses clinical risk factors with or without femoral neck bone mineral density (BMD) to predict absolute fracture risk. The clinical risk factors included in the algorithm include age, body mass index (BMI), previous fracture, parental history of hip fracture, glucocorticoid therapy, smoking, alcohol intake, rheumatoid arthritis, and secondary causes of osteoporosis. FRAX has been shown to have moderately good discrimination between fracture and nonfracture cases and reasonably close agreement between predicted and observed fracture frequency, particularly for hip fracture.[7,8] However, FRAX has not yet been shown to be useful in obese women. Higher BMD, BMI, and greater frequency of falls in obese women with fracture might affect its performance. In addition, the prevalence of obesity in the populations used to develop FRAX was 18.3%, whereas the current prevalence of obesity in the United States is 34% and it is 23% in Europe.[9,10]

This study evaluated the ability of FRAX with or without femoral neck BMD to predict fractures in obese and nonobese older postmenopausal women who participated in the Study of Osteoporotic Fractures. In this analysis, 6049 women were identified as having the required clinical risk factors and femoral neck BMD necessary for use of FRAX. Of these women, 18.5% were obese. Hip fractures, major osteoporotic fractures, and any clinical fractures were collected over mean follow-up of 9.03 years. Receiver operator curve analysis showed no difference between obese and nonobese women in fracture prediction by FRAX, with or without femoral neck BMD. Predicted hip fracture risk was lower than observed risk in both obese and nonobese women, especially when clinical risk factors and femoral neck BMD were both used, whereas predicted major osteoporotic fracture risk and observed risk were in close agreement in both groups. For hip fracture, FRAX with and without BMD were both useful in obese and nonobese women for threshold 10-year fracture probabilities in the range of 4% to 10%, although in obese women, FRAX plus BMD was better than FRAX alone. For major osteoporotic fractures, both FRAX models were useful in obese and nonobese women for threshold 10-year fracture probabilities in the range of 10% to 30%. For all clinical fractures, FRAX with or without BMD was not useful unless 10-year probability thresholds were greater than 30%. The study concluded that FRAX is useful in predicting hip and major osteoporotic fractures in obese postmenopausal women, especially when BMD is included.

These findings indicate that the FRAX fracture risk algorithm performs well in obese women. The results indicate that fracture risk estimates obtained in obese women using clinical risk factors plus BMD are better than fracture risk estimates obtained with clinical risk factors alone. It is not necessary to apply a correction factor to the risk estimate obtained because obese women have higher hip BMD and BMI than nonobese women. The positive and negative predictive values for FRAX with or without BMD are very similar between obese and non-obese women. The lower treatment rates for osteoporosis in obese women may reflect the belief that their higher BMD protects them from fractures. Clinical trials are needed to rigorously demonstrate that postmenopausal osteoporosis therapies work as well in obese women at increased risk of fracture as they do in nonobese women.

B. L. Clarke, MD

References

1. Premaor MO, Pilbrow L, Tonkin C, Parker RA, Compston J. Obesity and fractures in postmenopausal women. *J Bone Miner Res.* 2010;25:292-297.
2. Compston JE, Watts NB, Chapurlat R, et al; GLOW Investigators. Obesity is not protective against fracture in postmenopausal women: GLOW. *Am J Med.* 2011; 124:1043-1050.
3. Gnudi S, Sitta E, Lisi L. Relationship of body mass index with main limb fragility fractures in postmenopausal women. *J Bone Miner Metab.* 2009;27:479-484.
4. Prieto-Alhambra D, Premaor MO, Fina Avilés F, et al. The association between fracture and obesity is site-dependent: a population-based study in postmenopausal women. *J Bone Miner Res.* 2012;27:294-300.
5. Kanis JA, on behalf of the World Health Organization Scientific Group. *Assessment of Osteoporosis at the Primary Care Healthcare Level. Technical Report.* Sheffield, UK: Who Collaborating Centre for Metabolic Bone Disease. University of Sheffield; 2008; http://www.shef.ac.uk/FRAX.
6. Kanis JA, Johnell O, Oden A, Johansson H, McCloskey E. FRAX and the assessment of fracture probability in men and women from the UK. *Osteoporos Int.* 2008;19:385-397.
7. Donaldson MG, Palermo L, Schousboe JT, Ensrud KE, Hochberg MC, Cummings SR. FRAX and risk of vertebral fractures: the fracture intervention trial. *J Bone Miner Res.* 2009;24:1793-1799.
8. Ensrud KE, Lui LY, Taylor BC, et al; Study of Osteoporotic Fractures Research Group. A comparison of prediction models for fractures in older women: is more better? *Arch Intern Med.* 2009;169:2087-2094.
9. Flegal KM, Carroll MD, Ogden CL, Curtin LR. Prevalence and trends in obesity among US adults, 1999–2008. *JAMA.* 2010;303:235-241.
10. Finucane MM, Stevens GA, Cowan MJ, et al. National, regional, and global trends in body-mass index since 1980: systematic analysis of health examination surveys and epidemiological studies with 960 country-years and 9·1 million participants. *Lancet.* 2011;377:557-567.

Effectiveness of Teriparatide in Women Over 75 Years of Age with Severe Osteoporosis: 36-Month Results from the European Forsteo Observational Study (EFOS)

Walsh JB, Lems WF, Karras D, et al (St James's Hosp and Trinity College, Dublin, Ireland; VU Univ Hosp, Amsterdam, The Netherlands; Veterans Administration Hosp, Athens, Greece; et al)
Calcif Tissue Int 90:373-383, 2012

This predefined analysis of the European Forsteo Observational Study (EFOS) aimed to describe clinical fracture incidence, back pain, and health-related quality of life (HRQoL) during 18 months of teriparatide treatment and 18 months post-teriparatide in the subgroup of 589 postmenopausal women with osteoporosis aged ≥ 75 years. Data on clinical fractures, back pain (visual analogue scale, VAS), and HRQoL (EQ-5D) were collected over 36 months. Fracture data were summarized in 6-month intervals and analyzed using logistic regression with repeated measures. A repeated-measures model analyzed changes from baseline in back pain VAS and EQ-VAS. During the 36-month observation period, 87 (14.8 %) women aged ≥ 75 years sustained a total of 111 new fractures: 37 (33.3%) vertebral fractures and 74 (66.7%) nonvertebral fractures. Adjusted odds of fracture was decreased by 80 % in the 30 to <36—month interval compared with the first 6-month interval ($P < 0.009$). Although the older subgroup had higher back pain scores and poorer HRQoL at baseline than the younger subgroup, both age groups showed significant reductions in back pain and improvements in HRQoL postbaseline. In conclusion, women aged ≥ 75 years with severe postmenopausal osteoporosis treated with teriparatide in normal clinical practice showed a reduced clinical fracture incidence by 30 months compared with baseline. An improvement in HRQoL and, possibly, an early and significant reduction in back pain were also observed, which lasted for at least 18 months after teriparatide discontinuation when patients were taking other osteoporosis medication. The results should be interpreted in the context of an uncontrolled observational study.

▶ Age is a significant predictor of osteoporosis and fractures.[1,2] The risk of osteoporotic fracture is greater in older postmenopausal women than younger women, even when the bone mineral density (BMD) is the same.[3] The population of women older than 80 years of age is steadily increasing,[4] and it is currently estimated that this group contributes 30% of all fragility fractures and more than 60% of nonvertebral fractures.[5]

Evidence that osteoporosis drugs prevent fractures in postmenopausal women older than 80 years of age is limited. Most of this evidence has come from subgroup analyses of randomized controlled trials. Teriparatide was previously shown to reduce the absolute risk of new vertebral fractures by 9.9% (relative risk reduction of 65%), compared with calcium and vitamin D supplementation, in a subgroup of women 75 years of age or older followed in a large clinical trial for 19 months.[6]

This predefined analysis evaluated fracture outcomes, back pain, and health-related quality of life in postmenopausal women 75 years of age or older included in the European Forsteo Observational Study. Forsteo is the commercial name for teriparatide in Europe, which is called Forteo in the United States. A total of 589 postmenopausal women aged 75 or older in this observational clinical practice study were treated with teriparatide for 18 months, and then followed for 18 months on other osteoporosis treatment, and compared with a larger cohort of women less than 75 years of age in the study. During the 36-month observation period, 14.8% of the women 75 years of age or older had new clinical fractures, with one-third being vertebral fractures and the other two-thirds nonvertebral fractures. Among women 75 years of age or older, teriparatide reduced all clinical fractures by 80% in the 30- to 36-month interval compared with the first 6-month interval. Women in this older subgroup had higher back pain scores and poorer health-related quality of life at baseline as expected, but teriparatide treatment reduced back pain and improved health-related quality of life over the 36 months of follow-up. The study concluded that teriparatide reduced clinical fractures and improved back pain and health-related quality of life in postmenopausal women 75 years of age and older.

These findings provide good evidence that teriparatide treatment for up to 18 months reduced clinical fractures by 30 to 36 months compared with the first 6 months, with an improvement in health-related quality of life and early reduction in back pain symptoms that persisted for 18 months after discontinuation of teriparatide and initiation of other osteoporosis medication. Most women in the study had previously received other potent osteoporosis medication, and most were taking calcium and vitamin D supplementation. These findings indicate that teriparatide prevents fractures in elderly women at high risk of fracture when treated as part of a sequential regimen. The main limitation of this study is that it is a nonrandomized, uncontrolled observational study.

B. L. Clarke, MD

References

1. Albrand G, Munoz F, Sornay-Rendu E, DuBoeuf F, Delmas PD. Independent predictors of all osteoporosis-related fractures in healthy postmenopausal women: the OFELY study. *Bone*. 2003;32:78-85.
2. Finigan J, Greenfield DM, Blumsohn A, et al. Risk factors for vertebral and non-vertebral fracture over 10 years: a population-based study in women. *J Bone Miner Res*. 2008;23:75-85.
3. Siris ES, Brenneman SK, Barrett-Connor E, et al. The effect of age and bone mineral density on the absolute, excess, and relative risk of fracture in postmenopausal women aged 50−99: results from the National Osteoporosis Risk Assessment (NORA). *Osteoporos Int*. 2006;17:565-574.
4. United Nations Department of Economic and Social Affairs, Population Division, World Population Aging. 2007. www.un.org/esa/population/publications/WPA2007/wpp2007.htm. Accessed March 2, 2013.
5. Boonen S. Medical treatment of age-related osteoporosis: present and future. In: Duque G, Kiel DP, eds. *Osteoporosis in Older Persons-Pathophysiology and Therapeutic Approach*. Springer, London: 2009; 137-152.
6. Boonen S, Marin F, Mellstrom D, et al. Safety and efficacy of teriparatide in elderly women with established osteoporosis: bone anabolic therapy from a geriatric perspective. *J Am Geriatr Soc*. 2006;54:782-789.

Novel Osteoporosis Therapies

Six Months of Parathyroid Hormone (1–84) Administered Concurrently *Versus* Sequentially with Monthly Ibandronate Over Two Years: The PTH and Ibandronate Combination Study (PICS) Randomized Trial

Schafer AL, Sellmeyer DE, Palermo L, et al (Univ of California, San Francisco; Johns Hopkins Univ, Baltimore, MD; et al)
J Clin Endocrinol Metab 97:3522-3529, 2012

Context.—PTH therapy improves bone mineral density (BMD) and decreases fractures in postmenopausal osteoporosis, but cost and the burden of daily injections limit its use.

Objective.—We evaluated two novel approaches to the use of 6 months of PTH therapy over 2 yr.

Design, Setting, Participants, and Interventions.—We conducted a randomized, double-blinded trial of two combinations of daily PTH(1–84) and monthly ibandronate in 44 postmenopausal women with low bone mass. Participants received either 6 months of concurrent PTH and ibandronate, followed by 18 months of ibandronate (concurrent) or two sequential courses of 3 months of PTH followed by 9 months of ibandronate (sequential) over 2 yr.

Main Outcome Measures.—Bone turnover markers were measured. Areal and volumetric BMD were assessed by dual-energy x-ray absorptiometry and quantitative computed tomography, respectively.

Results.—Over 2 yr, areal BMD at the spine and hip increased similarly in both groups, with 7.5 and 8.2% increases in spine BMD in the concurrent and sequential arms, respectively (difference −0.6%, 95% confidence interval = −3.4–2.1%). Volumetric BMD also increased similarly between groups. With concurrent therapy, mean N-propeptide of type I collagen increased 75% between baseline and month 1 and then declined. With sequential therapy, the second 3-month PTH course increased N-propeptide of type I collagen markedly (209%), although to a lesser absolute degree than the first.

Conclusions.—Six months of PTH(1–84), used over 2 yr with a bisphosphonate in either of our dosing regimens increased BMD substantially. Short PTH courses may provide the benefits of anabolic osteoporosis therapy with reduced burden for patients.

▶ Parathyroid hormone (PTH) given as PTH 1-34 (teriparatide) or full-length PTH 1-84 stimulates an increase in bone mineral density (BMD) and significantly reduces fractures in women with postmenopausal osteoporosis.[1,2] These anabolic changes occur because PTH improves bone microarchitecture by increasing trabecular connectivity and cortical thickness, resulting in decreased skeletal fragility.[3] Because of the high cost and inconvenience of daily PTH injection therapy over 2 years, alternative protocols to administer PTH either sequentially or in combination are desirable. Previous trials have shown that combination therapy with continuous alendronate and PTH blunted the beneficial effects of teriparatide alone.[4,5] More recent studies suggest that less frequently dosed bisphosphonates may have different effects when used in combination with PTH.[6,7] Sequential therapy with short courses of PTH alternating with a bisphosphonate may be a useful way to increase BMD and reduce fractures for reduced cost and less inconvenience.

This study evaluated the effect of 2 combinations of daily PTH 1-84 and monthly ibandronate in 44 postmenopausal women with low BMD. Patients were randomized to receive either 6 months of concurrent PTH 1-84 plus ibandronate, followed by 18 months of ibandronate (concurrent) or 2 sequential courses of 3 months of PTH 1-84 followed by 9 months of ibandronate (sequential), over 2 years. Areal BMD by dual-energy x-ray, volumetric BMD by quantitative computed tomography, and markers of bone turnover were followed serially over the study period. The study showed that areal BMD at the spine and hip increased similarly in both groups, with 7.5% and 8.2% increases in spine BMD in the concurrent and sequential treatment groups, respectively. Volumetric BMD also increased similarly between groups. With concurrent therapy, mean serum P1NP increased 75% between baseline and month 1 and then declined. With sequential therapy, the second 3-month PTH 1-84 course increased P1NP by 209%, although to a lesser degree than during the first course. The study concluded that 6 months of PTH 1-84 distributed over 2 years with a bisphosphonate in either concurrent or sequential regimens increased BMD significantly, and that short courses of PTH 1-84 may provide significant anabolic benefits with reduced burden for patients.

These findings demonstrate that combination anabolic and antiresorptive therapy may have significant benefit in treatment of postmenopausal osteoporosis. The timing and sequence of PTH 1-84 in combination with a bisphosphonate appears to determine the skeletal outcomes. Combination therapy with concurrent or sequential PTH 1-84 and monthly ibandronate resulted in significantly increased lumbar spine areal and volumetric BMD and increased markers of bone formation. Given that subjects received PTH 1-84 only for 25% of the total study duration, this study shows that anabolic effects of PTH can be maximized and prolonged by use in combination with ibandronate. Future trials may show more attractive ways to use sequential or combination treatment with anabolic and antiresorptive therapies.

B. L. Clarke, MD

References

1. Neer RM, Arnaud CD, Zanchetta JR, et al. Effect of parathyroid hormone (1-34) on fractures and bone mineral density in postmenopausal women with osteoporosis. *N Engl J Med.* 2001;344:1434-1441.
2. Greenspan SL, Bone HG, Ettinger MP, et al. Effect of recombinant human parathyroid hormone (1-84) on vertebral fracture and bone mineral density in postmenopausal women with osteoporosis: a randomized trial. *Ann Intern Med.* 2007;146:326-339.
3. Dempster DW, Cosman F, Kurland ES, et al. Effects of daily treatment with parathyroid hormone on bone microarchitecture and turnover in patients with osteoporosis: a paired biopsy study. *J Bone Miner Res.* 2001;16:1846-1853.
4. Black DM, Greenspan SL, Ensrud KE, et al. The effects of parathyroid hormone and alendronate alone or in combination in postmenopausal osteoporosis. *N Engl J Med.* 2003;349:1207-1215.
5. Finkelstein JS, Hayes A, Hunzelman JL, et al. The effects of parathyroid hormone, alendronate, or both in men with osteoporosis. *N Engl J Med.* 2003;349:1216-1226.
6. Cosman F, Eriksen EF, Recknor C, et al. Effects of intravenous zoledronic acid plus subcutaneous teriparatide [rhPTH(1-34)] in postmenopausal osteoporosis. *J Bone Miner Res.* 2011;26:503-511.
7. Cosman F, Nieves J, Zion M, et al. Daily and cyclic parathyroid hormone in women receiving alendronate. *N Engl J Med.* 2005;353:566-575.

Differing Effects of PTH 1-34, PTH 1-84 and Zoledronic Acid on Bone Microarchitecture and Estimated Strength in Postmenopausal Women with Osteoporosis. An 18 Month Open-Labeled Observational Study using HR-pQCT

Hansen S, Hauge EM, Beck Jensen J-E, et al (Odense Univ Hosp, Denmark; Aarhus Univ Hosp, Denmark; Hvidovre Univ Hosp, Denmark)
J Bone Miner Res 28:736-745, 2013

Whereas the beneficial effects of intermittent treatment with parathyroid hormone (PTH) (intact PTH 1-84 or fragment PTH 1-34, teriparatide) on vertebral strength is well documented, treatment may not be equally effective in the peripheral skeleton. We used high resolution peripheral quantitative computed tomography (HR-pQCT) to detail effects on compartmental geometry, density and microarchicture as well as finite element (FE) estimated integral strength at the distal radius and tibia in postmenopausal osteoporotic women treated with PTH 1-34 (20 µg sc. daily, n = 18) or PTH 1-84 (100 µg sc. daily, n = 20) for 18 month in an open label, non-randomized study. A group of postmenopausal osteoporotic women receiving zoledronic acid (5 mg infusion once yearly, n = 33) was also included. Anabolic therapy increased cortical porosity in radius (PTH 1-34 32 ± 37%, PTH 1-84 39 ± 32%, both $p < 0.001$) and tibia (PTH 1-34 13 ± 27%, PTH 1-84 15 ± 22%, both $p < 0.001$) with corresponding declines in cortical density. With PTH 1-34 increases in cortical thickness in radius (2.0 ± 3.8%, $p < 0.05$) and tibia (3.8 ± 10.4%, $p < 0.01$) were seen. Trabecular number increased in tibia with both PTH 1-34 (4.2 ± 7.1%, $p < 0.05$) and PTH 1-84 (5.3 ± 8.3%, $p < 0.01$). Zoledronic acid did not impact cortical porosity at either site, but increased cortical thickness (3.0 ± 3.5%, $p < 0.01$), total (2.7 ± 2.5%, $p < 0.001$) and cortical density (1.5 ± 2.0%, $p < 0.01$) in tibia as well as trabecular volume fraction in radius (2.5 ± 5.1%, $p < 0.05$) and tibia (2.2 ± 2.2%, $p < 0.01$). FE estimated bone strength was preserved, but not increased, with PTH 1-34 and zoledronic acid at both sites, while it decreased with PTH 1-84 in radius (−2.8 ± 5.8%, $p < 0.05$) and tibia (−3.9 ± 4.8%, $p < 0.001$). Conclusively, divergent treatment-specific effects in cortical and trabecular bone were observed with anabolic and zoledronic acid therapy. The finding of decreased estimated strength with PTH 1-84 treatment was surprising and warrants confirmation.

▶ Both full-length parathyroid hormone (PTH) 1-84 and PTH 1-34 act as anabolic agents on the skeleton when given intermittently. PTH 1-34 (teriparatide) is approved for treatment of osteoporosis in the United States and other countries, whereas PTH 1-84 is approved for this indication in Europe and other countries. These agents both stimulate new bone formation with short-term or intermittent use and serve to increase bone mineral density and reduce vertebral fractures.[1] PTH 1-34 also reduces nonvertebral fractures, whereas PTH 1-84 does not.[1,2] Neither has been shown to reduce hip fractures. Both forms of PTH stimulate modeling-based bone formation on quiescent bone surfaces in addition to stimulating remodeling-based bone formation that occurs after bone resorption.[3] A previous study found that PTH 1-34 treatment for 18 months decreased cortical bone mineral density and trabecular thinning but preserved bone strength by high-resolution peripheral quantitative computed tomography (CT) scanning at the wrist and tibia.[4] Other studies have found that treatment with PTH 1-34 or 1-84 causes large increases in trabecular bone mineral density and vertebral strength by quantitative CT scanning.[5,6] The reasons for the differences in apparent site-specific effects of PTH 1-34 and PTH 1-84 are not clear.

This study evaluated 18 postmenopausal women treated with PTH 1-34, 20 μg subcutaneously each day for 18 months, and 20 postmenopausal women treated with PTH 1-84, 100 μg subcutaneously each day for 18 months, in an open-label, nonrandomized trial. A comparison group of 33 postmenopausal women treated with zoledronic acid 5 mg intravenously once yearly was included. High-resolution peripheral quantitative CT scanning of the radius and tibia showed that women treated with both forms of PTH had increased cortical porosity at both the radius and tibia, with decreased cortical bone mineral density. PTH 1-34 also caused small increases in cortical thickness at these sites. Trabecular number increased in the tibia with both forms of PTH. Zoledronic acid did not affect cortical porosity, but it increased cortical thickness, total bone density, and cortical bone density in the tibia as well as trabecular volume in both the radius and tibia. Finite element analysis of bone strength based on changes in these parameters showed that bone strength was preserved, but not increased, with PTH 1-34 and zoledronic acid at both sites, whereas small decreases were seen with PTH 1-84. The study concluded that anabolic and zoledronic acid therapies caused divergent effects on cortical and trabecular bone at the distal wrist and tibia, with preservation of estimated bone strength with PTH 1-34 and zoledronic acid but a mild decrease in estimated strength with PTH 1-84.

The results of this interesting study need to be confirmed because of the variance in treatment results with the 2 forms of PTH used compared with the findings with zoledronic acid. Both PTH 1-34 and PTH 1-84 caused an increase in cortical porosity and decrease in cortical bone density at the radius and tibia. Trabecular number in the tibia increased with both agents, as did cortical thickness in both the radius and tibia with PTH 1-34. Zoledronic acid did not change cortical porosity at the radius or tibia, whereas trabecular bone volume increased. Bone strength estimated by finite element analysis remained stable with PTH 1-34 and zoledronic acid, whereas PTH 1-84 caused bone strength to decrease at both the radius and tibia. Further study is required to establish whether PTH 1-34 and PTH 1-84 differ in terms of treatment effect on bone strength.

B. L. Clarke, MD

References

1. Neer RM, Arnaud CD, Zanchetta JR, et al. Effect of parathyroid hormone (1–34) on fractures and bone mineral density in postmenopausal women with osteoporosis. *N Engl J Med.* 2001;344:1434-1441.
2. Greenspan SL, Bone HG, Ettinger MP, et al. Effect of recombinant human parathyroid hormone (1–84) on vertebral fracture and bone mineral density in postmenopausal women with osteoporosis: a randomized trial. *Ann Intern Med.* 2007;146:326-339.

3. Ma YL, Zeng Q, Donley DW, et al. Teriparatide increases bone formation in modeling and remodeling osteons and enhances IGF-II immunoreactivity in postmenopausal women with osteoporosis. *J Bone Miner Res.* 2006;21:855-864.
4. Macdonald HM, Nishiyama KK, Hanley DA, Boyd SK. Changes in trabecular and cortical bone microarchitecture at peripheral sites associated with 18 months of teriparatide therapy in postmenopausal women with osteoporosis. *Osteoporos Int.* 2011;22:357-362.
5. Graeff C, Chevalier Y, Charlebois M, et al. Improvements in vertebral body strength under teriparatide treatment assessed in vivo by finite element analysis: results from the EUROFORS study. *J Bone Miner Res.* 2009;24:1672-1680.
6. Bauer DC, Garnero P, Bilezikian JP, et al. Short-term changes in bone turnover markers and bone mineral density response to parathyroid hormone in postmenopausal women with osteoporosis. *J Clin Endocrinol Metab.* 2006;91:1370-1375.

Effect of 12 Months of Whole-Body Vibration Therapy on Bone Density and Structure in Postmenopausal Women: A Randomized Trial

Slatkovska L, Alibhai SMH, Beyene J, et al (Mount Sinai Hosp, Ontario, Canada; Univ of Toronto, Ontario, Canada; McMaster Univ, Hamilton, Ontario, Canada)

Ann Intern Med 155:668-679, 2011

Background.—Although data from studies in animals demonstrated beneficial effects of whole-body vibration (WBV) therapy on bone, clinical trials in postmenopausal women showed conflicting results.

Objective.—To determine whether WBV improves bone density and structure.

Design.—A 12-month, single-center, superiority, randomized, controlled trial with 3 parallel groups. (ClinicalTrials.gov registration number: NCT00420940).

Setting.—Toronto General Hospital, Ontario, Canada.

Participants.—202 healthy postmenopausal women with bone mineral density (BMD) T-scores between -1.0 and -2.5 who were not receiving prescription bone medications.

Intervention.—Participants were randomly assigned to 1 of 3 groups (1:1:1 ratio) by using a block-randomization scheme and sealed envelopes. They were asked to stand on a low-magnitude (0.3 g) 90-Hz or 30-Hz WBV platform for 20 minutes daily or to serve as control participants; all participants received calcium and vitamin D.

Measurements.—Bone outcome assessors, who were blinded to group assignment, determined trabecular volumetric BMD and other measurements of the distal tibia and distal radius with highresolution peripheral quantitative computed tomography and areal BMD with dual-energy x-ray absorptiometry at baseline and at 12 months.

Results.—12 months of WBV therapy had no significant effect on any bone outcomes compared with no WBV therapy. For the primary outcome of tibial trabecular volumetric BMD, mean change from baseline was 0.4 mg/cm^3 (95% CI, -0.4 to 1.2 mg/cm^3) in the 90-Hz WBV group, -0.1 mg/cm^3 (CI, -1.0 to 0.8 mg/cm^3) in the 30-Hz WBV group, and -0.2 mg/cm^3 (CI, -1.1 to 0.6 mg/cm^3) in the control group ($P = 0.55$).

Changes in areal BMD at the femoral neck, total hip, and lumbar spine were also similar among the groups. Overall, low-magnitude WBV at both 90 and 30 Hz was well-tolerated.

Limitations.—Adherence to WBV ranged from 65% to 79%. Double-blinding was not possible.

Conclusion.—Whole-body vibration therapy at 0.3 *g* and 90 or 30 Hz for 12 months did not alter BMD or bone structure in postmenopausal women who received calcium and vitamin D supplementation.

▶ Whole-body vibration has been advocated as a nonpharmaceutical treatment for postmenopausal osteoporosis in recent years. Treatment of animal models with low-frequency vibration has been shown to increase bone formation rate, bone mineral density (BMD), trabecular structure, and cortical thickness. Recent randomized, controlled trials in humans have shown conflicting results.[1-3] This treatment involves standing on a motor-driven oscillating platform that produces vertical accelerations that are transmitted from the feet to the weight-bearing muscles and skeleton.[4] Transmission of whole-body vibration depends on the intensity of the vibration, knee-joint angle, distance of the skeletal site from the oscillating plate, and dampening of the vibration by the muscles and soft tissues.[5,6] Whole-body vibration is thought to cause osteogenic effects because of induced fluid shear forces during flow of bone tissue fluid in the canalicular network, leading to mechanical signal transduction via the Wnt signaling pathway in osteocytes.[7]

This study evaluated the effect of whole-body vibration in 202 healthy postmenopausal women with osteopenia but without fractures. Subjects were randomized to receive vibration at low-magnitude (0.3 g) 30-Hz or 90-Hz frequencies for 20 minutes each day with calcium and vitamin D supplementation, or calcium and vitamin D supplementation alone, for 1 year. The study showed no significant differences in the primary outcome of tibial volumetric BMD, or secondary outcomes of bone structure at the distal tibia or radius, or areal BMD at the lumbar spine or hip sites, between treatment groups over 12 months. Adherence to therapy ranged from 65% to 79%. The treatments were well tolerated. The study concluded that whole-body vibration for 1 year did not affect BMD or bone structure in healthy postmenopausal women treated with calcium and vitamin D supplementation.

These negative findings demonstrated that daily low-frequency vibration treatment for 1 year in healthy osteopenic postmenopausal women did not result in an improvement in BMD or bone structure. Previous studies showing benefit had smaller sample sizes, greater loss to follow-up, and did not provide calcium or vitamin D supplementation. It is possible that high-magnitude whole-body vibration treatment might have a different effect on skeletal outcomes, but this remains controversial. Two trials of high-frequency whole-body vibration showed a small benefit on areal hip BMD.[8,9] Limitations of this study include unsupervised administration of whole-body vibration therapy at home and the inability to blind the study. Further studies will be required to conclusively demonstrate benefit with this type of therapy.

B. L. Clarke, MD

References

1. Slatkovska L, Alibhai SM, Beyene J, Cheung AM. Effect of whole-body vibration on BMD: a systematic review and meta-analysis. *Osteoporos Int.* 2010;21:1969-1980.
2. Verschueren SM, Bogaerts A, Delecluse C, et al. The effects of whole-body vibration training and vitamin D supplementation on muscle strength, muscle mass, and bone density in institutionalized elderly women: a 6-month randomized, controlled trial. *J Bone Miner Res.* 2011;26:42-49.
3. Beck BR, Norling TL. The effect of 8 mos of twice-weekly low- or higher intensity whole body vibration on risk factors for postmenopausal hip fractures. *Am J Phys Med Rehabil.* 2010;89:997-1009.
4. Rauch F, Sievanen H, Boonen S, et al; International Society of Musculoskeletal and Neuronal Interactions. Reporting whole-body vibration intervention studies: recommendations of the International Society of Musculoskeletal Interactions. *J Musculoskelet Neuronal Interact.* 2010;10:193-198.
5. Kiiski J, Heinonen A, Järvinen TL, Kannus P, Sievänen H. Transmission of vertical whole body vibration to the human body. *J Bone Miner Res.* 2008;23:1318-1325.
6. Rubin C, Pope M, Fritton JC, Magnusson M, Hansson T, McLeod K. Transmissibility of 15-herz to 35-herz vibrations to the human hip and lumbar spine: determining the physiologic feasibility of delivering low-level anabolic mechanical stimuli to skeletal regions at greatest risk of fracture because of osteoporosis. *Spine (Phila Pa 1976).* 2003;28:2621-2627.
7. Ozcivici E, Luu YK, Adler B, et al. Mechanical signals as anabolic agents in bone. *Nat Rev Rheumatol.* 2010;6:50-59.
8. Gusi N, Raimundo A, Leal A. Low-frequency vibratory exercise reduces the risk of bone fracture more than walking: a randomized controlled trial. *BMD Musculoskelet Disord.* 2006;7:92.
9. Verschueren SM, Roelants M, Delecluse C, et al. Effect of 6-month whole body vibration training on hip density, muscle strength, an postural control in postmenopausal women: a randomized controlled pilot study. *J Bone Miner Res.* 2004;19:352-359.

Fracture Risk and Zoledronic Acid Therapy in Men with Osteoporosis

Boonen S, Reginster J-Y, Kaufman J-M, et al (Katholieke Universiteit Leuven, Belgium; Univ of Liege, Belgium; Ghent Univ, Belgium; et al)
N Engl J Med 367:1714-1723, 2012

Background.—Fractures in men are a major health issue, and data on the antifracture efficacy of therapies for osteoporosis in men are limited. We studied the effect of zoledronic acid on fracture risk among men with osteoporosis.

Methods.—In this multicenter, double-blind, placebo-controlled trial, we randomly assigned 1199 men with primary or hypogonadism-associated osteoporosis who were 50 to 85 years of age to receive an intravenous infusion of zoledronic acid (5 mg) or placebo at baseline and at 12 months. Participants received daily calcium and vitamin D supplementation. The primary end point was the proportion of participants with one or more new morphometric vertebral fractures over a period of 24 months.

Results.—The rate of any new morphometric vertebral fracture was 1.6% in the zoledronic acid group and 4.9% in the placebo group over the 24-month period, representing a 67% risk reduction with zoledronic acid (relative risk, 0.33; 95% confidence interval, 0.16 to 0.70; $P = 0.002$). As compared with men who received placebo, men who received zoledronic acid had fewer moderate-to-severe vertebral fractures ($P = 0.03$) and less height loss ($P = 0.002$). Fewer participants who received zoledronic acid had clinical vertebral or nonvertebral fractures, although this difference did not reach significance because of the small number of fractures. Bone mineral density was higher and bone-turnover markers were lower in the men who received zoledronic acid ($P < 0.05$ for both comparisons). Results were similar in men with low serum levels of total testosterone. The zoledronic acid and placebo groups did not differ significantly with respect to the incidence of death (2.6% and 2.9%, respectively) or serious adverse events (25.3% and 25.2%).

Conclusions.—Zoledronic acid treatment was associated with a significantly reduced risk of vertebral fracture among men with osteoporosis. (Funded by Novartis Pharma; ClinicalTrials.gov number, NCT00439647.)

▶ Osteoporosis affects men by causing significant morbidity and mortality related to fractures.[1,2] About 40% of fractures in adults older than 50 years of age occur in men,[3] and mortality after fracture is higher in men than women.[4] Previous studies in men demonstrated improvement in bone mineral density and markers of bone turnover without being powered for fracture reduction.[5-9] Men at risk for fracture are still not commonly identified or treated.[10] These issues have led to a need for randomized, controlled trials of osteoporosis treatment in men.

This double-blind, placebo-controlled trial randomized 1199 men 50 to 89 years of age with primary or hypogonadism-associated osteoporosis to receive zoledronic acid 5 mg or placebo intravenously at baseline and at 12 months. All subjects received calcium and vitamin D supplementation. The primary endpoint was the proportion of participants with 1 or more new morphometric vertebral fractures over 24 months. The rate of new vertebral morphometric fractures over 2 years was 1.6% in the zoledronic acid group and 4.9% in the placebo group, representing a 67% reduction in relative risk. Men in the zoledronic acid group had fewer moderate-to-severe vertebral fractures and less height loss. Fewer clinical or nonvertebral fractures were seen in the zoledronic acid group, but these were not statistically significant because of the small numbers of fractures. Bone mineral density increased, and markers of turnover decreased in the zoledronic acid group. Results were similar in men with primary or hypogonadism-associated osteoporosis. There was no difference in deaths or adverse events between the 2 groups. The study concluded that zoledronic acid reduced vertebral fractures in men with osteoporosis.

These findings demonstrate that 2 infusions of zoledronic acid over 2 years reduce the relative risk of new vertebral morphometric fractures in osteoporotic men by 67%. The results are similar to the findings with zoledronic acid in postmenopausal women with osteoporosis, where the reduction in relative risk was 72% at 2 years. These findings suggest that the antifracture effect of zoledronic acid is the same in men and women. Findings were similar in men with normal and mildly decreased testosterone levels. This study was not powered to show an effect on nonvertebral fractures. Further studies are needed to show antifracture efficacy of zoledronic acid and other osteoporosis agents in men.

B. L. Clarke, MD

References

1. Looker AC, Orwoll ES, Johnston CC Jr, et al. Prevalence of low femoral bone density in older U.S. adults from NHANES III. *J Bone Miner Res.* 1997;12:1761-1768.
2. Center JR, Nguyen TV, Schneider D, Sambrook PN, Eisman JA. Mortality after all major types of osteoporotic fracture in men and women: an observational study. *Lancet.* 1999;353:878-882.
3. Johnell O, Kanis JA. An estimate of the worldwide prevalence and disability associated with osteoporotic fractures. *Osteoporos Int.* 2006;17:1726-1733.
4. Haentjens P, Magaziner J, Colón-Emeric CS, et al. Meta-analysis: excess mortality after hip fracture among older women and men. *Ann Intern Med.* 2010;152:380-390.
5. Orwoll ES, Scheele WH, Paul S, et al. The effect of teriparatide [human parathyroid hormone (1–34)] therapy on bone density in men with osteoporosis. *J Bone Miner Res.* 2003;18:9-17.
6. Boonen S, Orwoll ES, Wenderoth D, Stoner KJ, Eusebio R, Delmas PD. Once-weekly risedronate in men with osteoporosis: results of a 2-year, placebo-controlled, double-blind, multicenter study. *J Bone Miner Res.* 2009;24:719-725.
7. Orwoll E, Ettinger M, Weiss S, et al. Alendronate for the treatment of osteoporosis in men. *N Engl J Med.* 2000;343:604-610.
8. Orwoll ES, Miller PD, Adachi JD, et al. Efficacy and safety of a once-yearly i.v. infusion of zoledronic acid 5 mg versus once-weekly 70-mg oral alendronate in the treatment of male osteoporosis: a randomized, multicenter, double-blind, active-controlled study. *J Bone Mineral Res.* 2010;25:2239-2250.
9. Orwoll ES, Binkley NC, Lewiecki EM, Gruntmanis U, Fries MA, Dasic G. Efficacy and safety of monthly ibandronate in men with low bone density. *Bone.* 2010;46:970-976.
10. Feldstein AC, Nichols G, Orwoll E, et al. The near absence of osteoporosis treatment in older men with fractures. *Osteoporos Int.* 2005;16:953-962.

Denosumab Treatment in Postmenopausal Women with Osteoporosis Does Not Interfere with Fracture-Healing: Results from the FREEDOM Trial
Adami S, FREEDOM Fracture-Healing Writing Group (Univ of Verona, Italy; et al)
J Bone Joint Surg Am 94:2113-2119, 2012

Background.—Fracture is the major complication of osteoporosis, and it allows the identification of individuals needing medical intervention for osteoporosis. After nonvertebral fracture, patients often do not receive osteoporosis medical treatment despite evidence that this treatment reduces the risk of subsequent fracture. In this preplanned analysis of the results of the three-year, placebo-controlled FREEDOM trial, we evaluated the effect of denosumab administration on fracture-healing to address theoretical concerns related to initiating or continuing denosumab therapy in patients presenting with a nonvertebral fracture.

Methods.—Postmenopausal women aged sixty to ninety years with osteoporosis were randomized to receive 60 mg of denosumab (n = 3902) or a placebo (n = 3906) subcutaneously every six months for three years. Investigators reported complications associated with a fracture or its management and with fracture-healing for all nonvertebral fractures that occurred during the study. Delayed healing was defined as incomplete fracture-healing six months after the fracture.

Results.—Six hundred and sixty-seven subjects (303 treated with denosumab and 364 who received a placebo) had a total of 851 nonvertebral fractures (386 in the denosumab group and 465 in the placebo group), including 199 fractures (seventy-nine in the denosumab group and 120 in the placebo group) that were treated surgically. Delayed healing was reported in seven subjects (two in the denosumab group and five in the placebo group), including one with subsequent nonunion (in the placebo group). Neither delayed healing nor nonunion was observed in any subject who had received denosumab within six weeks preceding or following the fracture. A complication associated with the fracture or intervention occurred in five subjects (2%) and twenty subjects (5%) in the denosumab and placebo groups, respectively (*p* = 0.009).

Conclusions.—Denosumab in a dose of 60 mg every six months does not seem to delay fracture-healing or contribute to other complications, even when it is administered at or near the time of the fracture.

▶ There is lingering concern that potent antiresorptive therapies that prevent fractures may delay fracture healing once fractures occur by decreasing bone resorption and bone formation required for the repair process. Osteoporotic fractures are associated with increased risk of subsequent fractures.[1-3] Most osteoporotic fractures are nonvertebral fractures, many of which require orthopedic repair. Most patients (70% to 80%) who have low-trauma fractures remain untreated for their osteoporosis,[4] despite their subsequent high risk of fractures.[5,6] Patients with hip fractures have a 20% risk of another fracture during the next 5 years.[5]

Denosumab is a new anti-RANK ligand monoclonal antibody that functions as a potent antiresorptive agent to prevent bone loss and fractures. This pre-planned analysis was designed to detect complications related to fracture healing caused by denosumab during the randomized, double-blind, placebo controlled FREEDOM Trial. This trial randomized 3902 postmenopausal women to denosumab 60 mg subcutaneously every 6 months and 3906 postmenopausal women to placebo every 6 months for 3 years. During the study, 667 women (386 in the denosumab group and 465 in the placebo group) had a total of 851 nonvertebral fractures that required surgical repair. Delayed healing was reported in 7 subjects, with 2 in the denosumab group and 5 in the placebo group. One patient in the placebo group had subsequent nonunion. Neither delayed healing nor nonunion was observed in any subject who received denosumab within 6 weeks proceeding or following fracture repair. A complication associated with fracture or fracture repair was seen in 5 (2%) subjects in the denosumab group and 20 (5%) subjects in the placebo group. The study concluded that denosumab 60 mg subcutaneously every 6 months did not appear to delay fracture healing or contribute to other complications, even when administered within 6 weeks of fracture.

These reassuring findings provide additional evidence that current US Food and Drug Administration—approved treatments for osteoporosis have no apparent adverse effects on fracture healing or postsurgical fracture repair. Because these agents potently suppress both bone resorption and bone formation required for fracture repair, they could potentially cause prolonged fracture healing or nonunion of fracture, especially if given closely around the time of fracture. Denosumab causes very rapid suppression of bone resorption and bone formation, more rapid than that caused by most currently available bisphosphonates. Nevertheless, there was no evidence of complications related to fracture or surgical repair of fracture.

B. L. Clarke, MD

References

1. Center JC, Biluc D, Nguyen TV, Eisman JA. Risk of subsequent fracture after low-trauma fracture in men and women. *JAMA*. 2007;297:387-394.
2. van Geel TA, van Helden S, Geusens PP, Winkens B, Dinant GJ. Clinical subsequent fractures cluster in time after first fractures. *Ann Rheum Dis*. 2009;68:22-102.
3. van Geel TA, Huntjens KM, van den Burgh JP, Dinant GJ, Geusens PP. Timing of subsequent fractures after an initial fracture. *Curr Osteoporos Rep*. 2010;8:118-122.
4. Andrade SE, Majumdar SR, Chan KA, et al. Low frequency of treatment of osteoporosis among postmenopausal women following a fracture. *Arch Intern Med*. 2003;163:2052-2057.
5. Colon-Emeric C, Kuchibhatia M, Pieper C, et al. The contribution of hip fracture to risk of subsequent fractures: data from two longitudinal studies. *Osteoporos Int*. 2003;14:879-883.
6. Klotzbuecher CM, Ross PD, Landsman PB, Abbott TA 3rd, Berger M. Patients with prior fractures have an increased risk of future fractures: a summary of the literature and statistical synthesis. *J Bone Miner Res*. 2000;15:721-739.

Metabolic Bone Disease

Effect of Cinacalcet on Cardiovascular Disease in Patients Undergoing Dialysis

The EVOLVE Trial Investigators (Stanford Univ School of Medicine, Palo Alto, CA; Denver Nephrology, CO; Instituto Nacional de Ciencias Médicas y Nutrición Salvador Zubirán, Mexico City; et al)
N Engl J Med 367:2482-2494, 2012

Background.—Disorders of mineral metabolism, including secondary hyperparathyroidism, are thought to contribute to extraskeletal (including vascular) calcification among patients with chronic kidney disease. It has been hypothesized that treatment with the calcimimetic agent cinacalcet might reduce the risk of death or nonfatal cardiovascular events in such patients.

Methods.—In this clinical trial, we randomly assigned 3883 patients with moderate-to-severe secondary hyperparathyroidism (median level of intact parathyroid hormone, 693 pg per milliliter [10th to 90th percentile, 363 to 1694]) who were undergoing hemodialysis to receive either cinacalcet or placebo. All patients were eligible to receive conventional therapy, including phosphate binders, vitamin D sterols, or both. The patients were followed for up to 64 months. The primary composite end point was the time until death, myocardial infarction, hospitalization for unstable angina, heart failure, or a peripheral vascular event. The primary analysis was performed on the basis of the intention-to-treat principle.

Results.—The median duration of study-drug exposure was 21.2 months in the cinacalcet group, versus 17.5 months in the placebo group. The primary composite end point was reached in 938 of 1948 patients (48.2%) in the cinacalcet group and 952 of 1935 patients (49.2%) in the placebo group (relative hazard in the cinacalcet group vs. the placebo group, 0.93; 95% confidence interval, 0.85 to 1.02; $P = 0.11$). Hypocalcemia and gastrointestinal adverse events were significantly more frequent in patients receiving cinacalcet.

Conclusions.—In an unadjusted intention-to-treat analysis, cinacalcet did not significantly reduce the risk of death or major cardiovascular events in patients with moderate-to-severe secondary hyperparathyroidism who were undergoing dialysis. (Funded by Amgen; EVOLVE ClinicalTrials.gov number, NCT00345839.)

▶ Patients with chronic kidney disease (CKD) have increased risk of cardiovascular death, especially those receiving renal replacement therapy. The risk of cardiovascular disease—related death in this group is increased by at least 10-fold compared with the general population.[1,2] A large number of risk factors have been identified as contributing to increased cardiovascular death, including disorders of bone and mineral metabolism—hyperphosphatemia, hypercalcemia, and secondary hyperparathyroidism.[3] Patients undergoing hemodialysis, increased serum phosphorus, calcium, parathyroid hormone, alkaline phosphatase, and fibroblast growth factor-23 have been associated with increased risk of death and cardiovascular events.[4-6] Disorders of mineral metabolism are thought to accelerate arterial calcification and decrease vascular compliance,[7,8] thereby leading to myocardial infarction (MI), congestive heart failure, and sudden death.

Cinacalcet (Sensipar) is a calcimimetic drug that acts as an allosteric activator of the calcium-sensing receptor on parathyroid cells, thereby reducing parathyroid hormone secretion. This drug has been approved for treatment of patients with secondary hyperparathyroidism resulting from CKD, parathyroid carcinoma, and severe primary hyperparathyroidism not able to undergo surgical intervention.

This large, prospective, clinical trial randomized 3883 subjects with moderate-to-severe secondary hyperparathyroidism receiving hemodialysis to receive cinacalcet or placebo for up to 64 months. Cinacalcet was given as add-on therapy to standard therapies that were continued, including phosphate binders, vitamin D analogues, or both. All cardiovascular endpoints were independently adjudicated. The study found that 48.5% of subjects on cinacalcet and 49.2% of those on placebo reached the primary composite endpoint of death, MI, hospitalization for unstable angina, heart failure, or a peripheral vascular event at 21.2 months and 17.5 months, respectively (relative hazard of cinacalcet vs placebo group 0.93; 95% confidence interval, 0.85 to 1.02; $P = .11$). Hypocalcemia and gastrointestinal side effects were more common in the cinacalcet group. The study concluded that cinacalcet did not significantly reduce the risk of death or cardiovascular events in patients with moderate-to-severe secondary hyperparathyroidism on hemodialysis.

This disappointing finding was interpreted by the investigators as nondefinitive. The nonsignificant primary composite endpoint risk reduction of 7% in the intention-to-treat analysis must be understood in context. Patients receiving hemodialysis are frequently frail and chronically ill, with expected mortality of 20.7% per year, and mean morbidity characterized by two hospitalizations for 12 hospital days per year. These patients commonly have cardiopulmonary, gastrointestinal, musculoskeletal, and neurocognitive symptoms, with a median pill burden of 19 per day. After adjustment for baseline characteristics, there was a nominally significant risk reduction of 12%. Nevertheless, in spite of reducing the rate of parathyroidectomy by more than 50%, cinacalcet was not shown to reduce death or cardiovascular endpoints. Further studies in the late-stage CKD population will be necessary to demonstrate therapies able to reduce mortality and cardiovascular death.

B. L. Clarke, MD

References

1. Go AS, Chertow GM, Fan D, McCulloch CE, Hsu CY. Chronic kidney disease and the risks of death, cardiovascular events, and hospitalization. *N Engl J Med.* 2004; 351:1296-1305.
2. Foley RN, Murray AM, Li S, et al. Chronic kidney disease and the risk for cardiovascular disease, renal replacement, and death in the United States Medicare population, 1998 to 1999. *J Am Soc Nephrol.* 2005;16:489-495.
3. Kidney Disease Improving Global Outcomes (KDIGO) CKD-MBD Work Group. KDIGO clinical practice guideline for the diagnosis, evaluation, prevention, and treatment of chronic kidney disease-mineral and bone disorder (CKD-MBD). *Kidney Int Suppl.* 2009;76:S1-S130.
4. Block GA, Klassem PS, Lazarus JM, Ofsthun N, Lowrie EG, Chertow GM. Mineral metabolism, mortality and morbidity in maintenance hemodialysis. *J Am Soc Nephrol.* 2004;15:2208-2218.
5. Floege J, Kim J, Ireland E, et al. Serum iPTH, calcium and phosphorus and the risk of mortality in a European haemodialysis population. *Nephrol Dial Transplant.* 2011;26:1948-1955.
6. Gutiérrez OM, Mannstadt M, Isakova T, et al. Fibroblast growth factor 23 and mortality among patients undergoing hemodialysis. *N Engl J Med.* 2008;359: 584-592.
7. Suzuki T, Yonemura K, Maruyama Y, et al. Impact of serum parathyroid hormone concentration and its regulatory factors on arterial stiffness in patients undergoing maintenance hemodialysis. *Blood Purif.* 2004;22:293-297.
8. London GM, Marchais SJ, Guérin AP, Métivier F. Arteriosclerosis, vascular calcifications and cardiovascular disease in uremia. *Curr Opin Nephrol Hypertens.* 2005;14:525-531.

Therapy of Hypoparathyroidism with PTH(1—84): A Prospective Four-Year Investigation of Efficacy and Safety

Cusano NE, Rubin MR, McMahon DJ, et al (Columbia Univ, NY)
J Clin Endocrinol Metab 98:137-144, 2013

Context.—PTH may be an effective treatment option for hypoparathyroidism, but long-term data are not available.

Objective.—We studied the effect of 4 yr of PTH(1—84) treatment in hypoparathyroidism.

Design.—Twenty-seven subjects were treated with PTH(1—84) for 4 yr, with prospective monitoring of calcium and vitamin D requirements, serum and urinary calcium, serum phosphorus, bone turnover markers, and bone mineral density (BMD).

Results.—Treatment with PTH(1—84) reduced supplemental calcium requirements by 37% ($P = 0.006$) and 1,25-dihydroxyvitamin D requirements by 45% ($P = 0.008$). Seven subjects (26%) were able to stop 1,25-dihydroxyvitamin D completely. Serum calcium concentration remained stable, and urinary calcium and phosphorus excretion fell. Lumbar spine BMD increased by 5.5 ± 9% at 4 yr ($P < 0.0001$). Femoral neck and total hip BMD remained stable. At 4 yr, distal radius BMD was not different from baseline. Bone turnover markers increased significantly, reaching a 3-fold peak from baseline values at 6-12 months ($P < 0.05$ for all), subsequently declining to steady-state levels at 30 months. Hypercalcemia was uncommon (11 episodes in eight subjects over 4 yr; 1.9% of all values), with most episodes occurring within the first 6 months and resolving with adjustment of supplemental calcium and vitamin D.

Conclusions.—PTH(1-84) treatment of hypoparathyroidism for up to 4 yr maintains the serum calcium concentration, while significantly reducing supplemental calcium and 1,25-dihydroxyvitamin D requirements. Lumbar spine BMD increases without significant changes at other sites. These data provide support for the safety and efficacy of PTH(1—84) therapy in hypoparathyroidism for up to 4 yr.

▶ Hypoparathyroidism is characterized by hypocalcemia, hyperphosphatemia, and decreased or absent parathyroid hormone (PTH).[1] It is the last classical endocrine disorder for which the missing hormone is not available for replacement therapy.[2] Patients are typically treated with calcium and vitamin D supplementation, but standard therapy typically leads to variable hypocalcemia, hypercalcemia, and hypercalciuria.[3] Long-term treatment with calcium and vitamin D supplementation may lead to kidney stones, renal dysfunction or failure, and soft-tissue calcifications.[4] New therapies for this chronic disorder are desperately needed.[5]

This study evaluated the effect of treatment of 27 patients with hypoparathyroidism with PTH 1 to 84 100 mcg (1-84) every other day for 4 years. Patients were followed prospectively for their calcium and vitamin D requirements, serum and urine calcium, serum phosphorus, bone turnover markers, and bone mineral density (BMD). Treatment with PTH (1-84) allowed significant reductions in calcium supplements by 37%, and 1,25-dihydroxyvitamin D (calcitriol) by 45%. Seven subjects (26%) were able to stop calcitriol completely. Serum calcium levels remained stable, and urine calcium and phosphorus decreased over time. Lumbar spine BMD increased over 4 years, whereas femoral neck and total hip BMD remained stable. At 4 years, distal radius BMD remained stable. Bone turnover markers increase significantly, peaking at 3-fold increases from baseline at 6 to 12 months, and then decreased to steady-state levels at 30 months. Hypercalciuria occurred infrequently on this regimen, with most episodes occurring within 6 months of the start of therapy, and normalizing with appropriate adjustment of calcium and vitamin D supplements. Patients tolerated PTH (1-84) without adverse events. The study concluded that long-term treatment of hypoparathyroidism with PTH (1-84) over 4 years maintains serum calcium in goal range, while allowing significant reduction in calcium and calcitriol supplementation, with decreased urine calcium and mildly increased lumbar spine BMD and stable hip BMD.

These findings provide the first evidence that long-term PTH (1-84) therapy over 4 years appears to be effective therapy for patients with chronic hypoparathyroidism. Besides maintaining mineral metabolism parameters in the desired goal range in spite of significantly reduced calcium and calcitriol supplementation, PTH (1-84) treatment returned markedly decreased markers of bone turnover to more normal levels after a short period of increased levels. Limitations of this study include every-other-day dosing of PTH (1-84), which does not resemble normal PTH kinetics. This study provides the first evidence regarding efficacy and safety of long-term PTH (1-84) in patients with chronic hypoparathyroidism.

B. L. Clarke, MD

References

1. Bilezikian JP, Khan A, Potts JT Jr, et al. Hypoparathyroidism in the adult: epidemiology, diagnosis, pathophysiology, target-organ involvement, treatment, and challenges for future research. *J Bone Miner Res.* 2011;26:2317-2337.
2. Shoback D. Clinical practice. Hypoparathyroidism. *N Engl J Med.* 2008;259:391-403.
3. Al-Azem H, Khan AA. Hypoparathyroidism. *Best Pract Res Clin Endocrinol Metab.* 2012;26:517-522.
4. Mitchell DM, Regan S, Cooley MR, et al. Long-term follow-up of patients with hypoparathyroidism. *J Clin Endocrinol Metab.* 2012;97:4507-4514.
5. Cusano NE, Rubin MR, Sliney J Jr, Bilezikian JP. Mini-review: new therapeutic options in hypoparathyroidism. *Endocrine.* 2012;41:410-414.

Miscellaneous

25(OH) Vitamin D Is Associated with Greater Muscle Strength in Healthy Men and Women

Grimaldi AS, Parker BA, Capizzi JA, et al (Hartford Hosp, CT; et al)
Med Sci Sports Exerc 45:157-162, 2013

Purpose.—The purpose of the study was to examine the relation between serum 25-hydroxy vitamin D (25(OH)D) levels and muscle strength in 419 healthy men and women over a broad age range (20—76 yr).

TABLE 3.—ANOVA Results Between Vitamin D and Strength for Between-Subject Effects when Age and Gender were Controlled (*F*-Statistics/*P* Value)

Test Type	Log Serum 25-Hydroxy Vitamin D	
	F	*P*
Handgrip		
Handgrip	0.087	0.77
Elbow		
Isometric extension APT	4.115	0.04
Isometric flexion APT	5.540	0.02
Isokinetic extension $60°s^{-1}$ APT	5.301	0.02
Isokinetic flexion $60°s^{-1}$ APT	6.906	0.01
Isokinetic extension $180°s^{-1}$ APT	8.133	0.01
Isokinetic flexion $180°s^{-1}$ APT	4.357	0.04
Knee		
Isometric extension APT	4.562	0.03
Isometric flexion APT	7.335	0.01
Isokinetic extension $60°s^{-1}$ APT	2.321	0.13
Isokinetic flexion $60°s^{-1}$ APT	5.668	0.02
Isokinetic extension $180°s^{-1}$ APT	2.468	0.12
Isokinetic flexion $180°s^{-1}$ APT	4.833	0.03

ANOVA results assessing the relation between vitamin D and strength variables when age and gender were controlled for in the model.

Methods.—Isometric and isokinetic strength of the arms and legs was measured using computerized dynamometry, and its relation to vitamin D was tested in multivariate models controlling for age, gender, resting HR, systolic blood pressure, diastolic blood pressure, body mass index, maximal oxygen uptake ($\dot{V}O_{2max}$,), physical activity counts, and season of vitamin D measurement.

Results.—Vitamin D was significantly associated with arm and leg muscle strength when controlling for age and gender. When controlling for other covariates listed previously, vitamin D remained directly related to both isometric and isokinetic arm strength but only to isometric leg strength.

Conclusion.—These data suggest that there may be a differential effect of vitamin D on upper and lower body strength. The mechanism for this difference remains unclear but could be related to differences in androgenic effects or to differences in vitamin D receptor expression. Our study supports a direct relation between vitamin D and muscle strength and suggests that vitamin D supplementation be evaluated to determine whether it is an effective therapy to preserve muscle strength in adults (Table 3).

▶ Vitamin D deficiency affects type II skeletal muscle fibers and is associated with muscle weakness (Grimaldi et al). Higher (as compared with lower) serum 25-hydroxy vitamin D (25(OH) D) concentrations have been associated with improved risks of cardiovascular disease, immune disorders, cancer, and muscle function in the elderly. In the study, 1% of the subjects had serum (25(OH) D) < 10 ng/mL, 7% between 10 and 20 ng/mL, 27% between 20 and 30 ng/dL and 65% with values > 30 ng/mL. The results were controlled for age and gender. The relationship between arm- and leg-muscle strength that favored arm over leg strength was not answered by the study. The authors' findings were corroborated by literature. They postulated that androgen effects might favor the arms over the legs as supported by the more profound effect of androgens on upper body development compared with the lower body.[1-4]

A. W. Meikle, MD

References

1. Goswami R, Vatsa M, Sreenivas V, et al. Skeletal muscle strength in young asian Indian females after vitamin d and calcium supplementation: a double-blind randomized controlled clinical trial. *J Clin Endocrinol Metab*. 2012;97:4709-4716.
2. Amstrup AK, Rejnmark L, Vestergaard P, et al. Vitamin D status, physical performance and body mass in patients surgically cured for primary hyperparathyroidism compared with healthy controls—a cross-sectional study. *Clin Endocrinol (Oxf)*. 2011;74:130-136.
3. Gilsanz V, Kremer A, Mo AO, Wren TA, Kremer R. Vitamin D status and its relation to muscle mass and muscle fat in young women. *J Clin Endocrinol Metab*. 2010;95:1595-1601.
4. Kukuljan S, Nowson CA, Sanders K, Daly RM. Effects of resistance exercise and fortified milk on skeletal muscle mass, muscle size, and functional performance in middle-aged and older men: an 18-mo randomized controlled trial. *J Appl Physiol*. 2009;107:1864-1873.

6 Adrenal Cortex

Adrenal Hormone Secretion and Pathology

Adrenal involvement in MEN1. Analysis of 715 cases from the Groupe d'étude des Tumeurs Endocrines database
Gatta-Cherifi B, Chabre O, Murat A, et al (Centre Hospitalier Universitaire de Bordeaux, Pessac, France; Centre Hospitalier Universitaire de Grenoble, France; Centre Hospitalier Universitaire, Nantes, France; et al)
Eur J Endocrinol 166:269-279, 2012

Objective.—Limited data regarding adrenal involvement in multiple endocrine neoplasia type 1 (MEN1) is available. We describe the characteristics of MEN1-associated adrenal lesions in a large cohort to provide a rationale for their management.

Methods.—Analysis of records from 715 MEN1 patients from a multicentre database between 1956 and 2008. Adrenal lesions were compared with those from a multicentre cohort of 144 patients with adrenal sporadic incidentalomas.

Results.—Adrenal enlargement was reported in 20.4% (146/715) of patients. Adrenal tumours (>10 mm in size) accounted for 58.1% of these cases (10.1% of the whole patient cohort). Tumours were bilateral and >40 mm in size in 12.5 and 19.4% of cases respectively. Hormonal hypersecretion was restricted to patients with tumours and occurred in 15.3% of them. Compared with incidentalomas, MEN1-related tumours exhibited more cases of primary hyperaldosteronism, fewer pheochromocytomas and more adrenocortical carcinomas (ACCs; 13.8 vs 1.3%). Ten ACCs occurred in eight patients. Interestingly, ACCs occurred after several years of follow-up of small adrenal tumours in two of the eight affected patients. Nine of the ten ACCs were classified as stage I or II according to the European Network for the Study of Adrenal Tumors. No evident genotype/phenotype correlation was found for the occurrence of adrenal lesions, endocrine hypersecretion or ACC.

Conclusions.—Adrenal pathology in MEN1 differs from that observed in sporadic incidentalomas. In the absence of relevant symptoms, endocrine biology can be restricted to patients with adrenal tumours and should focus on steroid secretion including the aldosterone–renin system. MEN1 is a high-risk condition for the occurrence of ACCs. It should be considered regardless of the size of the tumour.

▶ Adrenal cortical cancer (ACC) is a rare disease, whereas the incidental finding of an adrenal mass is more or less common. Multiple endocrine neoplasia (MEN1) is also a rather rare entity. Therefore, most of the current systematically obtained knowledge on the biological behavior of adrenal cortical tumors derives from the data obtained in patients who are not affected by the MEN1 syndrome.

Nonetheless, clinical experience from case reports and case series suggested that a higher fraction of MEN1-related adrenocortical tumors is malignant. This study documented that ACC is, by a factor of 10, more frequent in patients with MEN1 than in patients with incidentally discovered adrenal tumors. In addition, ACCs were diagnosed in adrenal lesions of a rather small size. Interestingly, metastases of neuroendocrine pancreatic tumors were also detected, including 2 of somatostatinomas and 1 of a gastrinoma.

Concerning hormone excess, it was found that hypersecretion of aldosterone or cortisol was more prevalent in patients with MEN1—associated adrenal lesions as compared with patients with incidentally discovered adrenal masses. Furthermore, in 2 cases with MEN1—related ACC, hyperandrogenemia was detected. However, a substantial number of patients had insufficient endocrine evaluation for hormone excess and, strictly speaking, MEN1—associated adrenal lesions are no incidentalomas. Therefore, the increased prevalence of hormonal abnormalities in MEN1 patients may not be surprising.

Last but not least, discussion arose on the genotype—phenotype correlation, and it was suggested that mutations in exon 2 carried an increased risk for the development of adrenal tumors. This was not the case in this large case series.

H. S. Willenberg, MD

Combination Chemotherapy in Advanced Adrenocortical Carcinoma
Fassnacht M, for the FIRM-ACT Study Group (Univ Hosp, Würzburg, Germany)
N Engl J Med 366:2189-2197, 2012

Background.—Adrenocortical carcinoma is a rare cancer that has a poor response to cytotoxic treatment.

Methods.—We randomly assigned 304 patients with advanced adrenocortical carcinoma to receive mitotane plus either a combination of etoposide (100 mg per square meter of body-surface area on days 2 to 4), doxorubicin (40 mg per square meter on day 1), and cisplatin (40 mg per square meter on days 3 and 4) (EDP) every 4 weeks or streptozocin (streptozotocin) (1 g on days 1 to 5 in cycle 1; 2 g on day 1 in subsequent cycles) every 3 weeks. Patients with disease progression received the alternative regimen as second-line therapy. The primary end point was overall survival.

Results.—For first-line therapy, patients in the EDP—mitotane group had a significantly higher response rate than those in the streptozocin—mitotane group (23.2% vs. 9.2%, $P < 0.001$) and longer median progression-free survival (5.0 months vs. 2.1 months; hazard ratio, 0.55;

95% confidence interval [CI], 0.43 to 0.69; *P* < 0.001); there was no significant between-group difference in overall survival (14.8 months and 12.0 months, respectively; hazard ratio, 0.79; 95% CI, 0.61 to 1.02; *P* = 0.07). Among the 185 patients who received the alternative regimen as second-line therapy, the median duration of progression-free survival was 5.6 months in the EDP–mitotane group and 2.2 months in the streptozocin–mitotane group. Patients who did not receive the alternative second-line therapy had better overall survival with first-line EDP plus mitotane (17.1 month) than with streptozocin plus mitotane (4.7 months). Rates of serious adverse events did not differ significantly between treatments.

Conclusions.—Rates of response and progression-free survival were significantly better with EDP plus mitotane than with streptozocin plus mitotane as first-line therapy, with similar rates of toxic events, although there was no significant difference in overall survival. (Funded by the Swedish Research Council and others; FIRM-ACT ClinicalTrials.gov number, NCT00094497.)

▶ This article reports on the first international randomized trial in adrenocortical cancer treatment (FIRM-ACT), a disease with an estimated incidence of 0.7 to 2.0 cases per 1 million population per year. It is an example showing how observation of different approaches and deficits in patient care is followed by a meeting of specialists and how their analysis leads to a trial that provides evidence for best patient management.[1] Although it formally established a first choice protocol of chemotherapy, this trial reached much further than that.

As a side effect, other studies were stimulated, and it was discovered that mitotane, a compound used in this trial, induces CYP3A4.[2] Interestingly, both doxorubicin and etoposide, drugs also used in this trial, are metabolized by the CYP3A4 pathway, too. Therefore, it was actually not shown whether mitotane is really beneficial in this form of treatment.

However, in so many centers around the world, the FIRM-ACT trial helped to build structures, brought patients to centers, gave birth to standard operating procedures, sourced tissue to reference pathologists, and made pathologists work hand-in-hand with clinicians. This trial created an amazing structure for patient care that is good for further large trials in such a rare disease.

Thus, this trial educated a generation of doctors and provided them with certitude for the design of treatment protocols. And it provided patients and their families with hope.

H. S. Willenberg, MD

References

1. Schteingart DE, Doherty GM, Gauger PG, et al. Management of patients with adrenal cancer: recommendations of an international consensus conference. *Endocr Relat Cancer.* 2005;12:667-680.
2. van Erp NP, Guchelaar HJ, Ploeger BA, Romijn JA, Hartigh Jd, Gelderblom H. Mitotane has a strong and a durable inducing effect on CYP3A4 activity. *Eur J Endocrinol.* 2011;164:621-626.

Activation of Cyclic AMP Signaling Leads to Different Pathway Alterations in Lesions of the Adrenal Cortex Caused by Germline PRKAR1A Defects versus Those due to Somatic GNAS Mutations

Almeida MQ, Azevedo MF, Xekouki P, et al (Nat Insts of Health, Bethesda, MD; et al)
J Clin Endocrinol Metab 97:E687-E693, 2012

Context.—The overwhelming majority of benign lesions of the adrenal cortex leading to Cushing syndrome are linked to one or another abnormality of the cAMP or protein kinase pathway. *PRKAR1A*-inactivating mutations are responsible for primary pigmented nodular adrenocortical disease, whereas somatic *GNAS* activating mutations cause macronodular disease in the context of McCune-Albright syndrome, ACTH-independent macronodular hyperplasia, and, rarely, cortisol-producing adenomas.

Objective and Design.—The whole-genome expression profile (WGEP) of normal (pooled) adrenals, *PRKAR1A-* (3) and *GNAS*-mutant (3) was studied. Quantitative RT-PCR and Western blot were used to validate WGEP findings.

Results.—MAPK and p53 signaling pathways were highly overexpressed in all lesions against normal tissue. *GNAS*-mutant tissues were significantly enriched for extracellular matrix receptor interaction and focal adhesion pathways when compared with *PRKAR1A*-mutant (fold enrichment 3.5, $P < 0.0001$ and 2.1, $P < 0.002$, respectively). *NFKB, NFKBIA,* and *TNFRSF1A* were higher in *GNAS*-mutant tumors ($P < 0.05$). Genes related to the *Wnt* signaling pathway (*CCND1, CTNNB1, LEF1, LRP5, WISP1,* and *WNT3*) were overexpressed in *PRKAR1A*-mutant lesions.

Conclusion.—WGEP analysis revealed that not all cAMP activation is the same: adrenal lesions harboring *PRKAR1A* or *GNAS* mutations share the downstream activation of certain oncogenic signals (such as MAPK and some cell cycle genes) but differ substantially in their effects on others.

▶ The question of how an adrenal cell can (over) produce cortisol in the absence of its trophic stimulus has led scientists to look for autoantibodies to the corticotropin receptor, for mutations in the corticotropin receptor or in the stimulatory subunit of the G-protein, for membrane receptors that may substitute for the corticotropin receptor, for alterations in enzymes to inactivate cyclic AMP, and for alterations in the protein kinase A proteins.

Mutations in the *GNAS* and *PRKAR1A* genes were identified as the molecular basis for McCune-Albright syndrome and Carney's complex, respectively. Although the first disorder leads to macronodular adrenal disease, the latter results in micronodular adrenal disease, although the same signaling pathway is altered. This group asked whether different gene expression profiles may account for the differences in clinical parameters and morphology of the adrenal lesions.

And yes, they found a number of similarities and differences in gene expression patterns (eg, RAB13 and EPAC-2 were higher in GNAS-positive lesions because they are activated by a cAMP-dependent but protein kinase A—independent mechanism).

It will be interesting to learn if there are differences in adrenal lesions when they have their origin in the expression of an ectopic receptor or in a mutation in the *GNAS* gene (proximal part of the same signaling pathway). Similarly, it is worth studying the molecular differences between Carney lesions resulting from the mutations in the *PRKAR1A* gene or phosphodiesterase 11A/8B defects (rather distal part of the same signaling pathway).

H. S. Willenberg, MD

Serum inhibin pro-αC is a tumor marker for adrenocortical carcinomas
Hofland J, Feelders RA, van der Wal R, et al (Erasmus Med Ctr, Rotterdam, The Netherlands; et al)
Eur J Endocrinol 166:281-289, 2012

Objective.—The insufficient diagnostic accuracy for differentiation between benign and malignant adrenocortical disease and lack of sensitive markers reflecting tumor load emphasize the need for novel biomarkers for diagnosis and follow-up of adrenocortical carcinoma (ACC).

Design.—Since the inhibin α-subunit is expressed within the adrenal cortex, the role of serum inhibin pro-αC as a tumor marker for ACC was studied in patients.

Methods.—Regulation of adrenal pro-αC secretion was investigated by adrenocortical function tests. Serum inhibin pro-αC levels were measured in controls ($n = 181$) and patients with adrenocortical hyperplasia ($n = 45$), adrenocortical adenoma (ADA, $n = 32$), ACC ($n = 32$), or non-cortical tumors ($n = 12$). Steroid hormone, ACTH, and inhibin A and B levels were also estimated in patient subsets.

Results.—Serum inhibin pro-αC levels increased by 16% after stimulation with ACTH ($P = 0.043$). ACC patients had higher serum inhibin pro-αC levels than controls (medians 733 vs 307 ng/l, $P < 0.0001$) and patients with adrenocortical hyperplasia, ADA, or non-adrenocortical adrenal tumors (148, 208, and 131 ng/l, respectively, $P = 0.0003$). Inhibin pro-αC measurement in ACC patients had a sensitivity of 59% and specificity of 84% for differentiation from ADA patients. Receiver operating characteristic analysis displayed areas under the curve of 0.87 for ACC vs controls and 0.81 for ACC vs ADA ($P < 0.0001$). Surgery or mitotane therapy was followed by a decrease of inhibin pro-αC levels in 10/10 ACC patients tested during follow-up ($P = 0.0065$).

Conclusions.—Inhibin pro-αC is produced by the adrenal gland. Differentiation between ADA and ACC by serum inhibin pro-αC is limited, but its levels may constitute a novel tumor marker for ACC (Fig 3).

▶ As stated in the introduction, the availability of a tumor marker specific for adrenal cortical cancer would be most welcome. In a recent article by the same group, the involvement of activin-inhibin-system in adrenal gland physiology and proliferation had been reviewed.[1] Along these lines, the inhibin pro-αC fragment was thought to constitute a good candidate protein worth being evaluated

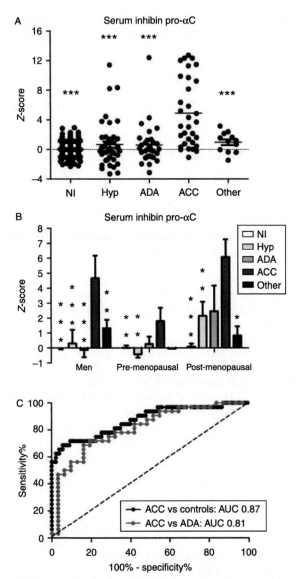

FIGURE 3.—Inhibin pro-αC levels after adjustment for gender and menopausal status. (A) Inhibin pro-αC levels after Z-score transformation in normal subjects (NI) and patients with adrenocortical hyperplasia (Hyp), adrenocortical adenoma (ADA), adrenocortical carcinoma (ACC), and non-cortical adrenal tumors (other). ***$P < 0.001$, compared with ACC. (B) Mean Z-scores of inhibin pro-αC levels, stratified by gender and menopausal status. ***$P < 0.001$, **$P < 0.01$, and *$P < 0.05$, compared with ACC. (C) ROC analysis of Z-scores of serum inhibin pro-αC levels. Patients with ACC ($n = 32$) were compared with control subjects ($n = 178$) or patients with ADA ($n = 32$). (Reprinted by permission from Macmillan Publishers Ltd: European Journal of Endocrinology. Hofland J, Feelders RA, van der Wal R, et al. Serum inhibin pro-αC is a tumor marker for adrenocortical carcinomas. *Eur J Endocrinol.* 2012;166:281-289, Copyright, 2012.)

along with other inhibins and markers of steroidogenesis, including cortisol after dexamethasone, sulfated DHEA, 11-deoxycortisol, and others.

Hofland et al were able to show that inhibin pro-αC levels were significantly higher in adrenocortical carcinoma patients as compared with patients with an adrenal adenoma, adrenal hyperplasia, or adrenal tumors of other histology (Fig 3). Nevertheless, the overlap between patients with adrenal cancers and other disease was high enough to reduce sensitivity and specificity substantially (Fig 3). Therefore, a prospective study will be necessary to show relapse or persistence of adrenal cortical cancer during clinical follow-up—after surgery, for example. In addition, this marker needs to be tested against urinary steroid profiling that seems to perform better, as recently documented by Arlt et al.[2]

H. S. Willenberg, MD

References

1. Hofland J, de Jong FH. Inhibins and activins: their roles in the adrenal gland and the development of adrenocortical tumors. *Mol Cell Endocrinol.* 2012;359: 92-100.
2. Arlt W, Biehl M, Taylor AE, et al. Urine steroid metabolomics as a biomarker tool for detecting malignancy in adrenal tumors. *J Clin Endocrinol Metab.* 2011;96: 3775-3784.

CT features and quantification of the characteristics of adrenocortical carcinomas on unenhanced and contrast-enhanced studies
Zhang HM, Perrier ND, Grubbs EG, et al (The Univ of Texas MD Anderson Cancer Ctr, Houston)
Clin Radiol 67:38-46, 2012

Aim.—To describe the morphological and contrast-agent washout characteristics of adrenocortical carcinomas (ACCs) on computed tomography (CT).

Materials and Methods.—Forty-one patients with histopathologically proven ACCs were retrospectively evaluated. The morphological characteristics of the ACCs were documented and compared with surgical and histopathological findings. The percentage of contrast agent enhancement washout (PEW) and relative PEW (RPEW) were calculated for 17 patients who had the combination of unenhanced, portal venous, and 15 min delayed phase images.

Results.—Characteristic imaging findings of ACCs included large size (38 of 41 tumours were >6 cm), well-defined margin with a thin enhancing rim (25 patients), and central stellate area of low attenuation on contrast-enhanced CT images (21 patients). Tumour extension into the inferior vena cava (IVC) with associated thrombus was identified on CT in six (14.6%) patients. Of 17 tumours evaluated, 12 (71%) had a PEW value of ≤60%, and 14 (82%) had an RPEW value of ≤40%.

Conclusion.—Large size, a well-defined margin with a thin enhancing rim, central low attenuation, and a predilection for extension into the IVC

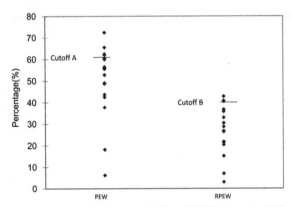

FIGURE 7.—Scatter-plot shows distribution of PEW and RPEW values for ACCs. "Cut-off A" is 60% and "cut-off B" is 40%, which are the PEW or RPEW thresholds commonly used in previous studies for distinguishing between adrenal adenomas and non-adenomas.[11-13] *Editor's Note*: Please refer to original journal article for full references. (Reprinted from Clinical Radiology. Zhang HM, Perrier ND, Grubbs EG, et al. CT features and quantification of the characteristics of adrenocortical carcinomas on unenhanced and contrast-enhanced studies. *Clin Radiol.* 2012;67:38-46, Copyright 2012, with permission from the Royal College of Radiologists.)

are typical morphological characteristics of ACC on CT. The contrast-washout characteristics of ACCs, in concordance with their malignant nature, share those of non-adenomas rather than adenomas (Fig 7).

▶ The next steps after the incidental discovery of an adrenal tumor on imaging studies frequently includes contrast-enhanced imaging studies. This is because the demonstration of a lipid-rich adrenal tumor with typical washout characteristics of contrast material is solid proof of an adrenal adenoma. However, in the majority of the studies, adrenal cortical adenomas are compared with metastasis to the adrenal gland and/or pheochromocytomas. But frequently, the question is whether the adrenal cortical tumor is a benign (adenoma) or malignant (carcinoma) lesion.

Zhang et al were able to analyze the radiological data of 41 patients with histo-pathologically proven adrenocortical carcinoma's. They found that 7% of the tumors were smaller than 6 cm, that a quarter of tumors were round or oval, and that three-quarters had well-defined margins. Although there were few foci with mature fat, malignant adrenocortical tumors showed unenhanced Houns-field units and contrast material washout characteristics of metastasis (Fig 7). Other features, including calcifications, lymphadenopathy, infiltration, or distant metastasis, were present in the minority of tumors.

This study is quite valuable because past studies have included a relatively small number of patients with adrenal carcinoma only.

H. S. Willenberg, MD

Cushing's Disease: Diagnosis and Treatment

[131I]Iodometomidate for Targeted Radionuclide Therapy of Advanced Adrenocortical Carcinoma
Hahner S, Kreissl MC, Fassnacht M, et al (Univ of Wuerzburg, Germany)
J Clin Endocrinol Metab 97:914-922, 2012

Context.—In advanced adrenocortical carcinoma (ACC), many patients have progressive disease despite standard treatment, indicating a need for new treatment options. We have shown high and specific retention of [123I]metomidate ([123I]IMTO) in ACC lesions, suggesting that labeling of metomidate with 131I offers targeted radionuclide therapy for advanced ACC.

Objective.—Safety and efficacy of radionuclide therapy with [131I] IMTO in advanced ACC.

Design/Setting.—This monocentric case series comprised 19 treatments in 11 patients with nonresectable ACC.

Patients and Intervention.—Between 2007 and 2010, patients with advanced ACC not amenable to radical surgery and exhibiting high uptake of [123I]IMTO in their tumor lesions were offered treatment with [131I] IMTO (1.6—20 GBq in one to three cycles of [131I]IMTO).

Main Outcome Measure.—Tumor response was assessed according to response evaluation criteria in solid tumors (RECIST version 1.1) criteria, and side effects were assessed by Common Toxicity Criteria (version 4.0).

Results.—Best response was classified as partial response in one case with a change in target lesions of −51% from baseline, as stable disease in five patients, and as progressive disease in four patients. One patient died 11 d after treatment with [131I]IMTO unrelated to radionuclide therapy. In patients responding to treatment, median progression-free survival was 14 months (range, 5—33) with ongoing disease stabilization in three patients at last follow-up. Treatment was well tolerated, but transient bone marrow depression was observed. Adrenal insufficiency developed in two patients.

Conclusions.—Radionuclide therapy with [131I]IMTO is a promising treatment option for selected patients with ACC, deserving evaluation in prospective clinical trials.

▶ Etomidate (and its derivate metomidate) was shown to have a strong affinity to 11beta-hydroxylase and can be used to label adrenocortical cells, including adrenocortical cancer (ACC).[1,2] Although this phenomenon is exploited for diagnostic purposes in 11C-metomidate positron emission tomography computed tomographies, this is the first study to investigate the therapeutic potential of metomidate linked to 131-iodine ([131I]IMTO).

Forty-nine patients with nonresectable ACC lesions were evaluated by [123I] IMTO single-photon emission computed tomography and were picked for a trial with [131I]IMTO when they showed high tracer uptake. Of them, 11 entered the study and 10 had complete data sets. The figure that was taken from the article shows partial response or stable disease in the majority of patients with few side effects. This is an impressive result because most of the patients underwent multiple therapies and surgical interventions before treatment with [^{131}I]IMTO. Also, the median of progression-free survival was greater than 1 year! In addition, 3 patients showed a durable stabilization in disease progression.

However, little more than one-sixth of the patients initially screened for this study carried a benefit from the treatment option with [^{131}I]IMTO, and further efforts of this kind are needed to meet the hopes of ACC patients. As a casual note, it may be interesting to study the causes why the majority of ACCs are not metomidate avid.

H. S. Willenberg, MD

References

1. de Jong FH, Mallios C, Jansen C, Scheck PA, Lamberts SW. Etomidate suppresses adrenocortical function by inhibition of 11 beta-hydroxylation. *J Clin Endocrinol Metab.* 1984;59:1143-1147.
2. Bergström M, Bonasera TA, Lu L, et al. In vitro and in vivo primate evaluation of carbon-11-etomidate and carbon-11-metomidate as potential tracers for PET imaging of the adrenal cortex and its tumors. *J Nucl Med.* 1998;39:982-989.

Primary Aldosteronism

KCNJ5 Mutations in European Families With Nonglucocorticoid Remediable Familial Hyperaldosteronism

Mulatero P, Tauber P, Zennaro MC, et al (Univ of Torino, Italy; Univ Regensburg, Germany; Paris Cardiovascular Res Ctr, France; et al)
Hypertension 59:235-240, 2012

Primary aldosteronism is the most frequent cause of endocrine hypertension. Three forms of familial hyperaldosteronism (FH) have been described, named FH-I to -III. Recently, a mutation of *KCNJ5* has been shown to be associated with FH-III, whereas the cause of FH-II is still unknown. In this study we searched for mutations in *KCNJ5* in 46 patients from 21 families with FH, in which FH-I was excluded. We identified a new germline G151E mutation in 2 primary aldosteronism—affected subjects from an Italian family and 3 somatic mutations in aldosterone-producing adenomas, T158A described previously as a germline mutation associated with FH-III, and G151R and L168R both described as somatic mutations in aldosterone-producing adenoma. The phenotype of the family with the G151E mutation was remarkably milder compared with the previously described American family, in terms of both clinical and biochemical parameters. Furthermore, patients with somatic *KCNJ5* mutations displayed a phenotype indistinguishable from that of sporadic primary aldosteronism. The functional characterization of the effects of the G151E mutation in vitro showed a profound alteration of the channel function, with loss of K$^+$ selectivity, Na$^+$ influx, and membrane depolarization. These alterations have been postulated to be responsible for voltage gate Ca^{2+} channel activation, increase in cytosolic calcium, and stimulation of aldosterone production and adrenal cell proliferation. In conclusion, we describe herein a new mutation in the KCNJ5 potassium channel associated with FH-III, responsible for marked alterations of channel function but associated with a mild clinical and hormonal phenotype.

▶ The discovery of mutations in the potassium channel KCNJ5 in patients with familial and sporadic forms of primary aldosteronism by the group of R. Lifton,[1] Yale, was a starter's gun for several consortia to study other families and patients with spontaneous forms of primary aldosteronism.

The contest brought scientists from all over the world together; inspired them to clone and mutate genes, establish assays, and perform functional experiments; passed them to different research journals along with their reviewers; and made them arrive with publications in early 2012, less than 1 year after the original report.[2-5] The competition was won by the European Network for the Study of Adrenal Tumors led by Paolo Mulatero, whose contribution showed that families believed to be affected by a polygenetic form of familial aldosteronism (type 2) may, in fact, have mutations in the KCNJ5 gene, sufficient to cause monogenetic disease.

However, the work of all consortia contributed to our conception about the clinical nature and frequency of KCNJ5 mutations in patients with primary aldosteronism. Soon, there may be substances available to target this potassium channel and come along with clinical studies that may lead to new diagnostic and treatment strategies for a subset of patients with primary aldosteronism.

H. S. Willenberg, MD

References

1. Choi M, Scholl UI, Yue P, et al. K+ channel mutations in adrenal aldosterone-producing adenomas and hereditary hypertension. *Science.* 2011;331:768-772.
2. Azizan EA, Murthy M, Stowasser M, et al. Somatic mutations affecting the selectivity filter of KCNJ5 are frequent in 2 large unselected collections of adrenal aldosteronomas. *Hypertension.* 2012;59:587-591.
3. Boulkroun S, Beuschlein F, Rossi GP, et al. Prevalence, clinical, and molecular correlates of KCNJ5 mutations in primary aldosteronism. *Hypertension.* 2012; 59:592-598.
4. Scholl UI, Nelson-Williams C, Yue P, et al. Hypertension with or without adrenal hyperplasia due to different inherited mutations in the potassium channel KCNJ5. *Proc Natl Acad Sci U S A.* 2012;109:2533-2538.
5. Åkerström T, Crona J, Delgado Verdugo A, et al. Comprehensive re-sequencing of adrenal aldosterone producing lesions reveal three somatic mutations near the KCNJ5 potassium channel selectivity filter. *PLoS One.* 2012;7:e41926.

Evaluation of the Sensitivity and Specificity of ^{11}C-Metomidate Positron Emission Tomography (PET)-CT for Lateralizing Aldosterone Secretion by Conn's Adenomas

Burton TJ, Mackenzie IS, Balan K, et al (Univ of Cambridge, UK; Addenbrooke's Hosp, Cambridge, UK)

J Clin Endocrinol Metab 97:100-109, 2012

Context.—Identification of unilateral aldosterone-producing (Conn's) adenomas has traditionally required lateralization by the invasive and technically difficult procedure of adrenal vein sampling (AVS). ^{11}C-metomidate, a potent inhibitor of adrenal steroidogenic enzymes, is a positron emission tomography (PET) radiotracer that is selectively accumulated by Conn's adenomas.

Objective.—The objective of the study was to compare the sensitivity and specificity of ^{11}C-metomidate PET-computed tomography (CT) against the current gold standard of AVS.

Design.—The design of the study was within-patient comparison of diagnostic techniques.

Setting.—The study was conducted at a single center-university teaching hospital.

Patients.—Thirty-nine patients with primary hyperaldosteronism (PHA) and five with nonfunctioning adenomas (incidentalomas) participated in the study.

Intervention(s).—The first six PHA patients were studied on three occasions to determine whether steroid pretreatment reduced ^{11}C-metomidate uptake by normal adrenal. Subsequent patients received dexamethasone for 3 d prior to injection of ^{11}C-metomidate 150−500 MBq.

Main Outcome Measure(s).—Maximum standardized uptake values (SUV$_{max}$) over regions of interest determined from 35−45 min after injection were measured.

Results.—Dexamethasone increased tumor to normal adrenal SUV$_{max}$ ratio by $25.6 \pm 5.0\% (P < 0.01)$. PET-CT visualized subcentimeter adenomas and distinguished hot from cold adenomas within a gland. In 25 patients with PHA and AVS lateralization to the side of an adenoma, SUV$_{max}$ overtumor (mean ± SEM) of 21.7 ± 1.6 was greater than over normal adrenal, 13.8 ± 0.6 ($P = 0.00003$); this difference was absent in 10 patients without lateralization on AVS ($P = 0.28$) and in four of five incidentalomas. On receiver-operator characteristics analysis, an SUV$_{max}$ ratio of 1.25:1 provided a specificity of 87% [95% confidence interval (69, 104)] and sensitivity of 76% (59, 93); in tumors with SUV$_{max}$ greater than 17, the specificity rose to 100%.

Conclusions.—[11]C-metomidate PET-CT is a sensitive and specific noninvasive alternative to AVS in the management of PHA.

▶ Adrenal venous sampling (AVS) is an invasive technique that may help to localize the source of aldosterone excess. It is recommended as the technique of choice to distinguish between unilateral or bilateral disease in primary aldosteronism, although it is cost-intensive (time and personal) and not necessarily successful. In addition, although there is vast clinical experience with this method, current calculation models are not substantiated by good arithmetic and data. Therefore, other techniques are most welcome to help with identifying the source of excess aldosterone secretion.

Etomidate was shown to have a strong affinity to steroidogenic enzymes that are of functional relevance,[1] and other groups developed this principle for use in positron emission tomography (PET) scans.[2,3] This study was performed to test ^{11}C-metomidate PET against AVS. This comparison is the major strength of this study. Burton et al found that ^{11}C-metomidate PET imaging was able to discriminate between unilateral or bilateral disease in the same way AVS did. Moreover, this functional ^{11}C-metomidate PET computed tomography (CT) seems to be even more sensitive because it picked up cases with aldosterone-producing adenomas in 1 adrenal, whereas AVS did not show lateralization. In addition, the authors, who state that medication interfering with AVS studies does not seem to play a major role, provided pretreatment with dexamethasone, and they also refer to spironolactone. However, concerning renin values, only a small number of patients received adequate antimineralocorticoid treatment. And only 1 patient with adequate control of mineralocorticoid excess was operated on. In fact, the authors defined patients as being true negative on metomidate PET-CT and AVS who actually may have restored aldosterone synthase activity in the normal tissue resulting from high renin (and angiotensin) values.

Nonetheless, this study seems to bring functional imaging for primary hyperaldosteronism very close to clinical routine. Patients and doctors will benefit from this approach.

H. S. Willenberg, MD

References

1. de Jong FH, Mallios C, Jansen C, Scheck PA, Lamberts SW. Etomidate suppresses adrenocortical function by inhibition of 11 beta-hydroxylation. *J Clin Endocrinol Metab.* 1984;59:1143-1147.
2. Bergström M, Bonasera TA, Lu L, et al. In vitro and in vivo primate evaluation of carbon-11-etomidate and carbon-11-metomidate as potential tracers for PET imaging of the adrenal cortex and its tumors. *J Nucl Med.* 1998;39:982-989.
3. Hennings J, Sundin A, Hägg A, Hellman P. 11C-metomidate positron emission tomography after dexamethasone suppression for detection of small adrenocortical adenomas in primary aldosteronism. *Langenbecks Arch Surg.* 2010;395:963-967.

Pattern of Adrenal Hormonal Secretion in Patients with Adrenal Adenomas: The Relevance of Aldosterone in Arterial Hypertension
Pappa T, Papanastasiou L, Kaltsas G, et al ("G Gennimatas" General Hosp, Athens, Greece; Natl Univ of Athens, Greece)
J Clin Endocrinol Metab 97:E537-E545, 2012

Context.—Approximately 10% of hypertensives are considered to exhibit autonomous aldosterone secretion (AAS). Although adrenal incidentalomas (AI) can be found in up to 19% of hypertensive individuals, data on the incidence of AAS in hypertensive patients with AI remain scarce.

Objective.—The aim was to study adrenal aldosterone (ALD) secretory pattern in patients with adrenal adenomas with and without arterial hypertension.

Design and Setting.—We conducted a case-control study in a tertiary general hospital.

Patients and Main Outcome Measures.—We investigated 72 normotensive subjects with normal adrenal morphology and 191 subjects divided in three groups: 46 normotensive individuals with an AI (NAI), 89 hypertensive patients with an AI (HAI), and 56 hypertensive patients with an adrenal adenoma identified after investigation for arterial hypertension (HAA). Evaluation of autonomous cortisol secretion was based on a low-dose dexamethasone suppression test. Autonomous ALD secretion was based on a modified saline infusion test (MSI). Normal cutoff levels were obtained from the control matched population.

Results.—Post-MSI ALD levels and the ALD/renin (REN) ratios were significantly elevated in HAI and HAA patients compared to NAI subjects. To evaluate the prevalence of AAS, we applied the combination of post-MSI ALD level and the ALD/REN ratio simultaneously (post-MSI cutoffs, ALD levels, 2.41 ng/dl; ALD/REN ratio, 0.35 ng/dl/μU/ml). Based on these cutoffs, 12% of NAI, 36.4% of HAI, and 54.2% of HAA patients had AAS. The prevalence of autonomous cortisol secretion did not differ among the three groups.

Conclusions.—Using a MSI test, we found a remarkably increased prevalence of AAS in hypertensive patients with adrenal adenomas, even when the latter represented an incidental finding.

▶ This group wanted to see whether hypertension is associated with autonomous aldosterone secretion in patients with an incidentally discovered adrenal adenoma. For comparison, they also tested patients with an incidentally discovered adrenal adenoma who did not have hypertension. However, the approach of this group is very noteworthy.

To exclude the influence of corticotropin on aldosterone secretion, cortisol is to be measured in patients subjected to the saline infusion test (SIT).[1] However, there are no data to guide interpretation of cortisol values during the SIT. Here, dexamethasone was given to patients beforehand (8 doses of 0.5 mg dexamethasone every 6 hours). This test was evaluated in normotensive individuals who did not have an adrenal tumor and a cut-off value for aldosterone after the test that was shown to be lower than proposed by an international guideline.[1] Interestingly, lower cut-off levels for aldosterone after SIT were also proposed by another group[2] and proposed for the fludrocortisone suppression test when it is combined with low-dose dexamethasone the evening before blood is drawn.[3] Thus, the approach of Pappa et al led to a more sensitive method in picking up autonomous aldosterone secretion.

To substantiate their findings, the authors treated patients who had autonomous aldosterone secretion with antimineralocorticoid drugs and showed a decline in blood pressure. However, they did not go so far as to demonstrate lateralized aldosterone secretion using adrenal venous sampling. The chances for picking up lateralization would have been good because every study patient had an adrenal tumor. In addition, autonomous aldosterone secretion was also found in 12% of normotensive patients with an incidentally discovered adrenal adenoma. So, the authors actually did not prove that the hypertension in such patients is caused by autonomous aldosterone secretion.

However, the authors were successful in developing a new sensitive test (that needs to be evaluated by different groups), and they showed that it is more likely to see autonomous aldosterone secretion in patients with an incidentally discovered adrenal adenoma and in patients who come for the evaluation of hypertension and have an adrenal adenoma.

H. S. Willenberg, MD

References

1. Funder JW, Carey RM, Fardella C, et al. Case detection, diagnosis, and treatment of patients with primary aldosteronism: an endocrine society clinical practice guideline. *J Clin Endocrinol Metab.* 2008;93:3266-3281.
2. Gouli A, Kaltsas G, Tzonou A, et al. High prevalence of autonomous aldosterone secretion among patients with essential hypertension. *Eur J Clin Invest.* 2011;41: 1227-1236.
3. Willenberg HS, Vonend O, Schott M, et al. Comparison of the saline infusion test and the fludrocortisone suppression test for the diagnosis of primary aldosteronism. *Horm Metab Res.* 2012;44:527-532.

7 Reproductive Endocrinology

Introduction

This year's selections include many citations related to pediatric endocrinology, hormonal action of estrogen and androgens, menopause, the influence of hormones on bone metabolism, polycystic ovary syndrome, aging, hypogonadism in men, and male hormone contraception.

PEDIATRICS

Pediatric reproductive endocrinology includes a manuscript by Harrington and Palmert, and they have established criteria for distinguishing between constitutional delay of growth and pubertal delay from isolated hypogonadotrophic hypogonadism.

REPRODUCTIVE FUNCTION IN FEMALES

Diaz et al report on Ethinyl estradiol-cyproterone acetate vs low-dose pioglitazone-flutamide-metformin for girls with androgen excess. They observed that these two methods of therapy produce comparable effects on androgens over one year of treatment. They differed in reversing inflammation, metabolic, and cardiovascular anomalies.

Administration of Kisspeptin might be an alternative therapeutic approach to restore fertility of hyperprolactinemic women who are intolerant to dopamine agonists as reported by Sonigo et al.

The hormonal effects of dehydroepiandrosterone-sulfate on various parameters have been studied, and the study by Gomez-Santos reports that DHEAS is useful for weight loss in obese post-menopausal women.

Grynber et al reported on the differential regulation of ovarian anti-mullerian hormone by estradiol through α and β estrogen receptors, and they observed that estradiol repressed the antil-mullerian hormone messenger RNAs in human granulosa cells which expressed a little more ERα and ERβ mRNA.

MENOPAUSE

The study by Wildman et al reported on whether sex hormone changes precede or follow an increase in body weight. They observed that the changes in body weight preceded the changes in sex hormones, rather than vice versa.

BONE HEALTH

The association of concurrent vitamin D and sex hormone deficiency with bone loss and fracture risk in men was associated with low vitamin D and low biological estradiol in association with high sex hormone binding globulin. This combination increased the risk of osteoporotic fractures in men in the aging study (Barrett-Connor et al).

POLYCYSTIC OVARIAN SYNDROME

A multicenter study Morin-Papunen et al evaluated whether Metformin improves pregnancy and live birth rates in women with polycystic ovary syndrome. They observed that Metformin was beneficial related to these parameters.

The evaluation of the insulin resistance in women with polycystic syndrome has been a matter of evaluation for many years. The study by Comerford et al observed that lean body mass and insulin resistance were associated in women with polycystic ovary syndrome rather than a degree of obesity, which is a little surprising.

Polycystic Ovary-Like Abnormalities have been observed in women with functional hypothalamic amenorrhea. Robin et al point out that it is important to make this distinction as we evaluate women with polycystic syndrome and sometimes misdiagnose them as having hypothalamic amenorrhea.

A genetic pattern for polycystic ovary syndrome has been sought for many years. Mutharasan et al did a fine mapping of chromosome 2p16.3 in Chinese polycystic ovary syndrome susceptibility locus. They observed two independent loci, the LH chorionic gonadotropin receptor, and the follicle-stimulating hormone receptor, that are likely to be important in the etiology of polycystic ovary syndrome regardless of ethnicity.

Microarray has become a popular technique for analyzing various gene disorders. This study by Kaur et al reports on the differential expression on granulosa cells with and without insulin resistance in identifying susceptibility genes through this network for linkage to diabetes mellitus, inflammation, cardiovascular disease, and infertility.

Fulghesu et al evaluated whether there is a dose response differential in women with polycystic ovary syndrome when treated with Metformin. Metformin dose was independent in their study.

HYPOGONADISM

Moskovic et al report that Clomiphene citrate is safe and effective for long-term management of hypogonadism and while this may be true for control of hypogonadism, careful study of the effects on bone would be very important during long-term in treatment with Clomiphene citrate.

Maiburg et al evaluated the genetic origin of Klinefelter syndrome and its effect on spermatogenesis.

Gregoriou et al evaluated the changes in hormonal profile and seminal parameters in men with the use of aromatase inhibitors, and they were able to observe that therapy increased fertility as well as testosterone to estradiol ratios. Aromatose inhibitors may be another method of treatment of men for hypogonadism to make them fertile and also to correct their testosterone levels.

Relating work stress on testosterone deficiency and andropause symptoms was evaluated by Hirokawa et al, and they observed that men with low testosterone levels had more psychological andropause symptoms than those with high levels.

CHORIONIC GONADAL DYSFUNCTION

Zacharin et al report on the recombinant follicle-stimulating hormone to human chorionic gonadotropin treatment in adolescents and young men with hypogonatropic hypogonadism, and they observed that this treatment was successful in normalizing testicular growth and improving spermatogenesis.

CONTRACEPTION IN MEN

There has long been an interest in male hormonal reversible contraception, and it has been studied by Ilani et al using the combination of testosterone and nestorone transdermal gels. The combination therapy was successful in reducing sperm concentration to less than one million per ml in 88.5% of men with minimal adverse effects from the therapy.

A. Wayne Meikle, MD

Bone Health in Men

The Association of Concurrent Vitamin D and Sex Hormone Deficiency With Bone Loss and Fracture Risk in Older Men: The Osteoporotic Fractures in Men (MrOS) Study
Barrett-Connor E, for the Osteoporotic Fractures in Men (MrOS) Research Group (Univ of California, San Diego; et al)
J Bone Miner Res 27:2306-2313, 2012

Low 25-hydroxyvitamin D (VitD), low sex hormones (SH), and high sex hormone binding globulin (SHBG) levels are common in older men. We tested the hypothesis that combinations of low VitD, low SH, and high SHBG would have a synergistic effect on bone mineral density (BMD), bone loss, and fracture risk in older men. Participants were a random subsample of 1468 men (mean age 74 years) from the Osteoporotic Fractures in Men Study (MrOS) plus 278 MrOS men with incident nonspine fractures studied in a case-cohort design. "Abnormal" was defined as lowest quartile for VitD (<20 ng/mL), bioavailable testosterone (BioT, <163 ng/dL), and bioavailable estradiol (BioE, <11 pg/mL); and highest quartile for SHBG (>59 nM). Overall, 10% had isolated VitD deficiency; 40% had only low SH or high SHBG; 15% had both SH/SHBG and VitD

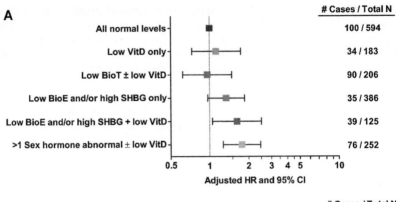

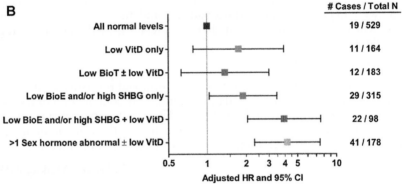

FIGURE 3.—Risk of nonspine fracture (*A*) and major osteoporotic fracture (*B*) by sex hormone/VitD groups: case-cohort sample. Adjusted for age, race, latitude of study site, season of blood draw, BMI, ever smoked, alcohol drinks per week, self-rated health condition, PASE score, kidney function (eGFR), and history of diabetes. VitD = vitamin D; BioE = bioavailable estradiol; BioT = bioavailable testosterone; SH = sex hormone. The proportion of men in each group was 34% normal, 11% low VitD only, 12% low BioT ± low VitD, 22% low BioE and/or high SHBG only, 7% low BioE and/or high SHBG + low VitD, and 14% >1 SH abnormality ± low VitD. (Reproduced from Journal of Bone and Mineral Research. Barrett-Connor E, for the Osteoporotic Fractures in Men (MrOS) Research Group. The association of concurrent vitamin D and sex hormone deficiency with bone loss and fracture risk in older men: the osteoporotic fractures in men (MrOS) study. *J Bone Miner Res.* 2012;27:2306-2313, with permission from the American Society for Bone and Mineral Research.)

abnormality; and 35% had no abnormality. Compared to men with all normal levels, those with both SH/SHBG and VitD abnormality tended to be older, more obese, and to report less physical activity. Isolated VitD deficiency, and low BioT with or without low VitD, was not significantly related to skeletal measures. The combination of VitD deficiency with low BioE and/or high SHBG was associated with significantly lower baseline BMD and higher annualized rates of hip bone loss than SH abnormalities alone or no abnormality. Compared to men with all normal levels, the multivariate-adjusted hazard ratio (95% confidence interval [CI]) for incident nonspine fracture during 4.6-year median follow-up was 1.2 (0.8–1.8) for low VitD alone; 1.3 (0.9–1.9) for low BioE and/or high

SHBG alone; and 1.6 (1.1–2.5) for low BioE/high SHBG plus low VitD. In summary, adverse skeletal effects of low sex steroid levels were more pronounced in older men with low VitD levels. The presence of low VitD in the presence of low BioE/high SHBG may contribute substantially to poor skeletal health (Fig 3).

▶ 25-Hydroxyvitamin D (25[OH]D) concentrations in serum < 20 ng/dL are observed commonly in elderly men. 25(OH)D contributes to bone health and could be a factor in hip fractures and bone loss in aging men. Although endogenous sex hormone declines in aging men, sex hormone binding globulin rises and affects free testosterone more than the total concentration. Estradiol is a better predictor of bone health in these men than androgens. In the Osteoporotic Fractures in Men Study of men with bone loss and fractures, the association of 25(OH)D, sex hormone, and osteoporotic fractures was investigated by Barrett-Connor et al. The combination of low 25(OH)D, low bio-estradiol, and high sex hormone–binding globulin were particularly deleterious to skeletal health. They found that more than 40% of older men with this combination of abnormalities exhibited higher rates of bone loss. An important finding was that 25(OH)D deficiency was only apparent in those men with low estradiol or high sex hormone–binding globulin. This study provides an impetus for further study and therapy to correct skeletal bone loss and fractures in older men.[1-5]

A. W. Meikle, MD

References

1. Barrett-Connor E, Laughlin GA, Li H, et al. The association of concurrent vitamin D and sex hormone deficiency with bone loss and fracture risk in older men: the osteoporotic fractures in men (MrOS) study. *J Bone Miner Res.* 2012;27: 2306-2313.
2. Blain H, Jaussent A, Thomas E, et al. Appendicular skeletal muscle mass is the strongest independent factor associated with femoral neck bone mineral density in adult and older men. *Exp Gerontol.* 2010;45:679-684.
3. Szulc P, Munoz F, Marchand F, Chapurlat R, Delmas PD. Rapid loss of appendicular skeletal muscle mass is associated with higher all-cause mortality in older men: the prospective MINOS study. *Am J Clin Nutr.* 2010;91:1227-1236.
4. Iannuzzi-Sucich M, Prestwood KM, Kenny AM. Prevalence of sarcopenia and predictors of skeletal muscle mass in healthy, older men and women. *J Gerontol A Biol Sci Med Sci.* 2002;57:M772-M777.
5. Taxel P, Fall PM, Albertsen PC, et al. The effect of micronized estradiol on bone turnover and calciotropic hormones in older men receiving hormonal suppression therapy for prostate cancer. *J Clin Endocrinol Metab.* 2002;87: 4907-4913.

Female Reproductive Function

Do Changes in Sex Steroid Hormones Precede or Follow Increases in Body Weight during the Menopause Transition? Results from The Study of Women's Health Across the Nation

Wildman RP, Tepper PG, Crawford S, et al (Albert Einstein College of Medicine, Bronx, NY; Univ of Pittsburgh Graduate School of Public Health, PA; Univ of Massachusetts, Worcester; et al)

J Clin Endocrinol Metab 97:E1695-E1704, 2012

Context.—Whether menopause-related changes in sex steroids account for midlife weight gain in women or whether weight drives changes in sex steroids remains unanswered.

Objective.—The objective of the study was to characterize the potential reciprocal nature of the associations between sex hormones and their binding protein with waist circumference in midlife women.

Design, Setting, and Participants.—The study included 1528 women (mean age 46 yr) with 9 yr of follow-up across the menopause transition from the observational Study of Women's Health Across the Nation.

Main Outcome Measures.—Waist circumference, SHBG, testosterone, FSH, and estradiol were measured.

Results.—Current waist circumference predicted future SHBG, testosterone, and FSH but not vice versa. For each SD higher current waist circumference, at the subsequent visit SHBG was lower by 0.04–0.15 SD, testosterone was higher by 0.08–0.13 SD, and $\log^2$ FSH was lower by 0.15–0.26 SD. Estradiol results were distinct from those above, changing direction across the menopause transition. Estradiol and waist circumference were negatively associated in early menopausal transition stages and positively associated in later transition stages (for each SD higher current waist circumference, future estradiol was lower by 0.15 SD in pre- and early perimenopause and higher by 0.38 SD in late peri- and postmenopause; *P* for interaction <0.001). In addition, they appeared to be reciprocal, with current waist circumference associated with future estradiol and current estradiol associated with future waist circumference. However, associations in the direction of current waist circumference predicting future estradiol levels were of considerably larger magnitude than the reverse.

Conclusions.—These Study of Women's Health Across the Nation data suggest that the predominant temporal sequence is that weight gain leads to changes in sex steroids rather than vice versa.

▶ It is well established that obesity becomes more prevalent in middle age. Wildman et al sought to determine if changes in sex steroid hormone antedate or follow increases in body weight during menopause. They considered potential causes such as aging and menopause transition. Obesity increases the risk of diabetes, cardiovascular disease, and certain cancers. They evaluated several models, but they concluded that there was a unidirectional relationship between waist circumference and body weight with sex hormone binding globulin (SHBG), testosterone, and follicle-stimulating hormone. Conversely, the relationship between waist girth and estradiol appeared to be bidirectional, indicating that estradiol concentrations might lead to changes in adiposity and adiposity might lead to changes in estradiol concentrations. Greater girth and weight predicted higher serum concentrations of testosterone. One postulation for the results was that low SHBG in obese women results in higher serum clearance of estradiol and lower circulating concentrations. The study has limitations in that the parameters selected might not have been the best and free hormone concentrations were not evaluated.[1-3]

A. W. Meikle, MD

References

1. Pasquali R. The hypothalamic-pituitary-adrenal axis and sex hormones in chronic stress and obesity: pathophysiological and clinical aspects. *Ann N Y Acad Sci.* 2012;1264:20-35.
2. Gambineri A, Tomassoni F, Munarini A, et al. A combination of polymorphisms in HSD11B1 associates with in vivo 11{beta}-HSD1 activity and metabolic syndrome in women with and without polycystic ovary syndrome. *Eur J Endocrinol.* 2011; 165:283-292.
3. Vicennati V, Pasqui F, Cavazza C, Pagotto U, Pasquali R. Stress-related development of obesity and cortisol in women. *Obesity (Silver Spring).* 2009;17:1678-1683.

Hyperprolactinemia-induced ovarian acyclicity is reversed by kisspeptin administration

Sonigo C, Bouilly J, Carré N, et al (Université Paris-Sud, France; et al)
J Clin Invest 122:3791-3795, 2012

Hyperprolactinemia is the most common cause of hypogonadotropic anovulation and is one of the leading causes of infertility in women aged 25—34. Hyperprolactinemia has been proposed to block ovulation through inhibition of GnRH release. Kisspeptin neurons, which express prolactin receptors, were recently identified as major regulators of GnRH neurons. To mimic the human pathology of anovulation, we continuously infused female mice with prolactin. Our studies demonstrated that hyperprolactinemia in mice induced anovulation, reduced GnRH and gonadotropin secretion, and diminished kisspeptin expression. Kisspeptin administration restored gonadotropin secretion and ovarian cyclicity, suggesting that kisspeptin neurons play a major role in hyperprolactinemic anovulation. Our studies indicate that administration of kisspeptin may serve as an alternative therapeutic approach to restore the fertility of hyperprolactinemic women who are resistant or intolerant to dopamine agonists.

▶ Hyperprolactinemia is a common cause of hypogonadotropic anovulation leading to infertility in reproductive-aged women. A direct effect of prolactin (PRL) on gonadotropin-releasing hormone (GnRH) release has been the presumed mechanism of action, but is not an established mechanism. Pulsatile administration of GnRH can reverse the hypogonadotropic hypogonadism in both genders and induce fertility. Kisspeptin neurons stimulate GnRH neurons and express PRL receptors.[1] These findings suggested to Sonigo et al that PRL affects the release of GnRH from the hypothalamus rather than having a direct effect on the pituitary or gonads. Further, the findings suggested that PRL affected upstream neurons, which affect GnRH neurons. In a mouse model with hyperprolactinemic anovulation, kisspeptin administration resulted in gonadotropin release and ovarian cyclicity, suggesting that kisspeptin neurons have substantial effects on reversing anovulation from PRL excess.[2] PRL inhibition of *Kiss1* gene expression and downstream suppression of GnRH and, consequently, gonadotropin secretion is the suggested mechanism for PRL excess–induced hypogonadism.[3,4] Kisspeptin might be considered an alternate therapy for those resistant or intolerant of dopamine agonist.[5]

A. W. Meikle, MD

References

1. George JT, Seminara SB. Kisspeptin and the hypothalamic control of reproduction: lessons from the human. *Endocrinology.* 2012;153:5130-5136.
2. Sonigo C, Bouilly J, Carré N, et al. Hyperprolactinemia-induced ovarian acyclicity is reversed by kisspeptin administration. *J Clin Invest.* 2012;122:3791-3795.
3. Sonigo C, Binart N. Overview of the impact of kisspeptin on reproductive function. *Ann Endocrinol (Paris).* 2012;73:448-458.
4. Topaloglu AK, Tello JA, Kotan LD, et al. Inactivating KISS1 mutation and hypogonadotropic hypogonadism. *N Engl J Med.* 2012;366:629-635.
5. Garcia-Galiano D, van Ingen Schenau D, Leon S, et al. Kisspeptin signaling is indispensable for neurokinin B, but not glutamate, stimulation of gonadotropin secretion in mice. *Endocrinology.* 2012;153:316-328.

Differential Regulation of Ovarian Anti-Müllerian Hormone (AMH) by Estradiol through α- and β-Estrogen Receptors

Grynberg M, Pierre A, Rey R, et al (Institut National de la Santé et de la Recherche Médicale, Clamart, France; Centro de Investigaciones Endocrinológicas, Buenos Aires, Argentina; et al)

J Clin Endocrinol Metab 97:E1649-E1657, 2012

Background.—Anti-Müllerian hormone (AMH) is a member of the TGF-β family, which limits follicle maturation. Recently serum AMH has been recognized as a useful diagnostic and prognostic tool in human reproductive endocrinology.

Objective.—The aim of this study was to investigate the regulation of human ovarian *AMH* by estradiol and FSH.

Methods.—AMH mRNA were quantified by real time RT-PCR in human granulosa cells (GC). AMH transcription was studied in KK1 GC cotransfected with estrogen receptors (ER)-β or ERα, and normal human AMH promoter-luciferase construct (hAMH-luc) or mutated AMH promoter reporter constructs. Binding sites for estradiol (estrogen response element half-site) and steroidogenic factor 1 were disrupted by targeted mutagenesis.

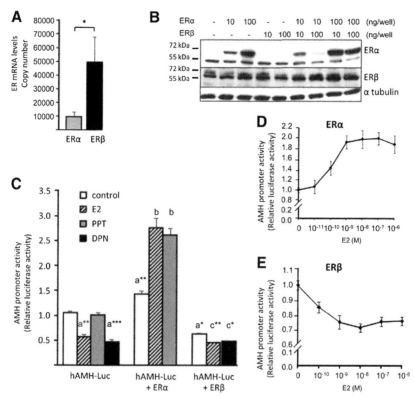

FIGURE 2.—Differential regulation of *AMH* transcription by estradiol through ERα and ERβ in KK1 GCs. A, Real-time RT-PCR analysis of *ER* expression in KK1 GC. Data were normalized to the housekeeping gene *HPRT*. Results were expressed in copy number and the levels of ERα and ERβ mRNA were compared using a Mann-Whitney *U* test. B, Western blotting analysis of ERα and ERβ in KK1 GC. C, Effect of over-expression of ERα or ERβ or/and ER agonists on hAMH-luc. KK1 cells were transfected with 1 μg/well of hAMH-luc and 100 ng/well of either *ERα* or *ERβ*. Luciferase activity was analyzed after 48 h of culture in control medium or with estradiol (E2) (10^{-6} M), PPT (10 nM), or DPN (10 nM). The relative light units of the first triplicate in control medium for hAMH-luc (hAMH-luc + ERα and hAMH-luc + ERβ) were fixed at one for each experiment, and the other results were normalized to this value (relative luciferase activity). Data shown correspond to the mean ± SEM of at least three experiments, each done in triplicate. Comparisons of means between different treatments were made by repeated measures ANOVA, followed by Dunnett *post hoc* test to compare all *vs.* controls (hAMH-luc, hAMH-luc + ERα, or hAMH-luc + ERβ in control medium). a, Significantly different from hAMH-luc; b, significantly different from hAMH-luc + ERα; c, significantly different from hAMH-luc + ERβ. D and E, Dose-response curves of estradiol effect on AMH transcription through ERα (D) or ERβ (E). KK1 cells were transfected with 1 μg/well of hAMH-luc and 100 ng/well of either *ERα* (D) or *ERβ* (E) plasmids. Luciferase activity was analyzed after 48 h of culture with increasing concentrations of estradiol (E2). The relative light units of the first triplicate in control medium for hAMH-luc + ERα or hAMH-luc + ERβ were fixed at one for each experiment, and the other results were normalized to this value (relative luciferase activity). Data shown correspond to the mean ± SEM of at least three experiments, each done in triplicate. *, $P < 0.05$; **, $P < 0.01$; ***, $P < 0.001$. (Reprinted from Grynberg M, Pierre A, Rey R, et al. Differential regulation of ovarian anti-müllerian hormone (AMH) by estradiol through α- and β-estrogen receptors. *J Clin Endocrinol Metab.* 2012;97:E1649-E1657; © 2012, with permission from the Author[s] and The Endocrine Society.)

The level of ER in GC was determined by quantitative RT-PCR and Western blotting.

Results.—In KK1 cells, estradiol up-regulated and inhibited hAMH-luc in the presence of ERα and ERβ respectively. Disruption of estrogen response element half-site and/or steroidogenic factor 1 binding sites did not modify ERβ-mediated effect of estradiol on hAMH-luc, whereas it affected that conveyed by ERα. The FSH enhancement of hAMH-luc was abolished by estradiol in cells overexpressing ERβ. When both ER were transfected, estradiol inhibited hAMH-luc or had no effect. Estradiol repressed AMH mRNAs in human GC, which express a little more ERα than ERβ mRNA.

Conclusions.—Our results show that AMH expression can be differentially regulated by estradiol depending on the ER and suggest that its decrease in GC of growing follicles, which mainly express ERβ, and during controlled ovarian hyperstimulation is due to the effect of estradiol (Fig 2).

▶ Anti-Müllerian hormone (AMH) is a member of the transforming growth factor-β family and is expressed in gonadal somatic cells. In females it is secreted by granulosa cells (GC) from the beginning of folliculogenesis to menopause, and it limits follicle maturation. Clinically, AMH is used as an indicator of ovarian GC tumors, a marker of ovarian follicular status, and it predicts ovarian response to controlled ovarian hyperstimulation. The regulation of ovarian AMH is not clear and the effects of follicle-stimulating hormone (FSH) and estradiol require further study, but FSH does have an inhibitory effect on AMH secretion.[1,2] Using AMH transcription in KK1 GC cotransfected with estrogen receptor ERα or ERβ and normal human AMH promoter-luciferase construct or mutated AMH promoter-reporter constructs, Grynberg et al observed differential regulation of ovarian AMH by estradiol. In the GC, they concluded that estradiol represses AMH expression when ERβ was in excess compared with ERα and that the apparent inhibitory effect of FSH on AMH expression was indirect and medicated through estradiol.[3-5]

A. W. Meikle, MD

References

1. Patrelli TS, Gizzo S, Sianesi N, et al. Anti-müllerian hormone serum values and ovarian reserve: can it predict a decrease in fertility after ovarian stimulation by ART cycles? *PLoS One.* 2012;7:e44571.
2. Bonilla-Musoles F, Castillo JC, Caballero O, et al. Predicting ovarian reserve and reproductive outcome using antimüllerian hormone (AMH) and antral follicle count (AFC) in patients with previous assisted reproduction technique (ART) failure. *Clin Exp Obstet Gynecol.* 2012;39:13-18.
3. Grzegorczyk-Martin V, Khrouf M, Bringer-Deutsch S, et al. Low circulating anti-Mullerian hormone and normal follicle stimulating hormone levels: which prognosis in an IVF program?. *Gynecol Obstet Fertil.* 2012;40:411-418.
4. Freour T, Masson D, Dessolle L, et al. Ovarian reserve and in vitro fertilization cycles outcome according to women smoking status and stimulation regimen. *Arch Gynecol Obstet.* 2012;285:1177-1182.
5. Zàrate A, Hernàndez-Valencia M, Austria E, Saucedo R, Hernàndez M. Diagnosis of premature menopause measuring circulating anti-Mullerian hormone. *Ginecol Obstet Mex.* 2011;79:303-307.

Polycystic Ovary-Like Abnormalities (PCO-L) in Women with Functional Hypothalamic Amenorrhea

Robin G, Gallo C, Catteau-Jonard S, et al (Université Lille Nord de France)
J Clin Endocrinol Metab 97:4236-4243, 2012

Context.—In the general population, about 30% of asymptomatic women have polycystic ovary-like abnormalities (PCO-L), *i.e.* polycystic ovarian morphology (PCOM) at ultrasound and/or increased anti-Müllerian hormone (AMH) serum level. PCOM has also been reported in 30—50% of women with functional hypothalamic amenorrhea (FHA).

Objective.—The aim of this study was to verify whether both PCOM and excessive AMH level indicate PCO-L in FHA and to elucidate its significance.

Design.—We conducted a retrospective analysis using a database and comparison with a control population.

Setting.—Subjects received ambulatory care in an academic hospital.

Patients.—Fifty-eight patients with FHA were compared to 217 control women with nonendocrine infertility and body mass index of less than 25 kg/m².

Interventions.—There were no interventions.

Main Outcome Measures.—We measured serum testosterone, androstenedione, FSH, LH, AMH, and ovarian area values. The antral follicle count (AFC) was used as a binary variable (*i.e.* negative or positive) because of the evolution of its sensitivity over the time of this study. The ability of these variables (except AFC) to detect PCO-L in both populations was tested by cluster analysis.

Results.—One cluster (cluster 2) suggesting PCO-L was detected in the control population (n = 52; 24%), whereas two such clusters were observed in the FHA population (n = 22 and n = 6; 38 and 10%; clusters 2 and 3, respectively). Cluster 2 in FHA had similar features of PCO-L as cluster 2 in controls, with higher prevalence of positive AFC (70%) and PCOM (70%), higher values of ovarian area and higher serum AMH (P < 0.0001 for all), and testosterone levels *(P < 0.01)* than in cluster 1. Cluster 3 in FHA was peculiar, with frankly elevated AMH levels. In the whole population (controls + FHA), PCO-L was significantly associated with lower FSH values (P < 0.0001).

Conclusion.—PCO-L in FHA is a frequent and usually incidental finding of unclear significance, as in controls. The association of PCO-L with hypothalamic amenorrhea should not lead to a mistaken diagnosis of PCOS.

▶ Polycystic ovary syndrome (PCOS) is a common disorder affecting women of reproductive age and is associated with androgenization, anovulation, and the metabolic syndrome. Robin et al make a link between functional hypothalamic amenorrhea (FHA), which is a frequent cause of anovulation, hypoestrogenism, and negative energy balance from excessive exercise leading to hypoinsulinism (in contrast to insulin resistance in PCOS). In FHA, luteinizing hormone levels tend to be higher than follicle-stimulating hormone levels as observed in PCOS. This also results in polycystic ovarian morphology (PCOM), which is observed in 30% to 50% of women with FHA. The presence of PCOM in women with FHA might lead to the mistaken diagnosis of PCOS. Another confounding finding in both disorders is that anti-Müllerian hormone (AMH) might be elevated in both, because AMH is the most common endocrine abnormality associated with PCOM. PCO-like disorder is also common in the general population. The authors observed the occurrence of PCOM in about 70% of women with FHA. Based on their study, they do not think that the association of PCO-like disorder with hypothalamic amenorrhea should be mistakenly diagnosed with PCOS.[1-5]

A. W. Meikle, MD

References

1. Dumesic DA, Abbott DH, Padmanabhan V. Polycystic ovary syndrome and its developmental origins. *Rev Endocr Metab Disord.* 2007;8:127-141.
2. Meczekalski B, Czyzyk A, Podfigurna-Stopa A, et al. Hypothalamic amenorrhea in a Camurati-Engelmann disease - a case report. *Gynecol Endocrinol.* 2013 Feb 1 [Epub ahead of print].
3. Santoro N. Update in hyper- and hypogonadotropic amenorrhea. *J Clin Endocrinol Metab.* 2011;96:3281-3288.
4. Caronia LM, Martin C, Welt CK, et al. A genetic basis for functional hypothalamic amenorrhea. *N Engl J Med.* 2011;364:215-225.
5. Scheid JL, De Souza MJ. Menstrual irregularities and energy deficiency in physically active women: the role of ghrelin, PYY and adipocytokines. *Med Sport Sci.* 2010;55:82-102.

Male Reproductive Function

The genetic origin of Klinefelter syndrome and its effect on spermatogenesis
Maiburg M, Repping S, Giltay J (Univ Med Ctr Utrecht, the Netherlands; Univ of Amsterdam, the Netherlands)
Fertil Steril 98:253-260, 2012

Klinefelter syndrome is the most prevalent chromosome abnormality and genetic cause of azoospermia in males. The availability of assisted reproductive technology (ART) has allowed men with Klinefelter syndrome to father their own genetic offspring. When providing ART to men with Klinefelter syndrome, it is important to be able to counsel them properly on both the chance of finding sperm and the potential effects on their offspring. The aim of this review is twofold: [1] to describe the genetic etiology of Klinefelter syndrome and [2] to describe how spermatogenesis occurs in men with Klinefelter syndrome and the consequences this has for children born from men with Klinefelter syndrome (Fig 1).

▶ In 1942, Harry Klinefelter described a syndrome (called Klinefelter syndrome [KS]) characterized by gynecomastia, small testes, and azoospermia. It characterized in 1959 with an additional X chromosome, typically 47 XXY, but also mosaic karyotypes that include an extra X chromosome. Malburg et al made a review of the genetic origin of KS. It affects about 1 500 to 11 000 men and is the most common

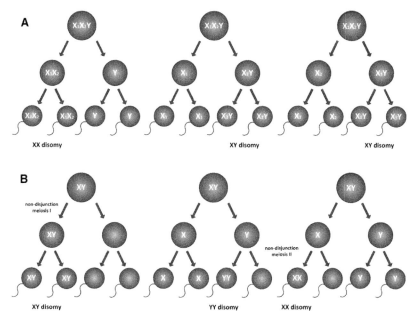

FIGURE 1.—Hypotheses on spermatogenesis in Klinefelter syndrome. (A) Meiosis of XXY cells. (B) Meiotic errors in 46,XY germ cells (testicular environment hypothesis). (Reprinted from Fertility and Sterility. Maiburg M, Repping S, Giltay J. The genetic origin of Klinefelter syndrome and its effect on spermatogenesis. *Fertil Steril.* 2012;98:253-260, Copyright 2012, with permission of the American Society for Reproductive Medicine.)

genetic cause of azoospermia. A premature separation of sister chromatids in meiosis I might be the most common cause of aneuploidy and could underlie the origin of nonmosaic XXY cases of either paternal or maternal origin.[1,2] X-chromosomes escaping inactivation have a higher expression in men with KS than normal men. The abundance of gene products might compromise testicular function and cause infertility. Men with KS are capable of making some sperm and fertility with in vitro fertilization. Although aneuploidy is common in sperm of men with KS, their children exhibit aneuploidy with 1100.[3,4] Even infertile men with normal karyotypes have a 2 to 10 times increased frequency of sperm aneuploidy compared with fertile controls. The strongest evidence for an altered testicular environment is that the patches of 46-XY spermatozoa stem cells are prone to increased aneuploidy.[5,6]

A. W. Meikle, MD

References

1. Vialard F, Bailly M, Bouazzi H, et al. The high frequency of sperm aneuploidy in Klinefelter patients and in non-obstructive azoospermia is due to meiotic errors in euploid spermatocytes. *J Androl.* 2012 [Epub ahead of print].
2. Bruining H, van Rijn S, Swaab H, et al. The parent-of-origin of the extra X chromosome may differentially affect psychopathology in Klinefelter syndrome. *Biol Psychiatry.* 2010;68:1156-1162.

3. Tüttelmann F, Gromoll J. Novel genetic aspects of Klinefelter's syndrome. *Mol Hum Reprod.* 2010;16:386-395.

4. Biselli JM, Machado FB, Zampieri BL, et al. Double aneuploidy (48,XXY,+21) of maternal origin in a child born to a 13-year-old mother: evaluation of the maternal folate metabolism. *Genet Couns.* 2009;20:225-234.

5. Chantot-Bastaraud S, Ravel C, Siffroi JP. Underlying karyotype abnormalities in IVF/ICSI patients. *Reprod Biomed Online.* 2008;16:514-522.

6. Wikström AM, Painter JN, Raivio T, Aittomäki K, Dunkel L. Genetic features of the X chromosome affect pubertal development and testicular degeneration in adolescent boys with Klinefelter syndrome. *Clin Endocrinol (Oxf).* 2006;65:92-97.

Changes in hormonal profile and seminal parameters with use of aromatase inhibitors in management of infertile men with low testosterone to estradiol ratios

Gregoriou O, Bakas P, Grigoriadis C, et al (Univ of Athens, Greece)
Fertil Steril 98:48-51, 2012

Objective.—To compare the effects of 2.5 mg letrozole with those of 1 mg anastrazole daily on the hormonal and semen profiles of a subset of infertile men with low T/E_2 ratios.

Design.—Prospective, nonrandomized study.

Setting.—Reproductive medicine clinic.

Patient(s).—The study group consisted of 29 infertile men with a low serum T/E_2 ratio (<10).

Intervention(s).—Patients were divided into two groups. Group A included 15 patients treated with 2.5 mg letrozole orally once daily for 6 months, and Group B consisted of 14 patients treated with 1 mg anastrazole orally every day for 6 months.

Main Outcome Measure(s).—Hormonal evaluation included measurement of serum FSH, LH, PRL, T, and E_2. In all sperm analyses

---

TABLE 1.—Results of Semen Analysis and Hormonal Tests Before and After 6 Months of Treatment with Letrozole 2.5 mg/d

Parameter	Before Treatment	After Treatment	P Value
Body mass index (kg/m²)	29.86 ± 2.53	30.1 ± 2.13	>.05
Testicular volume (mL)	14.89 ± 4.32	15.01 ± 4.30	.94
Serum FSH (mIU/mL)	8.35 ± 2.03	8.41 ± 1.95	.93
Serum LH (mIU/mL)	9.55 ± 1.84	9.28 ± 1.80	.69
Serum T (ng/dL)	275 ± 29	495 ± 65	<.001
Serum E_2 (pg/mL)	26.7 ± 1.75	14.98 ± 2.58	<.001
T/E_2 ratio	9 ± 0.2	36 ± 4.5	<.001
Ejaculate volume (ml)	2.85 ± 0.36	3.35 ± 0.20	.005
Sperm count ($\times 10^6$)	3.5 ± 1.43	5.19 ± 1.62	.001
Motility (%)	11.05 ± 2.48	22.13 ± 4.37	.001
TFSF[a] ($\times 10^6$)	1.71 ± 0.87	2.51 ± 1.09	.013

Note: Values are mean ± SE.
[a]TFSF was estimated by multiplying total sperm count ($\times 10^6$) by motility (%) and by morphology (%).

pretreatment and posttreatment total motile sperm counts (ejaculate volume × concentration × motile fraction) were evaluated.

Result(s).—The use of aromatase inhibitors (either letrozole or anastrazole) in cases of infertile men with low T/E_2 ratios improved both hormonal and semen parameters.

Conclusion(s).—This study suggests that some men with severe oligospermia, low T levels, and normal gonadotropin concentration may have a treatable endocrinopathy (Table 1).

▶ Aromatase converts testosterone to estradiol and androstenedione to estrone and is present in many tissues. Aromatase inhibitors have wide use in clinical medicine to inhibit unwanted estrogen effects on various estrogen responsive tissues. Estrogen is also important in bone health in both men and women and gonadotropin feedback. Aromatase inhibitors by reducing formation of estrogens are known to secondarily increase gonadotropins, which then enhance gonadal function in men with partial gonadotropin deficiency. Gregoriou et al determined whether aromatase inhibitors would transform infertile men with low testosterone to estradiol ratios to fertile men. As shown in Table 1, aromatase inhibitors did not significantly increase luteinizing hormone and follicle-stimulating hormone, but they did significantly elevate serum testosterone, ejaculate volume and sperm count. The study by Gregoriou et al has limitations. It was a relatively small study and there was no documentation on fertility outcomes. There is a concern of osteoporosis in men treated long-term with aromatase indicators.[1-5]

A. W. Meikle, MD

References

1. Saylam B, Efesoy O, Cayan S. The effect of aromatase inhibitor letrozole on body mass index, serum hormones, and sperm parameters in infertile men. *Fertil Steril.* 2011;95:809-811.
2. Cakan M, Aldemir M, Topcuoglu M, Altuğ U. Role of testosterone/estradiol ratio in predicting the efficacy of tamoxifen citrate treatment in idiopathic oligoasthenoteratozoospermic men. *Urol Int.* 2009;83:446-451.
3. Patry G, Jarvi K, Grober ED, Lo KC. Use of the aromatase inhibitor letrozole to treat male infertility. *Fertil Steril.* 2009;92:829.e1-829.e2.
4. Roth MY, Amory JK, Page ST. Treatment of male infertility secondary to morbid obesity. *Nat Clin Pract Endocrinol Metab.* 2008;4:415-419.
5. Pavlovich CP, King P, Goldstein M, Schlegel PN. Evidence of a treatable endocrinopathy in infertile men. *J Urol.* 2001;165:837-841.

Job demands as a potential modifier of the association between testosterone deficiency and andropause symptoms in Japanese middle-aged workers: A cross-sectional study

Hirokawa K, Taniguchi T, Fujii Y, et al (Baika Women's Univ, Ibaraki, Osaka, Japan; Okayama Prefectural Univ, kuboki Soja City, Japan; et al)
Maturitas 73:225-229, 2012

Objective.—The present study investigated whether job demands modify the association between low levels of testosterone and andropause symptoms.

Study Design.—Participants were Japanese middle-aged workers in a middle-size company. Blood samples were drawn to determine serum levels of testosterone. Participants completed a self-report questionnaire that included 5 items from the Job Content Questionnaire (JCQ) that assesses job demands, the Aging Males' Symptoms (AMS) scale as well as questions regarding health behaviors and history of disease. Analysis of data was limited to the 183 men who completed all components of the questionnaire and provided blood samples (mean age = 51.9 years, SD = 7.7, age range 34—67 years).

Main Outcome Measures.—The AMS which comprises three symptom sub-scales: somatic, psychological, and sexual.

Results.—Men with low testosterone levels (<349 ng/dL) had more psychological andropause symptoms than those with high levels. In men with high psychological job demands, compared to men with low job demands, testosterone levels were positively associated with the total score for andropause symptoms and scores for somatic and psychological symptoms.

Conclusions.—Level of job demands may intensify the effect of testosterone deficiency on andropause symptoms (Table 4).

▶ As men age, symptoms suggestive of hypogonadism manifest, including fatigue, low energy, depression, low libido, erectile dysfunction, and more fat and less muscle mass. Serum concentrations of testosterone decline as men age at about 1% per year. Andropause has been a common term used for this complex set of symptoms and gonadal function. Serum-free testosterone concentration declines more rapidly than total testosterone because sex hormone—binding globulin tends to increase as men age. The mechanism for andropause is not well defined, but it affects the hypothalamic-pituitary-gonadal axis. Some factors are known, such as obesity, sleep apnea, stress, and poor health. Hirokawa et al conducted a study in middle age Japanese men to determine if job stress was associated with testosterone deficiency and andropause symptoms. Testosterone deficiency allowed them to predict psychological symptoms in these men. Men with lower testosterone values had more depression than those with higher testosterone concentrations. The study has limitations in that symptoms and signs of hypogonadism were not assessed after testosterone replacement therapy.[1-3]

A. W. Meikle, MD

TABLE 4.—Results of Multiple Regression Analyses Stratified by Job Demand

	Total Score		Somatic Symptoms		Psychological Symptoms		Sexual Symptoms	
	Standardized-β	P	Standardized-β	P	Standardized-β	P	Standardized-β	P
Low job demands								
Testosterone deficiency (dummy as 1)	−0.01	0.919	−0.09	0.423	0.11	0.365	0.00	0.979
Age	0.25	0.040	0.17	0.175	0.11	0.357	0.39	0.001
F value	1.19	0.321	0.73	0.651	0.89	0.522	2.46	0.025
Durbin–Watson test	1.25		1.36		1.15		1.65	
Adjusted R-square	0.02		0.02		0.01		0.11	
High job demands								
Testosterone deficiency (dummy as 1)	0.24	0.015	0.27	0.005	0.23	0.018	0.12	0.222
Age	0.18	0.068	0.06	0.513	0.11	0.254	0.32	0.001
F value	2.88	0.009	3.86	0.001	2.22	0.039	3.15	0.005
Durbin–Watson test	1.29		1.36		1.43		1.56	
Adjusted R-square	0.12		0.17		0.08		0.13	

Standardized-betas were adjusted for BMI, sleep hours, smoking habits, and alcohol consumption.

References

1. Hansen AM, Larsen AD, Rugulies R, Garde AH, Knudsen LE. A review of the effect of the psychosocial working environment on physiological changes in blood and urine. *Basic Clin Pharmacol Toxicol.* 2009;105:73-83.
2. Ohlson CG, Söderfeldt M, Söderfeldt B, Jones I, Theorell T. Stress markers in relation to job strain in human service organizations. *Psychother Psychosom.* 2001; 70:268-275.
3. Theorell T, Harms-Ringdahl K, Ahlberg-Hultén G, Westin B. Psychosocial job factors and symptoms from the locomotor system—a multicausal analysis. *Scand J Rehabil Med.* 1991;23:165-173.

A New Combination of Testosterone and Nestorone Transdermal Gels for Male Hormonal Contraception

Ilani N, Roth MY, Amory JK, et al (Harbor-Univ of California, Los Angeles; Univ of Washington, Seattle; et al)
J Clin Endocrinol Metab 97:3476-3486, 2012

Context.—Combinations of testosterone (T) and nestorone (NES; a nonandrogenic progestin) transdermal gels may suppress spermatogenesis and prove appealing to men for contraception.

Objective.—The objective of the study was to determine the effectiveness of T gel alone or combined with NES gel in suppressing spermatogenesis.

Design and Setting.—This was a randomized, double-blind, comparator clinical trial conducted at two academic medical centers.

Participants.—Ninety-nine healthy male volunteers participated in the study.

Interventions.—Volunteers were randomized to one of three treatment groups applying daily transdermal gels (group 1: T gel 10 g + NES 0 mg/placebo gel; group 2: T gel 10 g + NES gel 8 mg; group 3: T gel 10 g + NES gel 12 mg).

Main Outcome Variable.—The main outcome variable of the study was the percentage of men whose sperm concentration was suppressed to 1 million/ml or less by 20–24 wk of treatment.

Results.—Efficacy data analyses were performed on 56 subjects who adhered to the protocol and completed at least 20 wk of treatment. The percentage of men whose sperm concentration was 1 million/ml or less was significantly higher for T + NES 8 mg (89%, $P < 0.0001$) and T + NES 12 mg (88%, $P = 0.0002$) compared with T + NES 0 mg group (23%). The median serum total and free T concentrations in all groups were maintained within the adult male range throughout the treatment period. Adverse effects were minimal in all groups.

Conclusion.—A combination of daily NES + T gels suppressed sperm concentration to 1 million/ml or less in 88.5% of men, with minimal adverse

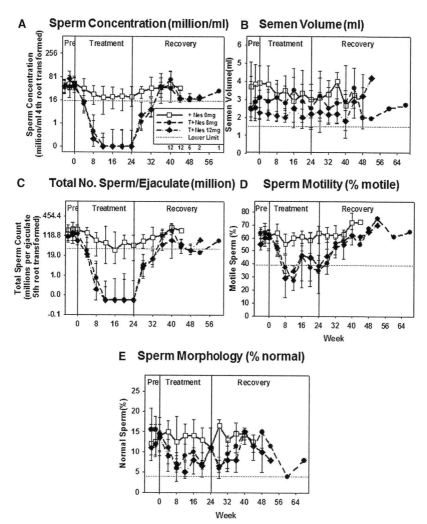

FIGURE 3.—Sperm concentration (A), semen volume (B), total sperm count per ejaculate (C), percentage motility (D), and percentage normal morphology (E) (median, 25th, and 75th percentile) in each treatment group during each assessment week in the pretreatment (PRE), treatment, and recovery periods. Note that a fourth root transformation was used for the sperm concentration (A) and the fifth root for total sperm count per ejaculate (C). Sperm motility and morphology were assessed only in samples with more than 5000 spermatozoa/ml. *Dotted lines* represent the lower reference range in adult men. (Reprinted from Ilani N, Roth MY, Amory JK, et al. A new combination of testosterone and nestorone transdermal gels for male hormonal contraception. *J Clin Endocrinol Metab.* 2012;97:3476-3486, Copyright © 2012, with permission from the Author[s] and The Endocrine Society.)

effects, and may be further studied as a male transdermal hormonal contraceptive (Fig 3).

▶ Female hormonal contraception has been available for many years, and studies of hormonal contraception for men have lagged behind. Male methods have often included withdrawal, condoms, and vasectomy and have not been well accepted.[1] Many of the male contraception studies have been supported by the World Health Organization. The approach of male contraception has employed testosterone generally by injection and oral or injectable progestin and has provided evidence of efficacy, safety, and reliable reversal. Ilani et al conducted a study of male hormonal contraception using a 10-g gel combining testosterone and Nestorone,[2] which does not have androgenic action. The study was a randomized, double-blind comparative trial. The efficacy was defined as sperm counts ≥1 million and was achieved in 88.5% of men. As with any testosterone preparation, a desired testosterone concentration requires titration. This was a short-term study, and long-term studies are needed. The cost of the therapy is another consideration and might be expensive; whether insurance carriers would approve the therapy remains uncertain.[3-7]

A. W. Meikle, MD

References

1. Ilani N, Roth MY, Amory JK, et al. A new combination of testosterone and nestorone transdermal gels for male hormonal contraception. *J Clin Endocrinol Metab.* 2012;97:3476-3486.
2. Mahmoud A, T'Sjoen G. Male hormonal contraception: where do we stand? *Eur J Contracept Reprod Health Care.* 2012;17:179-186.
3. Grimes DA, Lopez LM, Gallo MF, Halpern V, Nanda K, Schulz KF. Steroid hormones for contraception in men. *Cochrane Database Syst Rev.* 2012;(3): CD004316.
4. Chang Q, Liu Z, Ma WZ, et al. Drug synergistic antifertility effect of combined administration of low-dose gossypol with steroid hormones in rats. *Chin Med J (Engl).* 2011;124:1678-1682.
5. Ilani N, Swerdloff RS, Wang C. Male hormonal contraception: potential risks and benefits. *Rev Endocr Metab Disord.* 2011;12:107-117.
6. Griksiene R, Ruksenas O. Effects of hormonal contraceptives on mental rotation and verbal fluency. *Psychoneuroendocrinology.* 2011;36:1239-1248.
7. Nieschlag E. The struggle for male hormonal contraception. *Best Pract Res Clin Endocrinol Metab.* 2011;25:369-375.

Polycystic Ovary Syndrome

Lean mass and insulin resistance in women with polycystic ovary syndrome
Comerford KB, Almario RU, Kim K, et al (The Univ of California at Davis)
Metabolism 61:1256-1260, 2012

Insulin resistance is common in women with polycystic ovary syndrome (PCOS). Muscle is the major tissue utilizing glucose while excess adipose tissue relates to insulin resistance. Thus, body composition is likely to be an important regulator of insulin sensitivity. Thirty-nine PCOS patients (age: 29.9 ± 1.0 years; BMI: 33.8 ± 1.2 kg/m^2) participated in a cross sectional study. Body composition was measured by dual energy x-ray absorptiometry (DEXA). Insulin resistance and secretion were assessed using oral glucose tolerance test (OGTT) and frequently sampled intravenous glucose tolerance test (FS-IVGTT). In contrast with the conventional expectations, lean mass correlated directly ($P < .05$) with the insulin resistance measure HOMA ($r = 0.440$); and inversely with the insulin sensitivity index QUICKI ($r = -0.522$) independent of fat mass. In 11 pairs of subjects matched for fat mass (35.6 ± 2.2 and 35.6 ± 2.4 kg) but with discordant lean mass (52.8 ± 1.8 vs 44.4 ± 1.6 kg), those with higher lean mass had a higher glucose response during OGTT (AUC$_{Glucose}$; $P = .034$). In contrast, 17 pairs matched for lean mass (48.7 ± 1.7 and 48.9 ± 1.6 kg) but discordant for fat mass (43.3 ± 2.6 vs 30.3 ± 8.9 kg) showed no differences in insulin resistance parameters. These novel findings indicate that lean mass relates directly to insulin resistance in PCOS.

▶ Polycystic ovary syndrome (PCOS) commonly affects young women with obesity, insulin resistance, and dyslipidemia. Previously, the insulin resistance was attributed to excess adipose tissue.[1] Evidence indicates that impaired insulin responsiveness in PCOS might be related to skeletal muscle rather than adipose tissue.[2] Serum testosterone concentrations did not relate to insulin resistance.[3] Since lean body mass accounts for about 80% of insulin-dependent glucose uptake, muscle can have a substantial influence on insulin responsiveness in PCOS. Visceral adipose tissue also blunts insulin responsiveness along with lean muscle mass. The authors further speculate that skeletal muscle growth might be affected by increased blood insulin concentration, but muscle quality might also be important. The study does not answer the question of how these observations can provide therapies to reverse insulin resistance in PCOS. Another unanswered question is whether these observations are also operative in other disorders with insulin resistance. These observations might lead to a shift in insulin responsiveness in women with PCOS.

A. W. Meikle, MD

References

1. Mario FM, do Amarante F, Toscani MK, Spritzer PM. Lean muscle mass in classic or ovulatory PCOS: association with central obesity and insulin resistance. *Exp Clin Endocrinol Diabetes*. 2012;120(9):511-516.
2. Forrester-Dumont K, Galescu O, Kolesnikov A, et al. Hyperandrogenism does not influence metabolic parameters in adolescent girls with PCOS. *Int J Endocrinol*. 2012;2012:434830.
3. Stovall DW, Bailey AP, Pastore LM. Assessment of insulin resistance and impaired glucose tolerance in lean women with polycystic ovary syndrome. *J Womens Health (Larchmt)*. 2011;20:37-43.

Ethinyl Estradiol-Cyproterone Acetate *Versus* Low-Dose Pioglitazone-Flutamide-Metformin for Adolescent Girls with Androgen Excess: Divergent Effects on *CD163*, *TWEAK* Receptor, *ANGPTL4*, and *LEPTIN* Expression in Subcutaneous Adipose Tissue

Díaz M, Chacón MR, López-Bermejo A, et al (Univ of Barcelona, Esplugues, Spain; Univ Rovira i Virgili, Tarragona, Spain; Instituto de Salud Carlos III, Madrid, Spain; et al)

J Clin Endocrinol Metab 97:3630-3638, 2012

Objective.—The aim was to compare the effects of a traditional therapy (an oral estroprogestagen) to those of a novel treatment (a low-dose combination of generics) in adolescent girls with androgen excess.

Study Design and Methods.—In an open-label trial over 1 yr, 34 adolescents (age, 16 yr; body mass index, 23 kg/m^2) with hyperinsulinemic androgen excess and without pregnancy risk were randomized to receive daily ethinyl estradiol-cyproterone acetate (EE-CA; Diane 35 Diario) or a low-dose combination of pioglitazone 7.5 mg/d, flutamide 62.5 mg/d, and metformin 850 mg/d (PioFluMet). Markers of androgen excess, C-reactive protein, high molecular weight adiponectin, lipids, carotid intima media thickness, body composition (absorptiometry), abdominal fat partitioning (magnetic resonance imaging), and gene expression in longitudinal biopsies

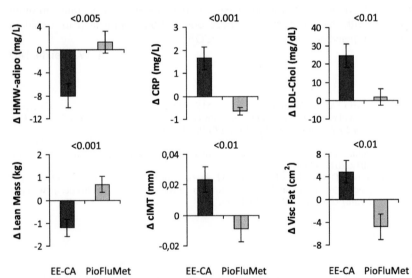

FIGURE 1.—Changes over 12 months in HMW-adiponectin (HMW-adipo), CRP, LDL-cholesterol, lean mass (by absorptiometry), cIMT, and visceral fat area (Visc Fat, by MRI) in adolescent girls with androgen excess treated with EE-CA (n = 17; *dark gray*) or low-dose PioFluMet (n = 17; *light gray*). Results are shown as mean and SEM. (Reprinted from Díaz M, Chacón MR, López-Bermejo A, et al. Ethinyl estradiol-cyproterone acetate versus low-dose pioglitazone-flutamide-metformin for adolescent girls with androgen excess: divergent effects on *CD163*, *TWEAK* receptor, *ANGPTL4*, and *LEPTIN* Expression in subcutaneous adipose tissue. *J Clin Endocrinol Metab.* 2012;97:3630-3638, © 2012, with permission from the Author[s] and The Endocrine Society.)

of sc adipose tissue at the abdominal level (RT-PCR) were assessed at baseline and after 1 yr.

Results.—EE-CA and low-dose PioFluMet reduced androgen excess comparably, but had divergent effects on C-reactive protein, high molecular weight adiponectin, lipids, carotid intima media thickness, lean mass, abdominal and visceral fat, and on the expression of *CD163*, leptin, TNF-like weak inducer of apoptosis receptor, and angiopoietin-like protein 4, respectively, related to macrophage activation, fat accretion, inflammation, and lipoprotein metabolism in adipose tissue. All these divergences pointed to a healthier condition on low-dose PioFluMet.

Conclusion.—EE-CA and PioFluMet are similarly effective in reversing androgen excess over 1 yr, but low-dose PioFluMet is superior in reversing inflammatory, metabolic, and cardiovascular anomalies that are often associated with androgen excess (Fig 1).

▶ In girls with polycystic ovary syndrome, there are 2 strategies for therapy for signs and symptoms associated with elevated androgen. This therapy has been directed at hirsutism, acne, and irregular menses. The standard approach for treatment of girls with polycystic ovary syndrome has been to use estrogen/progestin combinations or the inclusion of estrogen plus cyproterone acetate as an antiandrogen. Alternative approaches have been used to correct the underlying metabolic abnormalities, which often include hyperinsulinemia, insulin resistance, resulting normalization ovarian function, and attenuating the risk for subsequent diabetes and cardiovascular disease. In the latter approach, some sensitizing agents, such as metformin, have been used in combination with flutamide and pioglitazone.[1] The combination of pioglitazone, flutamide, and metformin were superior in reversing inflammatory abnormalities associated with androgen excess in these girls as reported by Diaz et al.[2] The study was the first to assess gene expression from subcutaneous adipose tissue nonobese polycystic ovary syndrome in adolescence. The main limitation of this study is the sparse amount of adipose tissue obtained. Further study is needed to determine the long-term efficacy and safety of these therapies in girls with polycystic ovary syndrome.[3-5]

A. W. Meikle, MD

References

1. Ibáñez L, Diaz M, Sebastiani G, et al. Treatment of androgen excess in adolescent girls: ethinylestradiol-cyproteroneacetate versus low-dose pioglitazone-flutamide-metformin. *J Clin Endocrinol Metab.* 2011;96:3361-3366.
2. Ibáñez L, Diaz M, López-Bermejo A, de Zegher F. Divergent effects of ethinylestradiol-drospirenone and flutamide-metformin on follistatin in adolescents and women with hyperinsulinemic androgen excess. *Gynecol Endocrinol.* 2011;27:197-198.
3. Ibáñez L, López-Bermejo A, Diaz M, Enriquez G, del Rio L, de Zegher F. Low-dose pioglitazone and low-dose flutamide added to metformin and oestro-progestagens for hyperinsulinaemic women with androgen excess: add-on benefits disclosed by a randomized double-placebo study over 24 months. *Clin Endocrinol (Oxf).* 2009;71:351-357.

4. Morales A, Morimoto S, Diaz L, Robles G, Diaz-Sánchez V. Endocrine gland-derived vascular endothelial growth factor in rat pancreas: genetic expression and testosterone regulation. *J Endocrinol.* 2008;197:309-314.

5. Ibáñez L, López-Bermejo A, Diaz M, Enriquez G, Valls C, de Zegher F. Pioglitazone (7.5 mg/day) added to flutamide-metformin in women with androgen excess: additional increments of visfatin and high molecular weight adiponectin. *Clin Endocrinol (Oxf).* 2008;68:317-320.

Metformin Improves Pregnancy and Live-Birth Rates in Women with Polycystic Ovary Syndrome (PCOS): A Multicenter, Double-Blind, Placebo-Controlled Randomized Trial

Morin-Papunen L, Rantala AS, Unkila-Kallio L, et al (Oulu Univ Hosp, Oys, Finland; Helsinki Univ Hosp, Finland; et al)

J Clin Endocrinol Metab 97:1492-1500, 2012

Background.—The role of metformin in the treatment of infertility in women with polycystic ovary syndrome (PCOS) is still controversial.

Objective and Outcomes.—We investigated whether metformin decreases the early miscarriage rate and improves the pregnancy rates (PR) and live-birth rates (LBR) in PCOS.

Methods.—This was a multicenter, randomized (1:1), double-blind, placebo-controlled study. Three hundred twenty women with PCOS and anovulatory infertility were randomized to metformin (n = 160, Diformin; obese women, 1000 mg two times daily; nonobese subjects, 500 mg + 1000 mg daily) or identical doses of placebo (n = 160). After 3 months' treatment, another appropriate infertility treatment was combined if

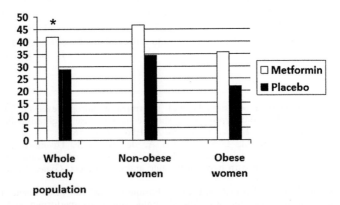

**P= 0.014 between the metformin and the placebo groups

FIGURE 3.—Live birth rates in the metformin and placebo groups in the whole population and in the nonobese and obese subjects. (Reprinted from Morin-Papunen L, Rantala AS, Unkila-Kallio L, et al. Metformin improves pregnancy and live-birth rates in women with polycystic ovary syndrome (PCOS): a multicenter, double-blind, placebo-controlled randomized trial. *J Clin Endocrinol Metab.* 2012;97:1492-1500, Copyright 2012, with permission from the Author[s] and The Endocrine Society.)

necessary. If pregnancy occurred, metformin/placebo was continued up to the 12th week.

Results.—Miscarriage rates were low and similar in the two groups (metformin 15.2% *vs.* placebo 17.9%, *P* = 0.8). Intent-to-treat analysis showed that metformin significantly improved PR and LBR (*vs.* placebo) in the whole study population (PR: 53.6 *vs.* 40.4%, *P* = 0.006; LBR: 41.9 *vs.* 28.8%, *P* = 0.014) and PR in obese women (49.0 *vs.* 31.4%, *P* = 0.04), and there was a similar trend in nonobese (PR: 58.6 *vs.* 47.6%, *P* = 0.09; LBR: 46.7 *vs.* 34.5%, *P* = 0.09) and in obese women with regard to LBR (35.7 *vs.* 21.9%, *P* = 0.07). Cox regression analysis showed that metformin plus standard infertility treatment increased the chance of pregnancy 1.6 times (hazard rate 1.6, 95% confidence interval 1.13–2.27).

Conclusion.—Obese women especially seem to benefit from 3 months' pretreatment with metformin and its combination thereafter with routine ovulation induction in anovulatory infertility (Fig 3).

▶ Metformin is commonly used to treat women with polycystic ovary syndrome (PCOS) to improve insulin sensitivity, reduce androgen effects, and improve fertility. Anovulation is common in women with PCOS, which affects approximately 5% to 10% of women of reproductive age. In addition, androgenic effects, such as hirsutism and acne, are commonly observed. More recent studies have focused on the improvement in the high rates of first trimester spontaneous abortions. In a randomized, double-blind study, Morin-Papunen et al observed that metformin not only improved pregnancy rates but also live birth rates in women with PCOS. The miscarriage rates were low in their population of infertile women with PCOS and did not change with metformin. Obese women were particularly benefited by the metformin therapy. A weakness of the study is that it did not assess a mechanism of action. A lower dose of metformin was used in nonobese women, which might have influenced the benefit in obese women.[1-5]

A. W. Meikle, MD

References

1. Tang T, Lord JM, Norman RJ, Yasmin E, Balen AH. Insulin-sensitising drugs (metformin, rosiglitazone, pioglitazone, D-chiro-inositol) for women with polycystic ovary syndrome, oligo amenorrhoea and subfertility. *Cochrane Database Syst Rev.* 2012;(5):CD003053.
2. Ghazeeri GS, Nassar AH, Younes Z, Awwad JT. Pregnancy outcomes and the effect of metformin treatment in women with polycystic ovary syndrome: an overview. *Acta Obstet Gynecol Scand.* 2012;91:658-678.
3. Crisosto N, Echiburú B, Maliqueo M, et al. Improvement of hyperandrogenism and hyperinsulinemia during pregnancy in women with polycystic ovary syndrome: possible effect in the ovarian follicular mass of their daughters. *Fertil Steril.* 2012;97:218-224.
4. Kjøtrød SB, Carlsen SM, Rasmussen PE, et al. Use of metformin before and during assisted reproductive technology in non-obese young infertile women with polycystic ovary syndrome: a prospective, randomized, double-blind, multi-centre study. *Hum Reprod.* 2011;26:2045-2053.
5. Vause TD, Cheung AP, Sierra S, et al. Ovulation induction in polycystic ovary syndrome: no. 242, May 2010. *Int J Gynaecol Obstet.* 2010;111:95-100.

Evidence for Chromosome 2p16.3 Polycystic Ovary Syndrome Susceptibility Locus in Affected Women of European Ancestry

Mutharasan P, Galdones E, Bernabé BP, et al (Northwestern Univ Feinberg School of Medicine, Chicago, IL; et al)

J Clin Endocrinol Metab 98:E185-E190, 2013

Context.—A previous genome-wide association study in Chinese women with polycystic ovary syndrome (PCOS) identified a region on chromosome 2p16.3 encoding the LH/choriogonadotropin receptor (*LHCGR*) and FSH receptor (*FSHR*) genes as a reproducible PCOS susceptibility locus.

Objective.—The objective of the study was to determine the role of the *LHCGR* and/or *FSHR* gene in the etiology of PCOS in women of European ancestry.

Design.—This was a genetic association study in a European ancestry cohort of women with PCOS.

Setting.—The study was conducted at an academic medical center.

Participants.—Participants in the study included 905 women with PCOS diagnosed by National Institutes of Health criteria and 956 control women.

Intervention.—We genotyped 94 haplotype-tagging single-nucleotide polymorphisms and two coding single-nucleotide polymorphisms mapping to the coding region of LHCGR and *FSHR* plus 20 kb upstream and downstream of the genes and test for association in the case control cohort and for association with nine quantitative traits in the women with PCOS.

Results.—We found strong evidence for an association of PCOS with rs7562215 ($P = 0.0037$) and rs10495960 ($P = 0.0046$). Although the marker with the strongest association in the Chinese PCOS genome-wide association study (rs13405728) was not informative in the European populations, we identified and genotyped three markers (rs35960650, rs2956355, and rs7562879) within 5 kb of rs13405728. Of these, rs7562879 was nominally associated with PCOS ($P = 0.020$). The strongest evidence for association mapping to *FSHR* was observed with rs1922476 ($P = 0.0053$). Furthermore, markers with the *FSHR* gene region were associated with FSH levels in women with PCOS.

Conclusions.—Fine mapping of the chromosome 2p16.3 Chinese PCOS susceptibility locus in a European ancestry cohort provides evidence for association with two independent loci and PCOS. The gene products *LHCGR* and *FSHR* therefore are likely to be important in the etiology of PCOS, regardless of ethnicity (Table 1).

▶ Polycystic ovary syndrome (PCOS) is associated with androgen excess, anovulation, obesity, insulin resistance, and an elevated risk of developing type 2 diabetes. A familial pattern of inheritance has been observed in many studies and susceptibility genes have also been reported. Mutharasan et al sought to determine if the luteinizing hormone/choriogonadotropin receptor (LHCGR) and/or follicle-stimulating hormone receptor (FSHR) plus 20 kb upstream and downstream was a cause of PCOS in women of European ancestry. They tested the association between 96 single-nucleotide polymorphisms mapping regions of

TABLE 1.—Results of Genetic Analyses

Trait	SNP	Allele	MAF[a]	Model 1 OR	Model 1 P Value	Model 2 OR	Model 2 P Value	Model 3 OR	Model 3 P Value	Model 4 OR	Model 4 P Value
Qualitative analysis											
LHCGR variants											
Case/control	rs7562215	T	0.069	0.71	0.013	0.72	0.044	0.56	0.0036	0.58	8.53×10^{-4}
Case/control	rs4319975	A	0.268	1.1	0.192	1.13	0.178	1.11	0.353	1.07	0.493
Case/control	rs10495960	A	0.158	1.31	0.0046	1.36	0.005	1.36	0.024	1.29	0.025
Case/control	rs4952923	G	0.193	1.22	0.022	1.29	0.012	1.26	0.07	1.17	0.125
Case/control	rs17326656	T	0.227	0.9	0.203	0.9	0.279	0.94	0.576	0.98	0.83
Case/control	rs4131886	G	0.264	0.93	0.336	0.94	0.501	0.97	0.811	1	0.996
Case/control	rs4519576	C	0.491	0.89	0.085	0.85	0.039	0.94	0.524	0.99	0.903
Case/control	rs35960650	T	0.349	1.11	0.127	1.15	0.103	1.2	0.078	1.11	0.218
Case/control	rs13405728[b]	NA	0.049	NA	NA	NA	NA	NA	NA	NA	NA
Case/control	rs2956355	T	0.093	1.08	0.492	0.96	0.754	0.88	0.45	1.01	0.916
Case/control	rs7562879	A	0.108	0.82	0.068	0.74	0.022	0.7	0.021	0.783	0.065
FSHR variants											
Case/control	rs6739570	T	0.066	1.37	0.038	1.5	0.019	1.36	0.162	1.26	0.202
Case/control	rs10205982	A	0.066	0.73	0.023	0.68	0.021	0.71	0.093	0.74	0.075
Case/control	rs17500266	G	0.46	0.88	0.061	0.88	0.11	0.83	0.07	0.85	0.061
Case/control	rs7591064	C	0.168	1.21	0.021	1.28	0.013	1.3	0.033	1.2	0.071
Case/control	rs11125188	T	0.487	0.87	0.048	0.85	0.041	0.77	0.012	0.82	0.019
Case/control	rs1922476	C	0.359	1.23	0.004	1.23	0.013	1.34	0.005	1.31	0.002
				Beta	P value	Beta	P value	Beta	P value	Beta	P value
Quantitative analysis											
FSH (mIU/ml)	rs17038320	T	0.164	−0.83	1.0×10^{-3}	−0.81	1.4×10^{-3}	−0.81	1.3×10^{-3}	−0.84	9.3×10^{-4}
FSH (mIU/ml)	rs17038059	T	0.195	−0.7	3.1×10^{-3}	−0.69	3.2×10^{-3}	−0.69	3.1×10^{-3}	−0.7	3.1×10^{-3}
FSH (mIU/ml)	rs17038141	A	0.159	−0.76	3.6×10^{-3}	−0.74	4.4×10^{-3}	−0.77	3.2×10^{-3}	−0.79	2.7×10^{-3}
TG (mg/dl)	rs7591064	C	0.168	−24	6.9×10^{-4}	−23	1.1×10^{-3}	−23	1.1×10^{-3}	−24	7.1×10^{-3}
TG (mg/dl)	rs4952931	G	0.42	−18	1.8×10^{-3}	−18	1.7×10^{-3}	−18	1.7×10^{-3}	−18	1.8×10^{-3}
TG (mg/dl)	rs17500266	G	0.46	18	1.9×10^{-3}	17	3.0×10^{-3}	17	3.2×10^{-3}	18	2.2×10^{-3}

Model 1, PCA adjusted; model 2, BMI and PCA adjusted; model 3, age, and PCA adjusted; model 4, age, BMI, and PCA adjusted. NA, Not available, did not genotype.
[a]Minor allele frequency in CEU.
[b]Chinese PCOS locus.

the LHCGR and FSHR. Their analysis identified 2 independent PCOS suscepti-bility loci that replicated findings in Chinese women, suggesting that the loci contribute to the PCOS phenotype in women of variable ethnicities. There are 3 known genes with reproductive function, LHCGR, FSHR, and GTE2A1L in the chromosome 2p16.3 region. Future studies are needed to match the phenotype with the genotype for this common reproductive disorder in females. This study further characterizes PCOS in women with different ethnicities.[1-5]

A. W. Meikle, MD

References

1. Urbanek M, Sam S, Legro RS, Dunaif A. Identification of a polycystic ovary syndrome susceptibility variant in fibrillin-3 and association with a metabolic phenotype. *J Clin Endocrinol Metab.* 2007;92:4191-4198.
2. Franks S. Candidate genes in women with polycystic ovary syndrome. *Fertil Steril.* 2006;86:S15.
3. Hickey TE, Legro RS, Norman RJ. Epigenetic modification of the X chromosome influences susceptibility to polycystic ovary syndrome. *J Clin Endocrinol Metab.* 2006;91:2789-2791.
4. Urbanek M, Woodroffe A, Ewens KG, et al. Candidate gene region for polycystic ovary syndrome on chromosome 19p13.2. *J Clin Endocrinol Metab.* 2005;90: 6623-6629.
5. Chen ZJ, Zhao H, He L, et al. Genome-wide association study identifies suscepti-bility loci for polycystic ovary syndrome on chromosome 2p16.3, 2p21 and 9q33.3. *Nat Genet.* 2011;43:55-59.

Differential Gene Expression in Granulosa Cells from Polycystic Ovary Syndrome Patients with and without Insulin Resistance: Identification of Susceptibility Gene Sets through Network Analysis
Kaur S, Archer KJ, Devi MG, et al (Univ of Delhi, India; Virginia Commonwealth Univ, Richmond; Gouri Hosps, Delhi, India; et al)
J Clin Endocrinol Metab 97:E2016-E2021, 2012

Context.—Polycystic ovary syndrome (PCOS) is a heterogeneous, genet-ically complex, endocrine disorder of uncertain etiology in women.

Objective.—Our aim was to compare the gene expression profiles in stimulated granulosa cells of PCOS women with and without insulin resis-tance *vs.* matched controls.

Research Design and Methods.—This study included 12 normal ovula-tory women (controls), 12 women with PCOS without evidence for insulin resistance (PCOS non-IR), and 16 women with insulin resistance (PCOS-IR) undergoing *in vitro* fertilization. Granulosa cell gene expression profiling was accomplished using Affymetrix Human Genome-U133 arrays. Differ-entially expressed genes were classified according to gene ontology using ingenuity pathway analysis tools. Microarray results for selected genes were confirmed by real-time quantitative PCR.

Results.—A total of 211 genes were differentially expressed in PCOS non-IR and PCOS-IR granulosa cells (fold change ≥ 1.5; $P \leq 0.001$) *vs.* matched

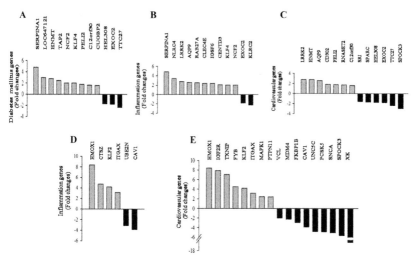

FIGURE 2.—Functional analysis of microarray data by IPA tools indicated differential expression ($P \leq 0.001$) of diabetes mellitus, inflammatory response, and cardiovascular disease genes in the granulosa cells of PCOS-IR (n = 4) (A–C) and PCOS non-IR (n = 3) subjects (D and E) *vs.* matched controls (n = 3). A, Histogram analysis of diabetes mellitus genes in PCOS-IR with at least 1.8-fold change in expression. B, Histogram analysis of inflammation response genes in PCOS-IR with at least 1.58-fold change in expression. C, Histogram analysis of cardiovascular disease genes in PCOS-IR with at least 1.59-fold change in expression. D, Histogram analysis of inflammation response genes in PCOS non-IR with at least 3.11-fold change in expression. E, Histogram analysis of cardiovascular disease genes in PCOS non-IR with at least 1.98-fold change in expression. (Reprinted from Kaur S, Archer KJ, Devi MG, et al. Differential gene expression in granulosa cells from polycystic ovary syndrome patients with and without insulin resistance: identification of susceptibility gene sets through network analysis. *J Clin Endocrinol Metab.* 2012;97:E2016-E2021, © 2012, with permission from the Author[s] and The Endocrine Society.)

controls. Diabetes mellitus and inflammation genes were significantly increased in PCOS-IR patients. Real-time quantitative PCR confirmed higher expression of NCF2 (2.13-fold), TCF7L2 (1.92-fold), and SER-PINA1 (5.35-fold). Increased expression of inflammation genes ITGAX (3.68-fold) and TAB2 (1.86-fold) was confirmed in PCOS non-IR. Different cardiometabolic disease genes were differentially expressed in the two groups. Decreased expression of CAV1 (-3.58-fold) in PCOS non-IR and SPARC (-1.88-fold) in PCOS-IR was confirmed. Differential expression of genes involved in TGF-β signaling (IGF2R, increased; and HAS2, decreased), and oxidative stress (TXNIP, increased) was confirmed in both groups.

Conclusions.—Microarray analysis demonstrated differential expression of genes linked to diabetes mellitus, inflammation, cardiovascular diseases, and infertility in the granulosa cells of PCOS women with and without insulin resistance. Because these dysregulated genes are also involved in oxidative stress, lipid metabolism, and insulin signaling, we hypothesize that these genes may be involved in follicular growth arrest and metabolic disorders associated with the different phenotypes of PCOS (Fig 2).

▶ Polycystic ovary syndrome (PCOS) is characterized by familial endocrine and metabolic disorders of unknown cause. The endocrine disorders include hyperandrogenism, ovulatory dysfunction, and polycystic ovaries. The frequent metabolic disorders are insulin resistance, obesity, dyslipidemia, and hypertension. Therefore, patients had increased risk of diabetes mellitus and cardiovascular disease. Kaur et al used a unique approach to ascertain genetic variants and recruited women undergoing ovarian stimulation to investigate abnormal expression of multiple genes of PCOS, insulin resistance, and cardiovascular disease in granulosa cells. They observed that PCOS patients compared with normal controls expressed significant differences in granulosa cell genes related to diabetes mellitus, inflammation, infertility in PCOS, and cardiovascular disease. The microarray approach yielded differences in gene expression in profiles of gonadotropin-stimulated granulosa cells of PCOS patients with or without insulin resistance. They postulated that because the deregulated genes were linked to oxidative stress, lipid metabolism and insulin signaling different genes might be involved in follicular growth arrest and metabolic disorders associated with various phenotypes of PCOS.[1-5]

A. W. Meikle, MD

References

1. Dai G, Lu G. Different protein expression patterns associated with polycystic ovary syndrome in human follicular fluid during controlled ovarian hyperstimulation. *Reprod Fertil Dev.* 2012;24:893-904.
2. Li Y, Liang XY. Effect of follicle stimulating hormone on the secretion of antimullerian hormone in the granulosa cells in patients with polycystic ovarian syndrome. *Zhonghua Fu Chan Ke Za Zhi.* 2012;47:5-8.
3. Qu F, Wang FF, Yin R, et al. A molecular mechanism underlying ovarian dysfunction of polycystic ovary syndrome: hyperandrogenism induces epigenetic alterations in the granulosa cells. *J Mol Med (Berl).* 2012;90:911-923.
4. Li Y, Wei LN, Liang XY. Follicle-stimulating hormone suppressed excessive production of antimullerian hormone caused by abnormally enhanced promoter activity in polycystic ovary syndrome granulosa cells. *Fertil Steril.* 2011;95: 2354-2358. 2358.e1.
5. Catteau-Jonard S, Jamin SP, Leclerc A, Gonzales J, Dewailly D, di Clemente N. Anti-Mullerian hormone, its receptor, FSH receptor, and androgen receptor genes are overexpressed by granulosa cells from stimulated follicles in women with polycystic ovary syndrome. *J Clin Endocrinol Metab.* 2008;93:4456-4461.

Is there a dose–response relationship of metformin treatment in patients with polycystic ovary syndrome? Results from a multicentric study
Fulghesu AM, Romualdi D, Di Florio C, et al (Università di Cagliari, Italy; Università Cattolica del Sacro Cuore, Rome, Italy; et al)
Hum Reprod 27:3057-3066, 2012

Study Question.—Do different dosages of metformin account for different clinical and biochemical outcomes in women with polycystic ovary syndrome (PCOS) and do basal anthropometric and metabolic characteristics of the patients provide any indications regarding the dose required to reach the target effect?

TABLE 5.—Hormonal and Metabolic Features of Patients Divided Into Responders and Non-Responders to Metformin Treatment

	Responder (89 pts)	Non-Responder (112 pts)	Significance (P)
Age (years)	22.74 ± 6.72	23.65 ± 6.49	NS
Weight (kg)	78.41 ± 20.24	72.68 ± 18.18	<0.05
BMI (kg/m^2)	30.08 ± 7.47	28.01 ± 6.72	<0.05
WHR	0.84 ± 0.09	0.82 ± 0.08	NS
Dose (mg)	1412.36 ± 331.26	1408.04 ± 309.65	NS
Dose/weight (mg/kg)	19.72 ± 4.46	20.21 ± 5.09	NS
Menses (no./6 months)	2.16 ± 1.38	3.35 ± 1.69	NS
ΔBMI (kg/m^2)	−1.03 ± 2.17	−1.07 ± 2.55	NS
ΔAUC-I (IU/l × 3 h)	−4836.22 ± 7196.71	−3375.39 ± 6930.95	NS
ΔHOMA	−0.99 ± 2.14	−1.26 ± 2.38	NS
ΔT (ng/ml)	−0.14 ± 0.31	0.01 ± 0.39	<0.05
FSH (mIU/ml)	5.22 ± 1.74	5.05 ± 1.34	NS
LH (mIU/ml)	6.60 ± 4.06	7.08 ± 4.25	NS
E2 (pg/ml)	39.71 ± 21.86	44.78 ± 32.17	NS
PRL (ng/ml)	17.33 ± 12.17	19.34 ± 12.40	NS
A (ng/ml)	2.98 ± 1.36	2.99 ± 1.29	NS
T tot (ng/ml)	0.70 ± 0.36	0.65 ± 0.34	NS
T free (ng/ml)	3.62 ± 3.61	4.64 ± 7.89	NS
SHBG (nmol/l)	37.01 ± 28.12	38.27 ± 25.69	NS
FAI	2.85 ± 2.41	2.52 ± 2.78	NS
F (ng/ml)	137.55 ± 45.27	141.64 ± 48.41	NS
17(OH)P (ng/ml)	1.30 ± 0.69	1.35 ± 0.80	NS
HOMA	3.65 ± 2.39	3.24 ± 2.29	NS
AUC-I (IU/l × 180 min)	19 200 ± 10 780	18 000 ± 9440	NS
HDL (mg/dl)	48.82 ± 12.13	49.90 ± 13.01	NS
LDL (mg/dl)	100.60 ± 26.71	105.44 ± 33.27	NS
Triglycerides (mg/dl)	95.27 ± 40.88	96.99 ± 60.37	NS
Total cholesterol (mg/dl)	168.58 ± 29.13	175.03 ± 37.01	NS

Responders exhibited an increase in menstrual frequency >2 cycles/year. BMI, body mass index; WHR, waist-to-hip ratio; SHBG, sex hormone-binding globulin; FAI, free androgen index; 17-OHP, 17 hydroxy-progesterone; AUC-I, area under the curve insulin (integrated plasma insulin during the glucose tolerance test); T, testosterone; T tot, total testosterone; E2, estradiol; A, androstenedione; PRL, prolactin; HOMA, homeostatic index [fasting insulin (μU/ml) × fasting glucose (mmol/l)/22, 5]; HDL, high-density lipoprotein; LDL, low-density lipoprotein; SHBG, sex hormone-binding globulin; FAI, free androgen index; 17-OHP, 17 hydroxyprogesterone. Values are mean ± SD.

Summary Answer.—Different doses of metformin exerted the same effects on clinical, biochemical and metabolic parameters in patients affected by PCOS.

What Is Known and What this Paper ADDS.—Since the insulin-sensitizing agents came into use in the management of PCOS, metformin has shown a positive benefits—risks ratio. Nonetheless, therapeutic schedules are not well standardized. This is the first study which systematically analyses the effect of different doses of metformin on clinical, hormonal and metabolic features of PCOS. On the basis of our results, higher doses are no more effective than lower doses.

Design.—A multicentric cohort prospective study. A total of 250 PCOS women were enrolled, 49 lost to follow-up. Menstrual cyclicity, hormonal assays, oral glucose tolerance test, lipid profile and ultrasonographic pelvic examination were evaluated at the baseline and after 6 months of metformin treatment at different doses (1000, 1500 and 1700 mg).

Participants and Setting.—A total of 201 PCOS patients completed the study without protocol violations in three university hospitals: seventy-three patients from Centre A (treated with metformin 500 mg twice a day), 60 patients from Centre B (treated with metformin 500 mg three times a day) and 68 patients from Centre C (treated with metformin 850 mg twice a day).

Main results and the Role of Chance.—Metformin exerted an overall positive effect on the clinical and endocrine-metabolic features of PCOS. The degree of these effects was independent of the administered dosage in every range of basal body mass index (BMI). When patients were stratified according to their insulinaemic status, scattered inter-doses differences were found in some of the outcome measures. Patients who exhibited an increase of >2 menstrual cycles/year were considered as responders to treatment. Responders had a higher basal BMI than non-responders and showed a greater reduction in plasma testosterone levels after metformin treatment, but other outcome measures did not differ significantly. Total insulin secretion in the 180 min following the glucose tolerance test before metformin treatment (basal AUC-I) was significantly correlated with the decrease in insulin secretion induced by metformin in both the whole group and in responders, but only correlated with the variation in the number of cycles in responders.

Bias, Confounding and Other Reasons for Caution.—The different doses were administered in different centres, and between-centre variation is a potential confounding factor.

Generalizability to Other Populations.—The paradigm of using the minimum effective dose of metformin could be pursued in other pathological conditions characterized by insulin resistance.

Study Funding/Competing Interest(s).—No funding or competing interests to declare (Table 5).

▶ Polycystic ovary syndrome (PCOS) is a very common disorder in females and has complex pathophysiology and clinical manifestations, which include hyperandrogenism, chronic anovulation, inappropriate gonadotropin secretion, and insulin resistance. The metabolic syndrome and diabetes are common in these women. Metformin has been used for years to treat the disorder with some success in inducing ovulation and fertility, and its benefits have been attributed to improved insulin sensitivity.[1] In a multicenter study, Fulghesu et al provided results on the dose-response relationship of metformin in treating PCOS. Although metformin improved clinical and endocrine—metabolic parameters, there was not a clear dose-response effect. The authors provided several possible mechanisms for the apparent lack of a dose response in women with PCOS. They felt that the interplay between metformin and ovarian autocrine and paracrine regulation of follicle growth and steroidogenesis were likely explanations for the failure to show a dose-response relationship. We need to learn more about the effects of metformin on these parameters.[2-4]

A. W. Meikle, MD

References

1. Palomba S, Falbo A, Di Cello A, Cappiello F, Tolino A, Zullo F. Does metformin affect the ovarian response to gonadotropins for in vitro fertilization treatment in patients with polycystic ovary syndrome and reduced ovarian reserve? A randomized controlled trial. *Fertil Steril.* 2011;96:1128-1133.
2. Weerakiet S, Sophonsritsuk A, Lertvikool S, Satirapot C, Leelaphiwat S, Jultanmas R. Randomized controlled trial of different doses of metformin for ovulation induction in infertile women with polycystic ovary syndrome. *J Obstet Gynaecol Res.* 2011;37:1229-1237.
3. Yasmin E, Glanville J, Barth J, Balen AH. Effect of dose escalation of metformin on clinical features, insulin sensitivity and androgen profile in polycystic ovary syndrome. *Eur J Obstet Gynecol Reprod Biol.* 2011;156:67-71.
4. Mathur R, Alexander CJ, Yano J, Trivax B, Azziz R. Use of metformin in polycystic ovary syndrome. *Am J Obstet Gynecol.* 2008;199:596-609.

Metabolic Syndrome

Differential effect of oral dehydroepiandrosterone-sulphate on metabolic syndrome features in pre- and postmenopausal obese women

Gómez-Santos C, Hernández-Morante JJ, Tébar FJ, et al (Univ of Murcia, Spain; Univ Hosp, Murcia, Spain)
Clin Endocrinol 77:548-554, 2012

Objective.—To analyze the effect in obese pre- and postmenopausal women of a daily dose of 100 mg dehydroepiandrosterone-sulphate (DHEA-S) provided over a period of 3 months as replacement therapy against metabolic syndrome.

Context.—Although DHEA-S appears to be effective against certain features of metabolic syndrome, its usefulness against this syndrome as a whole has not been evaluated to date.

Design/Patients.—A randomized, double-blind placebo-controlled trial was conducted involving 61 postmenopausal women, who received DHEA-S ($n = 41$) or placebo ($n = 20$) for 3 months. The effect of DHEA-S treatment on the same postmenopausal women was compared with the effects observed in a group of premenopausal women ($n = 20$).

Measurements.—Anthropometric measurements were taken at the beginning and at the end of the treatment. Similarly, different parameters that define metabolic syndrome and other cardiometabolic variables were determined.

Results.—Dehydroepiandrosterone-sulphate replacement produced weight loss in the obese women studied. Moreover, waist circumference, glucose and systolic and diastolic blood pressure, among other metabolic syndrome parameters, improved in the postmenopausal group, who showed a significant reduction in the total metabolic syndrome score ($P < 0.05$). In contrast, in premenopausal women, the effect of DHEA-S was limited to obesity parameters, and no effect was observed on metabolic syndrome components. No significant changes were evident in the placebo group.

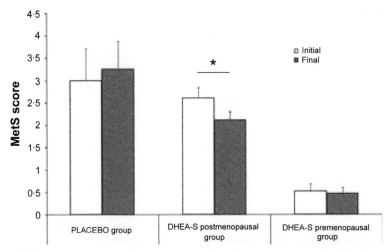

FIGURE 1.—Effect of, dehydroepiandrosterone-sulphate treatment in the three groups studied (placebo, prepostmenopausal women), in Metabolic syndrome, Metabolic syndrome (Score). Mean ± SEM. Differences between initial (filled square) and final (empty square) samples were tested with a paired Student's t-test. Single asterisk represents statistical significant differences, $P < 0.05$. (Reprinted from Gómez-Santos C, Hernández-Morante JJ, Tébar FJ, et al. Differential effect of oral dehydroepiandrosterone-sulphate on metabolic syndrome features in pre- and postmenopausal obese women. *Clin Endocrinol.* 2012;77:548-554, with acknowledgement of Wiley-Blackwell.)

Conclusions.—An oral dose of DHEA-S is useful for weight loss. In obese postmenopausal women, the hormone significantly improves plasma biochemical levels and anthropometric characteristics, leading to a better metabolic profile, which highlights the usefulness of this therapy against metabolic syndrome in this group of women (Fig 1).

▶ The metabolic syndrome is characterized by obesity, dyslipidemia, diabetes, and cardiovascular risk. In aging women, the metabolic syndrome increases and dehydroepiandrosterone-sulfate (DHEA-S) declines.[1] Studies have shown an inverse relationship between DHEA-S and obesity. An improvement of the metabolic syndrome related to effects on lipids and insulin sensitivity following DHEA-S administration has been inconsistent. In addition, some peptides related to obesity, including leptin, adiponectin, and ghrelin, have been shown to be related to DHEA-S. Gomez-Santos et al tested the hypothesis that oral DHEA-S therapy might affect obesity in pre- and postmenopausal women. They employed a randomized, double-blind, placebo-controlled, trial in both pre- and postmenopausal women. Although postmenopausal women had improvement in anthropometric and biochemical parameters of the metabolic syndrome, premenopausal women had a benefit of DHEA-S therapy but not in other parameters of the metabolic syndrome. Further study is needed to determine optimal dose of DHEA-S on these parameters and the long-term safety and benefit.[2-6]

A. W. Meikle, MD

References

1. Gómez-Santos C, Larqué E, Granero E, Hernández-Morante JJ, Garaulet M. Dehydroepiandrosterone-sulphate replacement improves the human plasma fatty acid profile in plasma of obese women. *Steroids.* 2011;76:1425-1432.
2. Labrie F. DHEA, important source of sex steroids in men and even more in women. *Prog Brain Res.* 2010;182:97-148.
3. Sutton-Tyrrell K, Zhao X, Santoro N, et al. Reproductive hormones and obesity: 9 years of observation from the Study of Women's Health Across the Nation. *Am J Epidemiol.* 2010;171:1203-1213.
4. Labrie F. Adrenal androgens and intracrinology. *Semin Reprod Med.* 2004;22: 299-309.
5. Gómez-Santos C, Hernández-Morante JJ, Tébar FJ, Granero E, Garaulet M. Differential effect of oral dehydroepiandrosterone-sulphate on metabolic syndrome features in pre- and postmenopausal obese women. *Clin Endocrinol (Oxf).* 2012;77:548-554.
6. Gomez-Santos C, Hernandez-Morante JJ, Margareto J, et al. Profile of adipose tissue gene expression in premenopausal and postmenopausal women: site-specific differences. *Menopause.* 2011;18:675-684.

Hypogonadism and Aging

Clomiphene citrate is safe and effective for long–term management of hypogonadism

Moskovic DJ, Katz DJ, Akhavan A, et al (Memorial Sloan Kettering Cancer Ctr, NY)
BJU Int 110:1524-1528, 2012

Objective.—• To assess the efficacy and safety of long-term clomiphene citrate (CC) therapy in symptomatic patients with hypogonadism (HG).

Patients and Methods.—• Serum T, oestradiol and luteinizing hormone (LH) were measured in patients who were treated with CC for over 12 months.

• Additionally, bone densitometry (BD) results were collected for all patients. Demographic, comorbidity, treatment and Androgen Deficiency in Aging Men (ADAM) score data were also recorded.

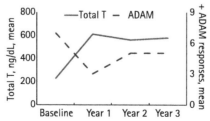

FIGURE 2.—Mean baseline and follow-up total T values as well as results of ADAM questionnaires quantifying the fraction of patients not reporting 'yes' for symptoms (defined as '+ response'). (Reprinted from Moskovic DJ, Katz DJ, Akhavan A, et al. Clomiphene citrate is safe and effective for long-term management of hypogonadism. *BJU Int.* 2012;110:1524-1528, with permission from British Journal of Urology International and John Wiley and Sons, www.interscience.wiley.com.)

• Comparison was made between baseline and post-treatment variables, and multivariable analysis was conducted to define predictors of successful response to CC.

• The main outcome measures were predictors of response and long-term results with long-term CC therapy in hypogonadal patients.

Results.—• The 46 patients (mean age 44 years) had baseline serum testosterone (T) levels of 228 ng/dL.

• Follow-up T levels were 612 ng/dL at 1 year, 562 ng/dL at 2 years, and 582 ng/dL at 3 years ($P < 0.001$).

• Mean femoral neck and lumbar spine BD scores improved significantly.

• ADAM scores (and responses) fell from a baseline of 7 to a nadir of 3 after 1 year.

• No adverse events were reported by any patients.

Conclusions.—• Clomiphene citrate is an effective long-term therapy for HG in appropriate patients.

• The drug raises T levels substantially in addition to improving other manifestations of HG such as osteopenia/osteoporosis and ADAM symptoms.

What's known on the subject? and What does the study add?

Clomiphene citrate (CC) has previously been documented to be efficacious in the treatment of hypogonadism. However little is known about the long term efficacy and safety of CC. Our study demonstrates that CC is efficacious after 3 years of therapy. Testosterone levels and bone mineral density measurement improved significantly and were sustained over this prolonged period. Subjective improvements were also demonstrated. No adverse events were reported (Fig 2).

▶ Hypogonadism, defined as low serum testosterone associated with characteristic symptoms, is a growing phenomenon in aging men. Men experience a decline of about 10% to 15% per decade of their serum testosterone. There are 2 forms of testosterone deficiency. Primary is caused by dysfunction gonad, whereas secondary hypogonadism is associated with dysfunction of a component of hypothalamic-pituitary-gonadal axis. There is a range of degrees of deficiency of testosterone in men with hypogonadism. In those with central deficiency, it has been shown that administration of antiestrogen can restore pituitary hormones and correct testosterone deficiency, improving fertility potential and symptoms. Moskovic et al report on use of clomiphene citrate for the treatment and management of long-term hypogonadism. In addition to improving serum testosterone levels, they also improved symptomatology and bone density.[1-3] Clomiphene citrate was well tolerated. A long-term efficacy study comparing transdermal testosterone replacement and clomiphene citrate was reported by Taylor and Levine, who observed that therapy increased testosterone 107% compared with 150% by transdermal testosterone. The authors propose that the mechanism of action is on disinhibition and central estrogen feedback that causes lowering testosterone levels in aging men; further studies are needed to confirm these observations and evaluate safety issues.[4]

A. W. Meikle, MD

References

1. Taylor F, Levine L. Clomiphene citrate and testosterone gel replacement therapy for male hypogonadism: efficacy and treatment cost. *J Sex Med.* 2010;7:269-276.
2. Ribeiro RS, Abucham J. Recovery of persistent hypogonadism by clomiphene in males with prolactinomas under dopamine agonist treatment. *Eur J Endocrinol.* 2009;161:163-169.
3. Shabsigh A, Kang Y, Shabsign R, et al. Clomiphene citrate effects on testosterone/estrogen ratio in male hypogonadism. *J Sex Med.* 2005;2:716-721.
4. Tan RS, Vasudevan D. Use of clomiphene citrate to reverse premature andropause secondary to steroid abuse. *Fertil Steril.* 2003;79:203-205.

8 Neuroendocrinology

ACTH

A 12-Month Phase 3 Study of Pasireotide in Cushing's Disease

Colao A, for the Pasireotide B2305 Study Group (Univ of Naples Federico II, Italy; et al)
N Engl J Med 366:914-924, 2012

Background.—Cushing's disease is associated with high morbidity and mortality. Pasireotide, a potential therapy, has a unique, broad somatostatin-receptor—binding profile, with high binding affinity for somatostatin-receptor subtype 5.

Methods.—In this double-blind, phase 3 study, we randomly assigned 162 adults with Cushing's disease and a urinary free cortisol level of at least 1.5 times the upper limit of the normal range to receive subcutaneous pasireotide at a dose of 600 μg (82 patients) or 900 μg (80 patients) twice daily. Patients with urinary free cortisol not exceeding 2 times the upper limit of the normal range and not exceeding the baseline level at month 3 continued to receive their randomly assigned dose; all others received an additional 300 μg twice daily. The primary end point was a urinary free cortisol level at or below the upper limit of the normal range at month 6 without an increased dose. Open-label treatment continued through month 12.

Results.—Twelve of the 82 patients in the 600-μg group and 21 of the 80 patients in the 900-μg group met the primary end point. The median urinary free cortisol level decreased by approximately 50% by month 2 and remained stable in both groups. A normal urinary free cortisol level was achieved more frequently in patients with baseline levels not exceeding 5 times the upper limit of the normal range than in patients with higher baseline levels. Serum and salivary cortisol and plasma corticotropin levels decreased, and clinical signs and symptoms of Cushing's disease diminished. Pasireotide was associated with hyperglycemia-related adverse events in 118 of 162 patients; other adverse events were similar to those associated with other somatostatin analogues. Despite declines in cortisol levels, blood glucose and glycated hemoglobin levels increased soon after treatment initiation and then stabilized; treatment with a glucose-lowering medication was initiated in 74 of 162 patients.

Conclusions.—The significant decrease in cortisol levels in patients with Cushing's disease who received pasireotide supports its potential use as a targeted treatment for corticotropin-secreting pituitary adenomas. (Funded by Novartis Pharma; ClinicalTrials.gov number, NCT00434148.)

▶ Cushing's disease is a rare disorder of chronic hypercortisolism caused by a corticotropin-secreting pituitary adenoma. The disorder is associated with central obesity, osteoporosis, arterial hypertension, insulin resistance, glucose intolerance, diabetes mellitus, dyslipidemia, cardiovascular disease, and increased mortality. Transsphenoidal surgery is the primary therapy in most patients, with remission rates of 65% to 90% when an expert pituitary surgeon operates.

The aim of this brilliant study was to investigate the treatment efficacy of pasireotide for the treatment of pituitary Cushing's disease. Pasireotide is a somatostatin analogue that targets 4 of the 5 somatostatin receptors, with highest affinity for subtype 5. This unique receptor-binding profile and the positive results found in a proof-of-concept study[1] provided the rationale for the present study. As shown in Fig 1 in the original article, the median urinary-free cortisol level decreased by approximately 50% by month 2 and remained stable in both groups. A normal urinary-free cortisol level was achieved more frequently in patients with baseline levels not exceeding 5 times the upper limit of the normal range than in patients with higher baseline levels (see Fig 2 in the original article). Importantly, the authors were also able to demonstrate positive effects on blood pressure, serum triglycerides and cholesterol, and body weight. As with other somatostatin analogues, the most common adverse events were related to transient gastrointestinal discomfort. In conclusion, pasireotide is the first (effective) drug for the medical treatment of pituitary Cushing's patients. This drug has been approved by the US Food and Drug Administration.

M. Schott, MD, PhD

Reference

1. Boscaro M, Ludlam WH, Atkinson B, et al. Treatment of pituitary-dependent Cushing's disease with the multireceptor ligand somatostatin analog pasireotide (SOM230): a multicenter, phase II trial. *J Clin Endocrinol Metab.* 2009;94:115-122.

General

Circulating Tumor Cells as Prognostic Markers in Neuroendocrine Tumors

Khan MS, Kirkwood A, Tsigani T, et al (Univ College London (UCL) Cancer Inst, UK; Cancer Res UK and UCL Cancer Trials Centre, UK)
J Clin Oncol 31:365-372, 2013

Purpose.—To determine the prognostic significance of circulating tumor cells (CTCs) in patients with neuroendocrine cancer.

Patients and Methods.—In this single-center prospective study, 176 patients with measurable metastatic neuroendocrine tumors (NETs) were recruited. CTCs were measured using a semiautomated technique based on immunomagnetic separation of epithelial cell adhesion molecule—expressing cells.

Results.—Overall, 49% patients had $\geq$ one CTC, 42% had $\geq$ two CTCs, and 30% had $\geq$ five CTCs in 7.5 mL blood. Presence of CTCs was associated with increased burden, increased tumor grade, and elevated serum chromogranin A (CgA). Using a 90-patient training set and 85-patient validation set, we defined a cutoff of < one or $\geq$ one as the optimal prognostic threshold with respect to progression-free survival (PFS). Applying this threshold, the presence of $\geq$ one CTC was associated with worse PFS and overall survival (OS; hazard ratios [HRs], 6.6 and 8.0, respectively; both $P < .001$). In multivariate analysis, CTCs remained significant when other prognostic markers, grade, tumor burden, and CgA were included. Within grades, presence of CTCs was able to define a poor prognostic subgroup. For grade 1, HRs were 5.0 for PFS ($P = .017$) and 7.2 for OS ($P = .023$); for grade 2, HRs were 3.5 for PFS ($P = .018$) and 5.2 for OS ($P = .036$)

Conclusion.—CTCs are a promising prognostic marker for patients with NETs and should be assessed in the context of clinical trials with defined tumor subtypes and therapy.

▶ Neuroendocrine tumors (NETs) comprise a heterogeneous group of tumors that arise most commonly from the gastrointestinal tract. The aim of the present study was to determine the prognostic significance of circulating tumor cells (CTCs) in patients with neuroendocrine cancer. The authors found a cutoff of 1 CTC or more as an optimal prognostic threshold with respect to progression-free survival (PFS) (see Fig 1 in the original article). Applying this threshold, the presence of 1 or more CTCs was associated with worse PFS and overall survival. This is the first study in NETs demonstrating the prognostic significance of CTCs. The identification of CTCs in NETs presents a number of opportunities such as the prediction of overall survival but also a prediction of therapy effects; therefore, this will have an important clinical implication in the future.

M. Schott, MD, PhD

Pituitary—General

MEN1 Gene Replacement Therapy Reduces Proliferation Rates in a Mouse Model of Pituitary Adenomas

Walls GV, Lemos MC, Javid M, et al (Churchill Hosp, Headington, Oxford, UK; et al)

Cancer Res 72:5060-5068, 2012

Multiple endocrine neoplasia type 1 (MEN1) is characterized by the combined occurrence of pituitary, pancreatic, and parathyroid tumors showing loss of heterozygosity in the putative tumor suppressor gene *MEN1*. This gene encodes the protein menin, the overexpression of which inhibits cell proliferation *in vitro*. In this study, we conducted a preclinical evaluation of *MEN1* gene therapy in pituitary tumors of $Men1^{+/-}$ mice, using a recombinant nonreplicating adenoviral serotype 5 vector that contained the murine *Men1* cDNA under control of a cytomegalovirus promoter (*Men1*.rAd5). Pituitary tumors in 55 *Men1*[+/−] female mice received a transauricular intratumoral injection of *Men1*.rAd5 or control treatments, followed by 5-bromo-2-deoxyuridine (BrdUrd) in drinking water for four weeks before magnetic resonance imaging (MRI) and immunohistochemical analysis. Immediate procedure-related and 4-week mortalities were similar in all groups, indicating that the adenoviral gene therapy was not associated with a higher mortality. Menin expression was higher in the *Men1*.rAd5-treated mice when compared with other groups. Daily proliferation rates assessed by BrdUrd incorporation were reduced significantly in *Men1*.rAd5-injected tumors relative to control-treated tumors. In contrast, apoptotic rates, immune T-cell response, and tumor volumes remained similar in all groups. Our findings establish that *MEN1* gene replacement therapy can generate menin expression in pituitary tumors, and significantly reduce tumor cell proliferation.

▶ Multiple endocrine neoplasia type 1 (MEN1), an autosomal dominant disorder, is characterized by the combined occurrence of tumors of the parathyroids, pancreatic islets (eg, gastrinomas and insulinomas) and anterior pituitary (eg, prolactinomas and somatotrophinomas). In addition, some patients with MEN1 develop adrenocortical tumors, foregut carcinoids, lipomas, meningiomas, facial angiofibromas, and collagenomas. Based on an established MEN1 mouse model, the authors explored the feasibility of in vivo MEN1 gene replacement. The authors show that in vivo expression of menin by use of a recombinant adenoviral vector in pituitary adenomas of MEN1 immunocompetent mice is effective in reducing tumor cell proliferation (Fig 4 in the original article) and is not associated with significant adverse effects or increased mortality (Fig 2 in the original article). This is absolutely an important study because it is a proof of concept for in vivo MEN1 gene replacement in reducing cell proliferation of anterior pituitary adenomas. Sometime in the future, this approach might also be applicable for MEN1 patients.

M. Schott, MD, PhD

Prolactin

Hyperprolactinemia-induced ovarian acyclicity is reversed by kisspeptin administration
Sonigo C, Bouilly J, Carré N, et al (Université Paris-Sud, France; et al)
J Clin Invest 122:3791-3795, 2012

Hyperprolactinemia is the most common cause of hypogonadotropic anovulation and is one of the leading causes of infertility in women aged 25–34. Hyperprolactinemia has been proposed to block ovulation through inhibition of GnRH release. Kisspeptin neurons, which express prolactin receptors, were recently identified as major regulators of GnRH neurons. To mimic the human pathology of anovulation, we continuously infused female mice with prolactin. Our studies demonstrated that hyperprolactinemia in mice induced anovulation, reduced GnRH and gonadotropin secretion, and diminished kisspeptin expression. Kisspeptin administration restored gonadotropin secretion and ovarian cyclicity, suggesting that kisspeptin neurons play a major role in hyperprolactinemic anovulation. Our studies indicate that administration of kisspeptin may serve as an alternative therapeutic approach to restore the fertility of hyperprolactinemic women who are resistant or intolerant to dopamine agonists

▶ Hyperprolactinemia is the most common cause of hypogonadotropic anovulation and represents a major etiology of infertility, with highest incidence in women 25 to 34 years of age. Gonadotropic deficiency has been proposed to result from direct suppression of prolactin (PRL) on gonadotropin-releasing hormone (GnRH) release, but evidence supporting this mechanism has never been provided. Because GnRH neurons are stimulated by kisspeptin (Kp) neurons, which unequivocally express PRL receptor,[1] the authors hypothesized that GnRH deficiency resulting from hyperprolactinemia is caused by reduced Kp input, which is now considered to be a primary gatekeeper governing reproduction. The authors now show that hyperprolactinemia in mice induces hypogonadotropic anovulation and diminished Kp expression (Fig 1 in the original article) and that peripheral Kp administration restores GnRH and gonadotropin secretion and ovarian cyclicity (Fig 2 in the original article). These data are consistent with the hypothesis that the anovulation of hyperprolactinemia is mediated through PRL inhibition of *Kiss1* gene expression and downstream diminution of GnRH and gonadotropin secretion. Kp neurons appear, therefore, to be the possible missing link between hyperprolactinemia and GnRH deficiency in mammals. As discussed by the authors, these findings suggest the possibility of therapeutic administration of Kp to hyperprolactinemic women who are resistant to dopamine agonists as a treatment for infertility.

M. Schott, MD, PhD

Reference

1. Smith JT, Li Q, Yap KS, et al. Kisspeptin is essential for the full preovulatory LH surge and stimulates GnRH release from the isolated ovine median eminence. *Endocrinology.* 2011;152:1001-1012.

9 Pediatric Endocrinology

Introduction

As always, this year's YEAR BOOK OF ENDOCRINOLGY offerings comprise an assemblage of topics and study designs. In the mix are randomized controlled trials, retrospective reviews, comparative analyses, and prospective studies. Also represented are a wide variety of scientific journals and research settings, which range from flagship endocrine to rather obscure orthodontia publications and from large community cohorts in Australia and the Netherlands to small groups of children with specific conditions in a subspecialty setting. Some of the articles provide welcome clarification of long-debated controversies, while others offer innovative discoveries that will immediately impact clinical care. Regardless, each was chosen on the basis of a significant contribution to the pursuit of knowledge and the provision of optimal clinical management of children with pediatric endocrine conditions.

The first two selections deal with very different aspects of growth hormone (GH) therapy in children with Prader-Willi syndrome (PWS). Approved for this indication in 2000, GH has been shown to be highly beneficial in improving linear growth and body composition in this patient population. The study described in selection No. 1 suggests that GH may also improve or at least prevent deterioration in subscales of cognition in these patients, although total IQ scores between treated and untreated groups did not differ. While hardly conclusive, this is an area that clearly merits additional study. Selection No. 2 is devoted to the equally important aspect of safety of GH therapy, which has been an issue of concern ever since reports of sudden death in children with PWS receiving GH surfaced. While the exact link between these tragic cases and GH has been inconclusive, this paper represents the first longitudinal follow-up of sleep-disordered breathing in children with PWS receiving GH therapy. While on balance highly reassuring, the study does remind us of a potentially vulnerable window shortly after initiation of treatment, reinforcing the current policy of careful surveillance surrounding GH therapy.

The next group of selections continues the theme of growth and extends it into the realm of over-nutrition as well. Selection No. 3 gives us what can reasonably be stated as the definitive answer regarding the impact of inhaled glucocorticoids on adult height. Although a statistically significant difference in adult height between the treated and placebo groups was seen, the discrepancy could be considered inconsequential. The next selection (No. 4) reports the phenomenon of extreme skeletal maturation in the setting of obesity, something that has long been recognized by pediatric endocrinologists but is scarcely found in the medical literature. Selection No. 5 also deals with obesity but approaches it from the standpoint of prevention using a universal, community-based early feeding intervention model. Simply teaching new mothers to respond to infant satiety cues resulted in a significant decrement in body mass index and rate of weight gain compared with the nonintervention group! The relationship between childhood weight trajectory and subsequent obesity is the focus of selection No. 6, which also relied on a community-based cohort using the enviably complete public health system in place in the Netherlands. Once again, we are reminded of the importance of preventive measures in early childhood as being perhaps the most efficacious tactic to stem the obesity tide.

The selections then move to the topic of thyroid disease, which is one of the most common reasons for referral to the pediatric endocrine clinic. Selection No. 7 nicely demonstrates the alteration in the hypothalamic-pituitary-thyroidal axis that seems to be ubiquitous in the setting of Down syndrome, and it offers a practical threshold of thyroid-stimulating hormone below which treatment is probably not warranted. Whether brand and generic levothyroxine are equivalent is the emphasis of selection No. 8, although the jury is still out on this important question. The last two of this year's selections pertain to puberty. While selection No. 9 purports to provide evidence for an earlier onset of puberty in boys, careful scrutiny of the results renders a sense of "No so fast!" in terms of making such a conclusion. Finally, selection No. 10 demonstrates that random, ultrasensitive luteinizing hormone does not revert to a prepubertal range in children being treated with a histrelin implant for central precocious puberty, which is an important issue for clinicians who are monitoring therapy to be aware of.

In conclusion, it is hoped that reading these YEAR BOOK selections will be both informative and enjoyable, will spark controversy and spur research, and will provide inspiration for the continued pursuit of intellectual inquiry and professional growth.

Erica Eugster, MD

Growth/Growth Hormone

Beneficial Effects of Growth Hormone Treatment on Cognition in Children with Prader-Willi Syndrome: A Randomized Controlled Trial and Longitudinal Study

Siemensma EPC, Tummers-de Lind van Wijngaarden RFA, Festen DAM, et al (Dutch Growth Res Foundation, Rotterdam, The Netherlands; et al)
J Clin Endocrinol Metab 97:2307-2314, 2012

Background.—Knowledge about the effects of GH treatment on cognitive functioning in children with Prader-Willi syndrome (PWS) is limited.

Methods.—Fifty prepubertal children aged 3.5 to 14 yr were studied in a randomized controlled GH trial during 2 yr, followed by a longitudinal study during 4 yr of GH treatment. Cognitive functioning was measured biennially by short forms of the WPPSI-R or WISC-R, depending on age. Total IQ (TIQ) score was estimated based on two subtest scores.

Results.—During the randomized controlled trial, mean SD scores of all subtests and mean TIQ score remained similar compared to baseline in GH-treated children with PWS, whereas in untreated controls mean subtest SD scores and mean TIQ score decreased and became lower compared to baseline. This decline was significant for the Similarities ($P = 0.04$) and Vocabulary ($P = 0.03$) subtests. After 4 yr of GH treatment, mean SD scores on the Similarities and Block design subtests were significantly higher than at baseline ($P = 0.01$ and $P = 0.03$, respectively), and scores on Vocabulary and TIQ remained similar compared to baseline. At baseline, children with a maternal uniparental disomy had a significantly lower score on the Block design subtest ($P = 0.01$) but a larger increment on this subtest during 4 yr of GH treatment than children with a deletion. Lower baseline scores correlated significantly with higher increases in Similarities ($P = 0.04$) and Block design ($P < 0.0001$) SD scores.

Conclusions.—Our study shows that GH treatment prevents deterioration of certain cognitive skills in children with PWS on the short term and significantly improves abstract reasoning and visuospatial skills during 4 yr of GH treatment. Furthermore, children with a greater deficit had more benefit from GH treatment.

▶ Short stature associated with Prader-Willi syndrome (PWS) has been an FDA-approved indication for growth hormone (GH) therapy for quite some time. Although the specific indication focuses on linear growth, the additional beneficial effects of GH on body composition and motor development in this population have long been touted. This randomized, controlled trial suggests that GH also improves cognition in children with PWS, or at least prevents deterioration in certain cognitive domains. Although this finding is intriguing, careful scrutiny of the results certainly raises some questions. Because the total IQ score of the GH-treated and untreated groups did not differ, one can't help but wonder whether the changes in subtest SD scores actually translated into meaningful differences in school performance or functions of daily living. Caution must also be used when discussing this type of study with parents of affected children who may be tempted to develop unreasonable expectations regarding the ability of GH to mitigate the IQ deficit intrinsic in the PWS phenotype. Lastly, additional studies that are not funded by pharmaceutical companies would be helpful in validating and expanding these results.

E. Eugster, MD

Longitudinal Evaluation of Sleep-Disordered Breathing in Children with Prader-Willi Syndrome during 2 Years of Growth Hormone Therapy

Al-Saleh S, Al-Naimi A, Hamilton J, et al (Univ of Toronto, Ontario, Canada; et al)
J Pediatr 162:263-268, 2013

Objective.—To review longitudinal polysomnography data to assess sleep-related disordered breathing (SRDB) before and up to 2 years after initiation of growth hormone (GH) therapy in children with Prader-Willi syndrome (PWS).

Study Design.—This was a retrospective review of systematic polysomnography evaluations performed in children with PWS before and at 6 weeks, 6 months, 1 year, and 2 years after initiation of GH therapy.

Results.—A total of 15 children with PWS were reviewed. At baseline, the median age was 3.7 years (range, 0.8-15.4 years), and the median body mass index percentile was 82.4 (range, 0-100). GH was discontinued in 2 of these 15 children owing to the occurrence of severe obstructive sleep apnea after 6 weeks of GH therapy. The remaining 13 children who were followed for up to 2 years on GH therapy demonstrated no statistically significant trends over time for any adverse sleep-related outcomes, specifically obstructive or central sleep apnea.

Conclusion.—In young children with PWS with known SRDB at baseline, the first few weeks after initiation of GH therapy may represent a vulnerable time for the development of significant SRDB. However, most children with PWS did not show significant changes in SRDB after 2 years of GH therapy. We conclude that long-term GH therapy appears to be safe after an initial period of increased risk in the context of SRDB in children with PWS (Fig 1).

▶ Growth hormone (GH) therapy has been shown to result in profound improvements in linear growth and body composition in children with Prader-Willi syndrome (PWS), which often translates into impressive functional gains in mobility and other aspects of daily life. However, enthusiasm has been tempered by reports of sudden death in children with PWS receiving GH therapy and the lingering concern of a direct link between GH and increased severity of obstructive sleep apnea in these patients. The situation is further complicated by the recognition that disordered sleep is ubiquitous in Prader-Willi patients and that the risk of sudden death associated with respiratory problems or infections exists regardless of GH therapy. In fact, many studies suggest that GH treatment may even decrease the mortality rate in this condition! Nevertheless, sleep studies prior to and following initiation of GH have become a standard of care for children with PWS. Although retrospective, this study adds the much-needed dimension of longitudinal follow-up regarding sleep-related disordered breathing in such children. The lack of any significant change in either the central apnea index or the obstructive apnea-hyperpnea index during a 2-year interval in 15 GH-treated children with PWS is highly reassuring. However, as seen in Fig 1, 2 young subjects experienced a worsening of sleep apnea after 6 weeks of treatment resulting in discontinuation of GH therapy. These results reinforce the

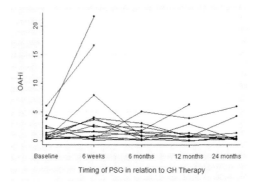

FIGURE 1.—OAHI in children with PWS during 2 years of GH therapy. There was no group trend for significant changes in OAHI in children with PWS on long-term GH therapy (*P* = .20). (Reprinted from Journal Pediatrics. Al-Saleh S, Al-Naimi A, Hamilton J, et al. Longitudinal evaluation of sleep-disordered breathing in children with Prader-Willi syndrome during 2 years of growth hormone therapy. *J Pediatr*. 2013;162:263-268, Copyright 2013, with permission from Elsevier.)

importance of careful surveillance in the context of GH treatment and the need for further investigation into the role of other factors, such as baseline adenotonsillar hypertrophy, baseline respiratory function, and environmental exposures like cigarette smoke. Such analyses in addition to large-scale, long-term controlled, prospective studies are clearly needed to resolve the ongoing debate.

E. Eugster, MD

Effect of Inhaled Glucocorticoids in Childhood on Adult Height
Kelly HW, for the CAMP Research Group (Univ of New Mexico, Albuquerque; et al)
N Engl J Med 367:904-912, 2012

Background.—The use of inhaled glucocorticoids for persistent asthma causes a temporary reduction in growth velocity in prepubertal children. The resulting decrease in attained height 1 to 4 years after the initiation of inhaled glucocorticoids is thought not to decrease attained adult height.

Methods.—We measured adult height in 943 of 1041 participants (90.6%) in the Childhood Asthma Management Program; adult height was determined at a mean (±SD) age of 24.9 ± 2.7 years. Starting at the age of 5 to 13 years, the participants had been randomly assigned to receive 400 µg of budesonide, 16 mg of nedocromil, or placebo daily for 4 to 6 years. We calculated differences in adult height for each active treatment group, as compared with placebo, using multiple linear regression with adjustment for demographic characteristics, asthma features, and height at trial entry.

Results.—Mean adult height was 1.2 cm lower (95% confidence interval [CI], −1.9 to −0.5) in the budesonide group than in the placebo group ($P = 0.001$) and was 0.2 cm lower (95% CI, -0.9 to 0.5) in the nedocromil group than in the placebo group ($P = 0.61$). A larger daily dose of inhaled glucocorticoid in the first 2 years was associated with a lower adult height (-0.1 cm for each microgram per kilogram of body weight) ($P = 0.007$). The reduction in adult height in the budesonide group as compared with the placebo group was similar to that seen after 2 years of treatment (-1.3 cm; 95% CI, -1.7 to -0.9). During the first 2 years, decreased growth velocity in the budesonide group occurred primarily in prepubertal participants.

Conclusions.—The initial decrease in attained height associated with the use of inhaled glucocorticoids in prepubertal children persisted as a reduction in adult height, although the decrease was not progressive or cumulative. (Funded by the National Heart, Lung, and Blood Institute and the National Center for Research Resources; CAMP ClinicalTrials.gov number, NCT00000575.)

▶ One of the most common questions asked by parents of slowly growing children is whether certain medications are the cause of their child's short stature. In particular, asthma medicines and attention deficit hyperactivity disorder medications are of special concern. Although many studies have attempted to investigate this issue, this one truly stands out because of its sample size, rigorous study design, and commendable retention rate. Despite previous conflicting results, this article provides what can safely be considered the definitive answer to this long-standing area of uncertainty, and the findings are mixed. On the one hand, as seen in Fig 2 in the original article, a highly statistically significant difference in adult height between the placebo and the budesonide group was seen. On the other hand, the difference was trivial (< 1/2 inch) and not likely to be significant in terms of quality of life or other meaningful measures. An important aspect of the findings was that prepubertal children appear to be most vulnerable to the suppressive growth effects of inhaled glucocorticoids. Therefore, whenever possible, it would seem prudent to minimize the dose and potency of these medications during this development period. When it is not, as the authors point out, the considerable benefits of well-controlled asthma surely outweigh the small decrement in adult height that may result from the use of inhaled glucocorticoids in children with reactive airway disease.

E. Eugster, MD

Skeletal maturation in obese patients
Giuca MR, Pasini M, Tecco S, et al (Univ of Pisa, Italy; Univ of L'Aquila, Italy)
Am J Orthod Dentofacial Orthop 142:774-779, 2012

Introduction.—The objective of this study was to compare skeletal maturation in obese patients and in subjects of normal weight to evaluate the best timing for orthopedic and orthodontic treatment. The null hypothesis was that obese and normal-weight patients show similar degrees of skeletal maturation.

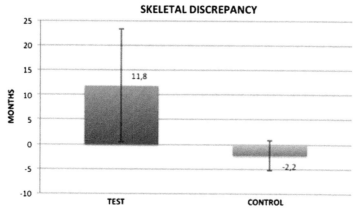

FIGURE.—Discrepancies between skeletal and chronologic ages in the test and control groups. (Reprinted from Giuca MR, Pasini M, Tecco S, et al. Skeletal maturation in obese patients. *Am J Orthod Dentofacial Orthop.* 2012;142:774-779, with permission from the American Association of Orthodontists.)

Methods.—The sample for this retrospective study consisted of 50 white patients (28 boys, 22 girls) whose x-rays (hand-wrist and lateral cephalometric radiographs) were already available. The test group included 25 obese patients (11 girls, 14 boys; average age, 9.8 ± 2.11 years), and the control group included 25 subjects of normal weight (11 girls, 14 boys; average age, 9.9 ± 2.5 years). Skeletal maturation was determined by using the carpal analysis method and the cervical vertebral maturation method.

Results.—According to the carpal analysis, there was a significant difference between skeletal and chronologic ages between the test group (11.8 ± 11.4 months) and the control group (−2.9 ± 3.1 months). Furthermore, the obese subjects exhibited a significantly higher mean cervical vertebral maturation score (2.8 ± 0.7) than did the control subjects (2 ± 0.6) ($P < 0.05$).

Conclusions.—Compared with the normal-weight subjects, the obese subjects showed a higher mean discrepancy between skeletal and chronologic ages according to the carpal analysis and had a significantly higher cervical vertebral maturation score. Thus, to account for the growth in obese patients with skeletal discrepancies, it might be necessary to perform examinations and dentofacial and orthopedic treatments earlier than in normal-weight subjects (Fig).

▶ This article is an example of how endocrinology overlaps with many seemingly disparate aspects of childhood growth and development. In this case, an article published in an orthodontics journal has highlighted something well known to pediatric endocrinologists worldwide, which is that exogenous obesity advances skeletal maturation. Indeed, it is not uncommon to find bone ages to be extraordinarily advanced (as much as + 5 standard deviations or more) in the setting of obesity, a phenomenon that prompts subspecialty referrals but is scarcely mentioned in standard textbooks. Therefore, although well recognized by experienced clinicians, a controlled study like this one, albeit quite small, is worth noting. As seen in the Fig, the obese group of children had a far greater discrepancy between bone age and chronological age than the nonobese group. Although the authors provide an interesting discussion regarding the purported role of leptin in driving skeletal advancement in the setting of obesity, a couple of important caveats regarding their findings deserve attention. One of these is the suggestion in the Results section that only the carpals were used for assessment of bone age using the Greulich and Pyle method. If so, this is concerning because convention has long held that the distal phalangeal epiphyses are the most sensitive part of the bone-age x-ray. An equally essential potential flaw is the lack of any information regarding the pubertal status of the subjects. Given their age, it is certainly possible that several were in central puberty or had physiologic adrenarche, both of which would obviously advance skeletal maturation. Regardless, this pilot study serves as useful corroboration of a long-held observation and will hopefully contribute to greater recognition of the pediatric obesity phenotype.

E. Eugster, MD

Miscellaneous

Evaluation of an intervention to promote protective infant feeding practices to prevent childhood obesity: outcomes of the NOURISH RCT at 14 months of age and 6 months post the first of two intervention modules
Daniels LA, Mallan KM, Battistutta D, et al (Queensland Univ of Technology, Brisbane, Australia; et al)
Int J Obes 1-7, 2012

Objective.—To evaluate a universal obesity prevention intervention, which commenced at infant age 4—6 months, using outcome data assessed 6 months after completion of the first of two intervention modules and 9 months from baseline.

Design.—Randomised controlled trial of a community-based early feeding intervention.

Subjects and Methods.—Six hundred and ninety-eight first-time mothers (mean age 30 ± 5 years) with healthy term infants (51% male) aged 4.3 ± 1.0 months at baseline. Mothers and infants were randomly allocated to self-directed access to usual care or to attend two group education modules, each delivered over 3 months, that provided anticipatory guidance on early feeding practices. Outcome data reported here were assessed at infant age 13.7 ± 1.3 months. Anthropometrics were expressed as z-scores (WHO reference). Rapid weight gain was defined as change in weight-for-age z-score (WAZ) of $> +0.67$. Maternal feeding practices were assessed via self-administered questionnaire.

Results.—There were no differences according to group allocation on key maternal and infant characteristics. At follow-up ($n = 598$ (86%)), the control group infants had higher BMI-for-age z-score (BMIZ) (0.42 ± 0.85 vs 0.23 ± 0.93, $P = 0.009$) and were more likely to show rapid weight gain from baseline to follow-up (odds ratio (OR) = 1.5, confidence interval (CI) 95% = 1.1–2.1, $P = 0.014$). Mothers in the control group were more likely to report using non-responsive feeding practices that fail to respond to infant satiety cues such as encouraging eating by using food as a reward (15% vs 4%, $P = 0.001$) or using games (67% vs 29%, $P < 0.001$).

Conclusions.—These results provide early evidence that anticipatory guidance targeting the 'when, what and how' of solid feeding can be effective in changing maternal feeding practices and, at least in the short term, reducing anthropometric indicators of childhood obesity risk. Analyses of outcomes at later ages are required to determine if these promising effects can be sustained.

▶ The track record of success in the treatment of children and adolescents with exogenous obesity worldwide is nothing short of dismal. Compounding the poor efficacy of the available therapeutic options are ubiquitous issues with high recidivism rates and failure to significantly alter entrenched familial and environmental lifestyle patterns. This constellation of obstacles demonstrates that, for the majority of obese pediatric patients, "the horse is already out of the barn" by the time medical attention for weight control is sought. Reinforcing the importance of obesity prevention is the well-established linear trajectory between the development of early-onset (under 2 years of age) overweight and subsequent body mass index during childhood and adolescence. Thus, this large Australian study is intrinsically appealing and intriguingly straightforward. By relying on that core principle of pediatrics known as "anticipatory guidance," the authors were able to demonstrate that merely educating new mothers on the practice of responsive feeding, which respects the infant's innate ability to self-regulate caloric intake, resulted in meaningful differences in indices of future obesity risk. Particular strengths of the study include the rigorous study design and impressive sample size. Only time will tell whether the protective leverage gained from interventions such as this one will be sustained. It may well be that a combination of approaches, including prenatal programming of taste preferences for healthy foods such as green vegetables, will be necessary in order to make inroads in the obesity epidemic. Ultimately, it is likely that common sense, rather than sexy strategies such as pharmacologic agents, will win the day.

E. Eugster, MD

Growth during Infancy and Childhood, and Adiposity at Age 16 Years: Ages 2 to 7 Years Are Pivotal

Liem ET, van Buuren S, Sauer PJJ, et al (Univ of Groningen, The Netherlands; Netherlands Organization for Applied Scientific Res TNO, Leiden)
J Pediatr 162:287-292.e2, 2013

Objective.—To assess the period during infancy and childhood in which growth is most associated with adolescent adiposity and the metabolic

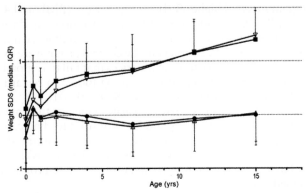

FIGURE 4.—Weight SDS in overweight/obese versus normal weight participants whose mothers did or did not smoke during pregnancy, by age. In the group whose mothers did not smoke, differences between the overweight/obese and normal weight participants are statistically significant at all time points (ie, $P \leq .005$). In the group whose mothers did smoke, differences between the overweight/obese and normal weight participants are statistically significant at all time points except age 0.5 year (ie, $P \leq .017$). ▽, Overweight/obese and smoking mother during pregnancy (n = 87); ■, overweight/obese and nonsmoking mother during pregnancy (n = 127); ●, normal weight and nonsmoking mother during pregnancy (n = 888); Δ, normal weight and smoking mother during pregnancy (n = 355). (Reprinted from Journal Pediatrics. Liem ET, van Buuren S, Sauer PJJ, et al. Growth during infancy and childhood, and adiposity at age 16 years: ages 2 to 7 years are pivotal. *J Pediatr.* 2013;162:287-292.e2, Copyright 2013, with permission from Elsevier.)

syndrome (MS) and whether this differs depending on maternal smoking during pregnancy.

Study Design.—A longitudinal population-based cohort study among 772 girls and 708 boys.

Results.—Weight gains between ages 2-4 years and ages 4-7 years were most strongly associated with higher body mass index (BMI), sum of skinfold measurements, body fat percentage, and waist circumference at age 16. A one SD increase in weight between ages 2-4 and 4-7 years was associated with increases in outcome measures of +0.82 to +1.47 SDs (all $P < .001$), and with a less favorable MS score. In children whose mothers smoked during pregnancy, the association of relative weight gain during ages 2-4 years with adolescent BMI was stronger than in children whose mothers did not smoke. For adolescent BMI, the increase was 0.42 SD higher ($P = .01$). This was similar for the other adiposity measures.

Conclusions.—Large relative increases in weight from ages 2 to 7 years are associated with adolescent adiposity and MS. This is more pronounced in adolescents whose mothers smoked during pregnancy (Fig 4).

▶ The association between weight trajectory in early childhood and the subsequent risk of being overweight or obese has been recognized for quite some time; thus, the basic tenet of this study is hardly novel. However, it is noteworthy for the very detailed and complete height and weight data derived from multiple measures in a large cohort (n = ~1500) of healthy children and for the inclusion of maternal smoking as a possible covariable. Only in the Netherlands could one conceive of such a high response rate and access to a public health system that is attended by 95% of the general population! The results of this study provide further ammunition for ongoing efforts aimed at the prevention of obesity that target mothers of preschool-aged children. As shown in Fig 4, maternal smoking during pregnancy was an independent risk factor for obesity and metabolic syndrome at age 16, even after adjustment for birth weight, which was lower on average in the exposed group. Although the authors suggest that smoking is a marker for other environmental factors that adversely impact health, recent studies have also implicated prenatal exposures in the genesis of epigenetic changes that promote a whole host of human ailments.[1] Thus, a multipronged approach that incorporates interventions geared toward both preconception and the early postnatal years will likely be needed.

E. Eugster, MD

Reference

1. Martínez JA, Cordero P, Campión J, Milagro FI. Interplay of early-life nutritional programming on obesity, inflammation and epigenetic outcomes. *Proc Nutr Soc.* 2012;71:276-283.

Hyperthyrotropinaemia in untreated subjects with Down's syndrome aged 6 months to 64 years: a comparative analysis
Meyerovitch J, Antebi F, Greenberg-Dotan S, et al (Schneider Children's Med Ctr of Israel, Petach Tikva; Clalit Health Services, Tel Aviv, Israel; et al)
Arch Dis Child 97:595-598, 2012

Objectives.—To determine whether an altered hypothalamic-pituitary-thyroid axis is inherent to Down's syndrome or if a high level of thyroid-stimulating hormone (TSH) is a feature in a subset of patients with Down's syndrome.

Design.—Comparative analysis.

Setting.—Major health maintenance organisation (3.8 million insured).

Patients.—A data warehouse search identified all subjects with Down's syndrome who attended Clalit Health Services in 2006 and were tested for TSH and free thyroxine (T4) level on the day of diagnosis (intention-to-treat population). The study group consisted of patients who were not diagnosed with thyroid disease or did not receive thyroid-modulating medication (n = 428). Their findings were compared with a control group of healthy age- and sex-matched subjects who were randomly selected from the general population.

Main Outcome Measures.—Distribution of free T4, TSH and total T3 levels.

Results.—The distribution plot for TSH showed a significant shift of the curve to higher values in the study group compared with the controls ($p \le 0.0001$). This finding held true on further analysis of the whole intention-to-treat population ($p < 0.006$). The free T4 distribution curve also shifted significantly to higher levels in patients with Down's syndrome ($p \leq 0.0001$).

Conclusions.—Down's syndrome is associated with higher TSH levels. The results suggest that hyperthyrotropinaemia is an innate attribute of chromosome 21 trisomy. Therefore, T4 treatment should not be contemplated in Down's Syndrome unless the TSH is >95th centile in the presence of normal-range free T4 levels.

▶ Pediatric endocrinologists have long debated the pros and cons of initiating treatment with levothyroxine in asymptomatic children with mild "compensated" hypothyroidism. Nowhere is this situation more frequently encountered than in children with Down syndrome (DS), who are notorious for mild biochemical abnormalities in thyroid-stimulating hormone (TSH) that often resolve spontaneously. Although studies conducted thus far have failed to demonstrate conclusive evidence of a deleterious effect of a mildly elevated TSH on growth and development in these children, many practitioners feel anxious withholding therapy, especially given the overlap between features of DS and symptoms of hypothyroidism. A major strength of this study is that it takes a population-based approach to address the question of what is intrinsically "normal" in pediatric patients with DS as compared with controls. The authors' results clearly indicate an altered set point of the hypothalamic–pituitary–thyroidal axis in DS, rather than evidence of autoimmune thyroiditis or other etiologies of hypothyroidism. Although the designation of a TSH of 9 or more as the threshold for treatment is arbitrary, it seems reasonable in the absence of other indicators of thyroid disease such as a goiter or positive antithyroid antibodies. As the authors point out, the precise underpinnings of this altered set point in the setting of trisomy 21 is an intriguing part of the puzzle that is as of yet unsolved.

E. Eugster, MD

Generic and Brand-Name L-Thyroxine Are Not Bioequivalent for Children With Severe Congenital Hypothyroidism

Carswell JM, Gordon JH, Popovsky E, et al (Harvard Med School, Boston, MA)
J Clin Endocrinol Metab 98:610-617, 2013

Context.—In the United States, generic substitution of levothyroxine (L-T$_4$) by pharmacists is permitted if the formulations aredeemedto be bioequivalent by the Federal Drug Administration, but there is widespread concern that the pharmacokinetic standard used is too insensitive.

Objective.—We aimed to evaluate the bioequivalence of a brand-name L-T$_4$ (Synthroid) and an AB-rated generic formulation (Sandoz, Princeton, NJ) in children with severe hypothyroidism.

Design.—This was a prospective randomized crossover study in which patients received 8 weeks of one L-T$_4$ formulation followed by 8 weeks of the other.

Setting.—The setting was an academic medical center.

Patients.—Of 31 children with an initial serum TSH concentration >100 mU/L, 20 had congenital hypothyroidism (CH), and 11 had auto-immune thyroiditis.

Main Outcome Measures.—The primary endpoint was the serum TSH concentration. Secondary endpoints were the free T_4 and total T_3 concentrations.

Results.—The serum TSH concentration was significantly lower after 8 weeks of Synthroid than after generic drug ($P = .002$), but thyroid hormone levels did not differ significantly. Subgroup analysis revealed that the difference in TSH was restricted to patients with CH ($P = .0005$). Patients with CH required a higher L-T_4 dose ($P < .0004$) and were younger ($P = .003$) butwerenot resistant to thyroid hormone; 15 of 16 CH patients had severe thyroid dysgenesis or agenesis on imaging. The response to generic vs brand-name preparation remained significant when adjusted for age.

Conclusions.—Synthroid and an AB-rated generic L-T_4 are not bioequivalent for patients with severe hypothyroidism due to CH, probably because of diminished thyroid reserve. It would therefore seem prudent not to substitute L-T_4 formulations in patients with severe CH, particularly in those <3 yr of age. Our results may have important implications for other severely hypothyroid patients in whom precise titration of L-T_4 is necessary.

▶ Few topics generate as much emotion and opinion as the issue of whether brand name pharmaceuticals are superior to their generic counterparts. Many families feel strongly that their child does better on one vs the other, and a decrease in compliance with medications has even been reported in association with a change in formulation. The situation is compounded by the frequent and indiscriminate switching of brand name to generic medications by pharmacists, often without the prescribing physician or patients' knowledge or consent. Therefore, a study like this is particularly welcome. Strengths of the study include the prospective, randomized design, the inclusion of only patients with severe hypothyroidism, and the efforts that were made to ensure compliance. Although the authors satisfactorily show that generic and brand levothyroxine were not bio-equivalent, support for some of their conclusions appears to be lacking. The suggestion that the reason a difference was seen in patients with congenital- but- not- acquired hypothyroidism was due to endogenous thyroid-hormone production in the latter group is questionable given the median thyroid-stimulating hormone (TSH) level of 254. While the average TSH level was statistically higher after 8 weeks on the generic drug, it appears that most of the subjects still had TSH levels in the normal range. Most importantly, this study offers no information to suggest that the difference noted between these preparations is clinically significant. In fact, a nearly simultaneously published article in the same journal suggests that it is not![1] Therefore, although one cannot necessarily endorse the authors' suggestion to only use brand name levothyroxine in infants with congenital hypothyroidism, this study does provide evidence for a policy long adhered to in the clinical setting: If a child is doing well on a particular brand of medication, there is no reason to change it. Conversely, if a switch is made, checking thyroid function tests sooner rather than later is the prudent course.

E. Eugster, MD

Reference

1. Lomenick JP, Wang L, Ampah SB, Saville BR, Greenwald FI. Generic levothyroxine compared with synthroid in young children with congenital hypothyroidism. *J Clin Endocrinol Metab.* 2013;98:653-658.

Secondary Sexual Characteristics in Boys: Data From the Pediatric Research in Office Settings Network

Herman-Giddens ME, Steffes J, Harris D, et al (Univ of North Carolina at Chapel Hill; American Academy of Pediatrics, Elk Grove Village, IL; et al)
Pediatrics 130:e1058-e1068, 2012

Background.—Data from racially and ethnically diverse US boys are needed to determine ages of onset of secondary sexual characteristics and examine secular trends. Current international studies suggest earlier puberty in boys than previous studies, following recent trend in girls.

Methods.—Two hundred and twelve practitioners collected Tanner stage and testicular volume data on 4131 boys seen for well-child care in 144 pediatric offices across the United States. Data were analyzed for prevalence and mean ages of onset of sexual maturity markers.

Results.—Mean ages for onset of Tanner 2 genital development for non-Hispanic white, African American, and Hispanic boys were 10.14, 9.14, and 10.04 years and for stage 2 pubic hair, 11.47, 10.25, and 11.43 years respectively. Mean years for achieving testicular volumes of ≥ 3 mL were 9.95 for white, 9.71 for African American, and 9.63 for Hispanic boys; and for ≥ 4 mL were 11.46, 11.75, and 11.29 respectively. African American boys showed earlier ($P < .0001$) mean ages for stage 2 to 4 genital development and stage 2 to 4 pubic hair than white and Hispanic boys. No statistical differences were observed between white and Hispanic boys.

Conclusions.—Observed mean ages of beginning genital and pubic hair growth and early testicular volumes were 6 months to 2 years earlier than in past studies, depending on the characteristic and race/ethnicity. The causes and public health implications of this apparent shift in US boys to a lower age of onset for the development of secondary sexual characteristics in US boys needs further exploration.

▶ This article represents the long-awaited companion piece to the landmark 1997 PROS study reporting an earlier onset of puberty in girls.[1] Although that study heralded years of vigorous debate that continues to this day, a secular trend of decreasing age of pubertal onset in girls is now accepted as a given by many. One of the enduring observations is that earlier puberty occurs particularly in overweight girls, whereas data suggest that the average age of puberty is unchanged in their normal-weight counterparts.[2] Much less information has been available about boys, although there has been an intriguing suggestion that being overweight is actually associated with a later age of pubertal onset than in the lean cohort.[3] Given the dearth of data on normal puberty in boys, this study is a valuable contribution. Particular strengths include the sample size, the inclusion of ethnic minorities and balanced representation of all US regions, and the use of testicular volume measurements in the assessment of pubertal status. The investigators took great pains to ensure the validity of the various measures, which is also to be commended. That being said, the results are internally inconsistent and raise a number of questions that make it difficult to come away with a resounding conclusion. One issue is that genital Tanner staging is notoriously subjective. In fact, many pediatric endocrinologists have abandoned its use entirely for this reason. The assessment of pubic hair, although much more reliable, does not necessarily imply central pubertal onset, as premature adrenarche is extremely common in the general population and more so in ethnic minorities than in whites. The most precise indicator of hypothalamic–pituitary–gonadal axis activation in boys is a testicular volume ≥ 4 mL, which was reached approximately 6 months earlier than classically referenced. However, it was statistically later in African-American boys than in the other groups, which was exactly the opposite of the other measures. And despite the observation of earlier pubic hair and genital development, there were no differences between the groups at age of Tanner 5 pubic hair and genital development, which was also no different from the original report by Marshall and Tanner.[4] So, what are we to conclude? As the authors point out, there are intrinsic flaws in a cross-sectional design, and additional longitudinal studies are needed to confirm or refute these results. In addition, determining testicular volumes in conjunction with other secondary sexual characteristics, such as pubic hair, would be invaluable in indicating whether the observed changes are indeed manifestations of central pubertal onset.

E. Eugster, MD

References

1. Herman-Giddens ME, Slora EJ, Wasserman RC, et al. Secondary sexual characteristics and menses in young girls seen in office practice: a study from the Pediatric Research in Office Settings network. *Pediatrics*. 1997;99:505-512.
2. Walvoord EC. The timing of puberty: is it changing? Does it matter? *J Adolesc Health*. 2010;47:433-439.
3. Lee JM, Kaciroti N, Appugliese D, Corwyn RF, Bradley RH, Lumeng JC. Body mass index and timing of pubertal initiation in boys. *Arch Pediatr Adolesc Med*. 2010;164:139-144.
4. Marshall WA, TAnner JM. Variations in the pattern of pubertal changes in boys. *Arch Dis Child*. 1970;45:13-23.

Random Luteinizing Hormone Often Remains Pubertal in Children Treated with the Histrelin Implant for Central Precocious Puberty

Lewis KA, Eugster EA (Indiana Univ School of Medicine, Indianapolis)
J Pediatr 2012 [Epub ahead of print]

Objective.—To investigate the use of random ultrasensitive (US) luteinizing hormone (LH) levels to monitor children being treated with a histrelin implant for central precocious puberty (CPP).

Study Design.—This was a prospective, uncontrolled, observational study at a pediatric endocrinology tertiary center. Thirty-three children (26 girls; mean age 7.2 ± 2.5 years) treated with a histrelin implant for CPP were enrolled. A random US LH measurement was obtained at 6 months, and a gonadotropin-releasing hormone analog stimulation test was performed at 12 months. Clinic visits occurred at baseline and at 6-month intervals.

Results.—In 59% of the patients (17 of 29), the 6-month random US LH exceeded the prepubertal range of ≤0.3 IU/L. In contrast, gonadotropin-releasing hormone analog stimulation tests revealed complete hypothalamic-pituitarygonadal axis suppression (peak LH <4 IU/L) in all 31 patients who underwent testing. US LH levels were highly correlated with peak stimulated LH levels. The mean peak stimulated LH level was higher in patients with a pubertal random LH than in those with a prepubertal random LH (1.2 ± 0.5 IU/L vs 0.5 ± 0.1 IU/L; *P* < .01). No patient had clinical evidence of pubertal progression.

Conclusion.—The random US LH level does not revert to a prepubertal range in more than one-half of patients with a histrelin implant and documented hypothalamic-pituitary-gonadal axis suppression. Long-term studies are needed to elucidate the optimal strategy for monitoring treatment in children with CPP.

▶ It's interesting to think about the way that assumptions sometimes trickle down into clinical practice and become widely accepted without a solid foundation. The discovery that a previously held belief is erroneous might occur as the result of a critical and deliberate re-examination or by happenstance. In this case, it appears to have been the latter. In designing a prospective study involving the histrelin implant for the treatment of central precocious puberty, the authors jumped on the popular bandwagon of using random ultrasensitive (US) luteinizing hormone (LH) values as a surrogate for degree of suppression of the hypothalamic-pituitary-gonadal (HPG) axis. This concept has been endorsed by a multidisciplinary consensus conference[1] and has become common practice at some institutions. Anecdotally, a US LH greater than the prepubertal range has been interpreted as indicative of treatment failure and used as cause for increasing the dose of monthly depot-leuprolide. What a surprise, then, to find that nearly half of these subjects had random US LH levels in the pubertal range, despite complete HPG axis suppression on GnRHa stimulation testing! Although random values were highly correlated with peak stimulated ones, the threshold for a random US LH that would indicate lack of suppression of the axis has not yet been identified. Until it is, use of this particular test for the purposes of monitoring of GnRHa therapy is of questionable utility. Regardless, it is refreshing to have a new development in the realm of clinical care that should decrease costs and lead to less testing.

E. Eugster, MD

Reference

1. Carel J, Eugster EA, Rogol A, et al; ESPE-LWPES GnRH Analogs Consensus Conference Group. Consensus statement on the use of gonadotropin-releasing hormone analogs in children. *Pediatrics*. 2009;123:e752-e762.

Addition of recombinant follicle-stimulating hormone to human chorionic gonadotropin treatment in adolescents and young adults with hypogonadotropic hypogonadism promotes normal testicular growth and may promote early spermatogenesis

Zacharin M, Sabin MA, Nair VV, et al (Royal Children's Hosp and Univ of Melbourne, Parkville, Victoria, Australia; Sanjay Gandhi Postgraduate Inst of Med Sciences, Lucknow, India)

Fertil Steril 98:836-842, 2012

Objective.—To assess the effect on spermatogenesis of adding recombinant follicle-stimulating hormone (FSH) to human chorionic gonadotropin (hCG) treatment protocols for adolescent/young adult males with hypogonadotropic hypogonadism (HH).

Design.—Observational descriptive study.

Setting.—Outpatient clinics.

Patient(s).—Nineteen males with hypogonadotropic hypogonadism, aged 14.5 to 31.0 years.

Intervention(s).—Treatment with either hCG treatment alone (n = 9; group 1) or in combination with recombinant FSH (n = 10; group 2), over 6 to 9 months.

Main Outcome Measure(s).—Combined testicular volume (CTV) and testosterone, inhibin B, semen/urine analysis at 6 to 9 months.

Result(s).—There were no differences between the two groups in baseline variables or changes in CTV with treatment. Despite this, evidence of spermatogenesis was present in all group 2 patients by 9 months (range 0.2 to 15×10^6/mL) compared with three of nine patients in group 1 (range 0 to $<1 \times 10^6$/mL). Whole group and subgroup analyses did not demonstrate any statistically significant correlations between age at onset of treatment and either CTV or sperm count.

Conclusion(s).—The addition of recombinant FSH to hCG treatment protocols in adolescent/young adult HH males results in normal testicular growth and may hasten induction of spermatogenesis.

▶ Adolescents with hypogonadotropic hypogonadism (HH) are often treated initially with exogenous androgen therapy, which has been associated with infertility in many. Exogenous human chorionic gonadotropin (hCG) has been successful in initiating and maintaining spermatogenesis in many men with HH.[1] Follicle-stimulating hormone (FSH) therapy has benefited fertility in men treated with hCG. In addition, childhood exposure to FSH might improve subsequent spermatogenesis.[2,3] Zacharin et al sought to determine if the addition of FSH to hCG benefits spermatogenesis in adolescents and young adult men with HH who had no prior therapy with testosterone. They observed that the combination of hCG/FSH resulted in normal testicular growth and possibly benefited spermatogenesis.[4,5] The timing of the combination therapy is critical and further study is needed to complete the recommendation. The authors did not find a good correlation with inhibin B concentrations and sperm production in young males and recommended that early induction is considered best to promote earlier appearance of sperm and conception.

A. W. Meikle, MD

References

1. Giagulli VA, Triggiani V, Corona G, et al. Effectiveness of gonadotropin administration for spermatogenesis induction in hypogonadotropic hypogonadism: a possible role of androgen receptor CAG repeat polymorphism and therapeutic measures. *Endocr Metab Immune Disord Drug Targets.* 2012;12:236-242.
2. Sinisi AA, Esposito D, Bellastella G, et al. Efficacy of recombinant human follicle stimulating hormone at low doses in inducing spermatogenesis and fertility in hypogonadotropic hypogonadism. *J Endocrinol Invest.* 2010;33:618-623.
3. Warne DW, Decosterd G, Okada H, Yano Y, Koide N, Howles CM. A combined analysis of data to identify predictive factors for spermatogenesis in men with hypogonadotropic hypogonadism treated with recombinant human follicle-stimulating hormone and human chorionic gonadotropin. *Fertil Steril.* 2009;92:594-604.
4. Sinisi AA, Esposito D, Maione L, et al. Seminal anti-Müllerian hormone level is a marker of spermatogenic response during long-term gonadotropin therapy in male hypogonadotropic hypogonadism. *Hum Reprod.* 2008;23:1029-1034.
5. Raivio T, Wikström AM, Dunkel L. Treatment of gonadotropin-deficient boys with recombinant human FSH: long-term observation and outcome. *Eur J Endocrinol.* 2007;156:105-111.

Distinguishing Constitutional Delay of Growth and Puberty from Isolated Hypogonadotropic Hypogonadism: Critical Appraisal of Available Diagnostic Tests
Harrington J, Palmert MR (The Univ of Toronto, Ontario, Canada)
J Clin Endocrinol Metab 97:3056-3067, 2012

Context.—Determining the etiology of delayed puberty during initial evaluation can be challenging. Specifically, clinicians often cannot distinguish

TABLE 3.—Studies that have Used hCG Stimulation Tests and Inhibin B to Diagnose HH

Study	First Author, Year (Ref.)	Test Protocol	No. of Subjects	HH Age (yr)	Testes Volume or Length
	hCG stimulation test				
1	Dunkel, 1985 (32)	hCG 5000 IU/m² on d 1, 3, 8, 10; serum T on d 1 and 15	19 males (12 IHH, 7 MPHD)	17.4 (12.5 −23.4)	3.9 ml (0.8 −9.6)
2	Kauschansky, 2002 (42)	hCG 1500 IU on d 1, 3, 5; serum T on d 1 and 7	19 males	16.1 (14 −18)	1−3 ml
3	Degros, 2003 (43)	hCG 5000 IU on d 1; serum T on d 1 and 3	13 males	19.9 (±3.3)	2.7 (±1.6) ml
4	Martin, 2005 (55)	Multiple hCG regimens used	9 males	15.7 (±1.6)	1.8 (±0.4) cm
5	Segal, 2009 (20)	hCG 1500 IU. Short hCG test (n = 38): hCG on d 1, 3, 4. Serum T on d 1 and 5. Extended hCG test (n = 31): hCG on d 1, 3, 4, 9, 12, 16, 19. Serum T on d 1, 5, 20.	14 males	12.7 (10.6 −16.9)	1.7 (1−3) ml
	Inhibin B				
6	Coutant, 2010 (17)[a]	Basal inhibin B levels	31 males (16 IHH, 15 MPHD)	HH: 16 (14.3; 17.0) MPHD: 15 (14.6; 15.1)	<3 ml in 16 males, 3−6 ml in 15 males
7	Adan, 2010 (65)	Basal inhibin B levels	13 males with IHH	15 (13−18.7)	2.6 (1.0−6.0) ml

Data are expressed as mean (SD or range) unless otherwise specified. To convert µg/liter of testosterone to nmol/liter, multiply by 3.5. T, Testosterone; PPV, positive predictive value; NPV, negative predictive value.
Editor's Note: Please refer to original journal article for full references.
[a]Data are expressed as median (25th; 75th percentiles).

constitutional delay of growth and puberty (CDGP) from isolated hypogonadotropic hypogonadism (IHH), with definitive diagnosis of IHH awaiting lack of spontaneous puberty by age 18 yr. However, the ability to make a timely, correct diagnosis has important clinical implications.

Objective.—The aim was to describe and evaluate the literature regarding the ability of diagnostic tests to distinguish CDGP from IHH.

Evidence Acquisition.—A PubMed search was performed using key words "puberty, delayed" and "hypogonadotropic hypogonadism," and citations within retrieved articles were reviewed to identify studies that assessed the utility of basal and stimulation tests in the diagnosis of delayed puberty. Emphasis was given to a test's ability to distinguish prepubertal adolescents with CDGP from those with IHH.

Evidence Synthesis.—Basal gonadotropin and GnRH stimulation tests have limited diagnostic specificity, with overlap in gonadotropin levels between adolescents with CDGP and IHH. Stimulation tests using more potent GnRH agonists and/or human chorionic gonadotropin may have better discriminatory value, but small study size, lack of replication of diagnostic thresholds, and prolonged protocols limit clinical application. A single inhibin B level in two recent studies demonstrated good differentiation between groups.

Conclusion.—Distinguishing IHH from CDGP is an important clinical issue. Basal inhibin B may offer a simple, discriminatory test if results from recent studies are replicated. However, current literature does not allow for recommendation of any diagnostic test for routine clinical use, making this an important area for future investigation (Table 3).

▶ By age 14, boys are expected to begin puberty as indicated by testicular development. Delayed puberty can be caused by many disorders, including hypergonadotropic hypogonadism, gonadal toxicity from chemotherapy, pituitary and testicular conditions, and many others. Distinguishing constitutional delay of growth and puberty (CDGP) from idiopathic hypogonadotropic hypogonadism (IHH) is an important management issue.[1,2] Basal and stimulated gonadotropin and gonadotropin-releasing hormone (GnRH) stimulated testing has yielded inconclusive diagnostic accuracy. Extended tests using human chorionic gonadotropin (hCG) resulted in improved positive predictive values to 92%. Improved diagnostic sensitivity has been reported with a combination of GnRH and hCG. Inhibin A is a glycoprotein hormone secreted by Sertoli cells of the testes and participates in the negative feedback of follicle-stimulating hormone. The review by Harrington and Palmert provided evidence for a simple, discriminatory test using serum inhibin B concentrations. A single inhibin B concentration of 35 pg/mL or less has 93% positive predictive values to diagnose those with IHH vs CDGP. However, further testing is needed to determine the best approach for correct diagnoses of these disorders.[3-5]

A. W. Meikle, MD

References

1. Wohlfahrt-Veje C, Andersen HR, Jensen TK, Grandjean P, Skakkebaek NE, Main KM. Smaller genitals at school age in boys whose mothers were exposed to non-persistent pesticides in early pregnancy. *Int J Androl.* 2012;35:265-272.
2. Ankarberg-Lindgren C, Westphal O, Dahlgren J. Testicular size development and reproductive hormones in boys and adult males with Noonan syndrome: a longitudinal study. *Eur J Endocrinol.* 2011;165:137-144.
3. Adan L, Lechevalier P, Couto-Silva AC, et al. Plasma inhibin B and antimüllerian hormone concentrations in boys: discriminating between congenital hypogonadotropic hypogonadism and constitutional pubertal delay. *Med Sci Monit.* 2010;16: CR511-CR517.
4. Coutant R, Biette-Demeneix E, Bouvattier C, et al. Baseline inhibin B and anti-Mullerian hormone measurements for diagnosis of hypogonadotropic hypogonadism (HH) in boys with delayed puberty. *J Clin Endocrinol Metab.* 2010;95: 5225-5232.
5. Marcus KA, Sweep CG, van der Burgt I, Noordam C. Impaired Sertoli cell function in males diagnosed with Noonan syndrome. *J Pediatr Endocrinol Metab.* 2008;21:1079-1084.

Article Index

Chapter 1: Diabetes

Basal Insulin and Cardiovascular and Other Outcomes in Dysglycemia   1

Association of Weight Status With Mortality in Adults With Incident Diabetes   3

Altered MAPK Signaling in Progressive Deterioration of Endothelial Function in Diabetic Mice   4

Association Between Coronary Vascular Dysfunction and Cardiac Mortality in Patients With and Without Diabetes Mellitus   5

Inverse relation of body weight and weight change with mortality and morbidity in patients with type 2 diabetes and cardiovascular co-morbidity: An analysis of the PROactive study population   6

Relationship between HbA$_{1c}$ levels and risk of cardiovascular adverse outcomes and all-cause mortality in overweight and obese cardiovascular high-risk women and men with type 2 diabetes   7

Management of hyperglycaemia in type 2 diabetes: a patient-centered approach. Position statement of the American Diabetes Association (ADA) and the European Association for the Study of Diabetes (EASD)   9

A Clinical Trial to Maintain Glycemic Control in Youth with Type 2 Diabetes   11

Large-scale association analysis provides insights into the genetic architecture and pathophysiology of type 2 diabetes   12

DNA methylation profiling identifies epigenetic dysregulation in pancreatic islets from type 2 diabetic patients   13

A metagenome-wide association study of gut microbiota in type 2 diabetes   13

Early Loss of the Glucagon Response to Hypoglycemia in Adolescents With Type 1 Diabetes   14

Glucagon regulates its own synthesis by autocrine signaling   15

Glucose activates free fatty acid receptor 1 gene transcription via phosphatidylinositol-3-kinase-dependent O-GlcNAcylation of pancreas-duodenum homeobox-1   16

Neonatal β Cell Development in Mice and Humans Is Regulated by Calcineurin/NFAT   17

Metabolic manifestations of insulin deficiency do not occur without glucagon action   18

Glucagonocentric restructuring of diabetes: a pathophysiologic and therapeutic makeover   19

TAK-875 versus placebo or glimepiride in type 2 diabetes mellitus: a phase 2, randomised, double-blind, placebo-controlled trial   20

Targeting VEGF-B as a novel treatment for insulin resistance and type 2 diabetes   21

The Effects of TAK-875, a Selective G Protein-Coupled Receptor 40/Free Fatty Acid 1 Agonist, on Insulin and Glucagon Secretion in Isolated Rat and Human Islets   22

Cardiovascular benefits and diabetes risks of statin therapy in primary prevention: an analysis from the JUPITER trial   23

Amorfrutins are potent antidiabetic dietary natural products   25

A Multiple-Ascending-Dose Study to Evaluate Safety, Pharmacokinetics, and Pharmacodynamics of a Novel GPR40 Agonist, TAK-875, in Subjects With Type 2 Diabetes   26

Ectopic expression of glucagon receptor in skeletal muscles improves glucose homeostasis in a mouse model of diabetes   27

Chapter 2: Lipoproteins and Atherosclerosis

Remnant Cholesterol as a Causal Risk Factor for Ischemic Heart Disease   30

Low HDL Cholesterol and the Risk of Diabetic Nephropathy and Retinopathy: Results of the ADVANCE Study   32

Effects of *trans* fatty acids on glucose homeostasis: A meta-analysis of randomized, placebo-controlled clinical trials   34

Efficacy and safety of a microsomal triglyceride transfer protein inhibitor in patients with homozygous familial hypercholesterolaemia: a single-arm, open-label, phase 3 study   36

Effects of AMG 145 on Low-Density Lipoprotein Cholesterol Levels: Results From 2 Randomized, Double-Blind, Placebo-Controlled, Ascending-Dose Phase 1 Studies in Healthy Volunteers and Hypercholesterolemic Subjects on Statins   39

Efficacy and Safety of Eicosapentaenoic Acid Ethyl Ester (AMR101) Therapy in Statin-Treated Patients With Persistent High Triglycerides (from the ANCHOR Study)   45

Effect of *Ezetimibe* on Major Atherosclerotic Disease Events and All-Cause Mortality   49

Atorvastatin with or without an Antibody to PCSK9 in Primary Hypercholesterolemia   52

Apolipoprotein B Synthesis Inhibition With Mipomersen in Heterozygous Familial Hypercholesterolemia: Results of a Randomized, Double-Blind, Placebo-Controlled Trial to Assess Efficacy and Safety as Add-On Therapy in Patients With Coronary Artery Disease   54

The effects of lowering LDL cholesterol with statin therapy in people at low risk of vascular disease: meta-analysis of individual data from 27 randomised trials   59

Dysfunctional High-Density Lipoprotein in Patients on Chronic Hemodialysis   64

Altered Activation of Endothelial Anti-and Proapoptotic Pathways by High-Density Lipoprotein from Patients with Coronary Artery Disease: Role of High-Density Lipoprotein—Proteome Remodeling   67

Impact of low-density lipoprotein to high-density lipoprotein ratio on aortic arch atherosclerosis in unexplained stroke   71

Chapter 3: Obesity

A Trial of Sugar-Free or Sugar-Sweetened Beverages and Body Weight in Children   76

A Randomized Trial of Sugar-Sweetened Beverages and Adolescent Body Weight   77

Natural killer T cells in adipose tissue prevent insulin resistance   79

History of weight cycling does not impede future weight loss or metabolic improvements in postmenopausal women ... 81

Translating the Diabetes Prevention Program Lifestyle Intervention for Weight Loss Into Primary Care: A Randomized Trial ... 82

Metabolically healthy obesity and risk of all-cause and cardiovascular disease mortality ... 84

Myths, Presumptions, and Facts about Obesity ... 86

Trends in mild, moderate, and severe stunting and underweight, and progress towards MDG 1 in 141 developing countries: a systematic analysis of population representative data ... 89

Sugar-Sweetened Beverages and Genetic Risk of Obesity ... 91

Obesity phenotype and incident hypertension: a prospective community-based cohort study ... 93

Bariatric Surgery Results in Cortical Bone Loss ... 94

The Effect of Excess Weight Gain With Intensive Diabetes Mellitus Treatment on Cardiovascular Disease Risk Factors and Atherosclerosis in Type 1 Diabetes Mellitus: Results From the Diabetes Control and Complications Trial/ Epidemiology of Diabetes Interventions and Complications Study (DCCT/EDIC) study ... 96

AMP-Activated Protein Kinase α1 Protects Against Diet-Induced Insulin Resistance and Obesity ... 98

Short-Term Caloric Restriction Normalizes Hypothalamic Neuronal Responsiveness to Glucose Ingestion in Patients With Type 2 Diabetes ... 100

Alterations in Gastrointestinal, Endocrine, and Metabolic Processes After Bariatric Roux-en-Y Gastric Bypass Surgery ... 101

Chapter 4: Thyroid

Thyroid Dysfunction and Autoantibodies in Early Pregnancy Are Associated with Increased Risk of Gestational Diabetes and Adverse Birth Outcomes ... 106

A TSHR-LH/CGR Chimera that Measures Functional Thyroid-Stimulating Autoantibodies (TSAb) Can Predict Remission or Recurrence in Graves' Patients Undergoing Antithyroid Drug (ATD) Treatment ... 108

Efficacy and Safety of Three Different Cumulative Doses of Intravenous Methylprednisolone for Moderate to Severe and Active Graves' Orbitopathy ... 110

Serum Antithyroglobulin Antibodies Interfere with Thyroglobulin Detection in Fine-Needle Aspirates of Metastatic Neck Nodes in Papillary Thyroid Carcinoma ... 113

Correlation between the Number of Lymph Node Metastases and Lung Metastasis in Papillary Thyroid Cancer ... 114

Role of TSH in the Spontaneous Development of Asymmetrical Thyroid Carcinoma in Mice with a Targeted Mutation in a Single Allele of the Thyroid Hormone-β Receptor ... 116

Somatic *RAS* Mutations Occur in a Large Proportion of Sporadic *RET*-Negative Medullary Thyroid Carcinomas and Extend to a Previously Unidentified Exon ... 117

Activation of the mTOR Pathway in Primary Medullary Thyroid Carcinoma and Lymph Node Metastases ... 119

Vandetanib in Patients With Locally Advanced or Metastatic Medullary Thyroid
Cancer: A Randomized, Double-Blind Phase III Trial   120

Maternal Thyroid Hormone Parameters during Early Pregnancy and Birth Weight:
The Generation R Study   122

Fetal Free Thyroxine Concentrations in Pregnant Women with Autoimmune
Thyroid Disease   123

Preoperative Diagnosis of Benign Thyroid Nodules with Indeterminate Cytology   125

Generation of functional thyroid from embryonic stem cells   127

Genome-wide analysis of thyroid hormone receptors shared and specific functions
in neural cells   131

Thyroid hormone triggers the developmental loss of axonal regenerative capacity
via thyroid hormone receptor α1 and krüppel-like factor 9 in Purkinje cells   134

Thyroid hormone is required for hypothalamic neurons regulating cardiovascular
functions   138

Tetrac Can Replace Thyroid Hormone During Brain Development in Mouse
Mutants Deficient in the Thyroid Hormone Transporter Mct8   141

Higher Free Thyroxine Levels Predict Increased Incidence of Dementia in Older
Men: The Health In Men Study   142

Hyperthyroid-associated osteoporosis is exacerbated by the loss of TSH signaling   144

Chapter 5: Calcium and Bone Metabolism

Serum 25-Hydroxyvitamin D Concentration and Risk for Major Clinical Disease
Events in a Community-Based Population of Older Adults: A Cohort Study   152

Associations of dietary calcium intake and calcium supplementation with
myocardial infarction and stroke risk and overall cardiovascular mortality in the
Heidelberg cohort of the European Prospective Investigation into Cancer and
Nutrition study (EPIC-Heidelberg)   154

Long term calcium intake and rates of all cause and cardiovascular mortality:
community based prospective longitudinal cohort study   156

Vitamin D with Calcium Reduces Mortality: Patient Level Pooled Analysis of
70,528 Patients from Eight Major Vitamin D Trials   158

Vitamin D Therapy and Cardiac Structure and Function in Patients With Chronic
Kidney Disease: The PRIMO Randomized Controlled Trial   160

A Pooled Analysis of Vitamin D Dose Requirements for Fracture Prevention   162

Dose Response to Vitamin D Supplementation in Postmenopausal Women:
A Randomized Trial   164

Increasing Occurrence of Atypical Femoral Fractures Associated With
Bisphosphonate Use   166

Incidence of Atypical Nontraumatic Diaphyseal Fractures of the Femur   169

Changes in bone mineral density and body composition during pregnancy and
postpartum. A controlled cohort study   171

Effect of Alendronate for Reducing Fracture by FRAX Score and Femoral Neck
Bone Mineral Density: The Fracture Intervention Trial   173

Oral bisphosphonates reduce the risk of clinical fractures in glucocorticoid-induced osteoporosis in clinical practice — 175

A Retrospective Study Evaluating Frequency and Risk Factors of Osteonecrosis of the Jaw in 576 Cancer Patients Receiving Intravenous Bisphosphonates — 178

Inflammatory Eye Reactions in Patients Treated With Bisphosphonates and Other Osteoporosis Medications: Cohort Analysis Using a National Prescription Database — 180

Effect of denosumab on bone mineral density and biochemical markers of bone turnover: 8-year results of a phase 2 clinical trial — 182

Skeletal Histomorphometry in Subjects on Teriparatide or Zoledronic Acid Therapy (SHOTZ) Study: A Randomized Controlled Trial — 185

Predictive Value of FRAX for Fracture in Obese Older Women — 187

Effectiveness of Teriparatide in Women Over 75 Years of Age with Severe Osteoporosis: 36-Month Results from the European Forsteo Observational Study (EFOS) — 189

Six Months of Parathyroid Hormone (1–84) Administered Concurrently *Versus* Sequentially with Monthly Ibandronate Over Two Years: The PTH and Ibandronate Combination Study (PICS) Randomized Trial — 191

Differing Effects of PTH 1-34, PTH 1-84 and Zoledronic Acid on Bone Microarchitecture and Estimated Strength in Postmenopausal Women with Osteoporosis. An 18 Month Open-Labeled Observational Study using HR-pQCT — 194

Effect of 12 Months of Whole-Body Vibration Therapy on Bone Density and Structure in Postmenopausal Women: A Randomized Trial — 196

Fracture Risk and Zoledronic Acid Therapy in Men with Osteoporosis — 198

Denosumab Treatment in Postmenopausal Women with Osteoporosis Does Not Interfere with Fracture-Healing: Results from the FREEDOM Trial — 200

Effect of Cinacalcet on Cardiovascular Disease in Patients Undergoing Dialysis — 202

Therapy of Hypoparathyroidism with PTH(1–84): A Prospective Four-Year Investigation of Efficacy and Safety — 205

25(OH) Vitamin D Is Associated with Greater Muscle Strength in Healthy Men and Women — 206

Chapter 6: Adrenal Cortex

Adrenal involvement in MEN1. Analysis of 715 cases from the Groupe d'étude des Tumeurs Endocrines database — 209

Combination Chemotherapy in Advanced Adrenocortical Carcinoma — 210

Activation of Cyclic AMP Signaling Leads to Different Pathway Alterations in Lesions of the Adrenal Cortex Caused by Germline PRKAR1A Defects versus Those due to Somatic GNAS Mutations — 212

Serum inhibin pro-αC is a tumor marker for adrenocortical carcinomas — 213

CT features and quantification of the characteristics of adrenocortical carcinomas on unenhanced and contrast-enhanced studies — 215

[131I]Iodometomidate for Targeted Radionuclide Therapy of Advanced Adrenocortical Carcinoma — 217

KCNJ5 Mutations in European Families With Nonglucocorticoid Remediable
Familial Hyperaldosteronism 218

Evaluation of the Sensitivity and Specificity of ^{11}C-Metomidate Positron Emission
Tomography (PET)-CT for Lateralizing Aldosterone Secretion by Conn's
Adenomas 220

Pattern of Adrenal Hormonal Secretion in Patients with Adrenal Adenomas: The
Relevance of Aldosterone in Arterial Hypertension 221

Chapter 7: Reproductive Endocrinology

The Association of Concurrent Vitamin D and Sex Hormone Deficiency With Bone
Loss and Fracture Risk in Older Men: The Osteoporotic Fractures in Men (MrOS)
Study 227

Do Changes in Sex Steroid Hormones Precede or Follow Increases in Body Weight
during the Menopause Transition? Results from The Study of Women's Health
Across the Nation 230

Hyperprolactinemia-induced ovarian acyclicity is reversed by kisspeptin
administration 231

Differential Regulation of Ovarian Anti-Müllerian Hormone (AMH) by Estradiol
through α- and β-Estrogen Receptors 232

Polycystic Ovary-Like Abnormalities (PCO-L) in Women with Functional
Hypothalamic Amenorrhea 235

The genetic origin of Klinefelter syndrome and its effect on spermatogenesis 236

Changes in hormonal profile and seminal parameters with use of aromatase
inhibitors in management of infertile men with low testosterone to estradiol ratios 238

Job demands as a potential modifier of the association between testosterone
deficiency and andropause symptoms in Japanese middle-aged workers: A cross-
sectional study 240

A New Combination of Testosterone and Nestorone Transdermal Gels for Male
Hormonal Contraception 242

Lean mass and insulin resistance in women with polycystic ovary syndrome 244

Ethinyl Estradiol-Cyproterone Acetate *Versus* Low-Dose Pioglitazone-Flutamide-
Metformin for Adolescent Girls with Androgen Excess: Divergent Effects on
CD163, *TWEAK* Receptor, *ANGPTL4*, and *LEPTIN* Expression in Subcutaneous
Adipose Tissue 246

Metformin Improves Pregnancy and Live-Birth Rates in Women with Polycystic
Ovary Syndrome (PCOS): A Multicenter, Double-Blind, Placebo-Controlled
Randomized Trial 248

Evidence for Chromosome 2p16.3 Polycystic Ovary Syndrome Susceptibility Locus
in Affected Women of European Ancestry 250

Differential Gene Expression in Granulosa Cells from Polycystic Ovary Syndrome
Patients with and without Insulin Resistance: Identification of Susceptibility Gene
Sets through Network Analysis 252

Is there a dose—response relationship of metformin treatment in patients with
polycystic ovary syndrome? Results from a multicentric study 254

Differential effect of oral dehydroepiandrosterone-sulphate on metabolic syndrome features in pre- and postmenopausal obese women — 257

Clomiphene citrate is safe and effective for long—term management of hypogonadism — 259

Chapter 8: Neuroendocrinology

A 12-Month Phase 3 Study of Pasireotide in Cushing's Disease — 263

Circulating Tumor Cells as Prognostic Markers in Neuroendocrine Tumors — 264

MEN1 Gene Replacement Therapy Reduces Proliferation Rates in a Mouse Model of Pituitary Adenomas — 265

Hyperprolactinemia-induced ovarian acyclicity is reversed by kisspeptin administration — 266

Chapter 9: Pediatric Endocrinology

Beneficial Effects of Growth Hormone Treatment on Cognition in Children with Prader-Willi Syndrome: A Randomized Controlled Trial and Longitudinal Study — 270

Longitudinal Evaluation of Sleep-Disordered Breathing in Children with Prader-Willi Syndrome during 2 Years of Growth Hormone Therapy — 272

Effect of Inhaled Glucocorticoids in Childhood on Adult Height — 273

Skeletal maturation in obese patients — 274

Evaluation of an intervention to promote protective infant feeding practices to prevent childhood obesity: outcomes of the NOURISH RCT at 14 months of age and 6 months post the first of two intervention modules — 276

Growth during Infancy and Childhood, and Adiposity at Age 16 Years: Ages 2 to 7 Years Are Pivotal — 277

Hyperthyrotropinaemia in untreated subjects with Down's syndrome aged 6 months to 64 years: a comparative analysis — 279

Generic and Brand-Name L-Thyroxine Are Not Bioequivalent for Children With Severe Congenital Hypothyroidism — 280

Secondary Sexual Characteristics in Boys: Data From the Pediatric Research in Office Settings Network — 282

Random Luteinizing Hormone Often Remains Pubertal in Children Treated with the Histrelin Implant for Central Precocious Puberty — 284

Addition of recombinant follicle-stimulating hormone to human chorionic gonadotropin treatment in adolescents and young adults with hypogonadotropic hypogonadism promotes normal testicular growth and may promote early spermatogenesis — 285

Distinguishing Constitutional Delay of Growth and Puberty from Isolated Hypogonadotropic Hypogonadism: Critical Appraisal of Available Diagnostic Tests — 286

Author Index

A

Adami S, 200
Adams AL, 169
Akhavan A, 259
Al Ghuzlan A, 117
Al-Naimi A, 272
Al-Saleh S, 272
Alegakis D, 106
Alexander EK, 125
Alfonso H, 142
Alibhai SMH, 196
Almario RU, 244
Almeida MQ, 212
Amory JK, 242
Andersson C, 7
Anderwald C-H, 101
Antebi F, 279
Antonica F, 127
Appelbaum E, 160
Archer KJ, 252
Aronis KN, 34
Astrup A, 86
Avci HX, 134
Avenell A, 158
Azevedo MF, 212

B

Bakas P, 238
Balan K, 220
Baliram R, 144
Ballantyne CM, 45
Baloch ZW, 125
Barrett-Connor E, 227
Bartalena L, 110
Battistutta D, 276
Bays HE, 45
Beck Jensen J-E, 194
Benn M, 30
Benoît G, 131
Bergenstal RM, 9
Berglund ED, 18
Bernabé BP, 250
Beyene J, 196
Biggs ML, 3
Bischoff-Ferrari HA, 162
Boichard A, 117
Boonen S, 198
Bouilly J, 231, 266
Bulsara MK, 14
Burant CF, 20

Burton TJ, 220
Buse JB, 9

C

Cai Z, 13
Cairns R, 6
Canepa Escaro F, 49
Cao J, 144
Capizzi JA, 206
Carnethon MR, 3
Carré N, 231, 266
Carrelli A, 94
Carswell JM, 280
Casazza K, 86
Caterson ID, 7
Catteau-Jonard S, 235
Cerrone D, 108
Chabre O, 209
Chacón MR, 246
Chatonnet F, 131
Cherrington AD, 19
Cho GY, 93
Chomitz VR, 77
Chu AY, 91
Chubb SAP, 142
Clark EM, 180
Colao A, 263
Comerford KB, 244
Crawford S, 230
Croux L, 117
Cuchel M, 36
Cunha DA, 13
Cusano NE, 205

D

Daniels LA, 276
de Boer IH, 152
De Chavez PJD, 3
de Groot JC, 25
de Ruyter JC, 76
Dedeurwaerder S, 13
Dell RM, 169
Dempster DW, 185
Devi MG, 252
Di Florio C, 254
Dias CS, 39
Díaz M, 246
Doehner W, 6
Donaldson MG, 173

Dralle H, 114
Dufour R, 54

E

Ebbeling CB, 77
Eiken PA, 180
Ensrud KE, 173
Erdmann E, 6
Eugster EA, 284

F

Falkevall A, 21
Fassnacht M, 210, 217
Feelders RA, 213
Feldman HA, 77
Ferdaoussi M, 16
Festen DAM, 270
Fontaine KR, 86
Foster CR, 5
Foster-Schubert KE, 81
Fujii Y, 240
Fulghesu AM, 254

G

Gagel RF, 120
Gagne C, 54
Galdones E, 250
Gallagher JC, 164
Gallo C, 235
Gatta-Cherifi B, 209
Geller ML, 182
Georgiou V, 106
Giltay J, 236
Giuca MR, 274
Giuliani C, 108
Gómez-Santos C, 257
Goodyer WR, 17
Gordon JH, 280
Greenberg-Dotan S, 279
Greene DF, 169
Gregoriou O, 238
Grigoriadis C, 238
Grimaldi AS, 206
Grubbs EG, 215
Grynberg M, 232
Gu X, 17

Gudovic A, 123
Guyot R, 131

H

Hagberg CE, 21
Hahner S, 217
Hamer M, 84
Hamilton J, 272
Han JM, 113
Hanotin C, 52
Hansen S, 194
Harii N, 108
Harrington J, 286
Harris D, 282
Hauge EM, 194
Hayek S, 49
Herman-Giddens ME, 282
Hernández-Morante JJ, 257
Hirokawa K, 240
Hofland J, 213
Horlait S, 175
Horn S, 141
Huang A, 4
Huang F, 27
Huckabay S, 178

I

Ikizler TA, 64
Ilani N, 242
Imayama I, 81
Inzucchi SE, 9

J

Javid M, 265
Jeon MJ, 113
Johnston RJ, 14

K

Kaaks R, 154
Kaltsas G, 221
Kang JH, 91
Karakosta P, 106
Karras D, 189
Kasprzyk DF, 127
Kastelein JJ, 45
Katz DJ, 259

Kaufman J-M, 198
Kaur S, 252
Kebede M, 16
Kelly HW, 273
Kennedy GC, 125
Kersseboom S, 141
Khan MS, 264
Khan SM, 34
Kim K, 244
Kim SH, 93
Kirkwood A, 264
Kreissl MC, 217

L

Lazovic G, 123
Lebrun C, 134
Lee SK, 93
Lee Y, 18
Leibiger B, 15
Leifke E, 26
Lemos MC, 265
Lems WF, 189
Levin G, 152
Lewiecki EM, 182
Lewis KA, 284
Li K, 154
Li Y, 13
Liem ET, 277
Linseisen J, 154
Liu Y, 17
López-Bermejo A, 246
Lyons DJ, 138

M

Ma J, 82
MacFadyen JG, 23
Machens A, 114
Mackenzie IS, 220
Maharaj A, 27
Maiburg M, 236
Mallan KM, 276
Mancini A, 16
Mantzoros CS, 34
Marcinak J, 20
Mason C, 81
Masud T, 158
Mayerl S, 141
McClung MR, 182
McKenney JM, 52
McMahon DJ, 205
Medici M, 122

Mehlem A, 21
Meier RPH, 166
Melhus H, 156
Meyerovitch J, 279
Michaëlsson K, 156
Mittag J, 138
Moede T, 15
Molinolo AA, 119
Møller UK, 171
Morin-Papunen L, 248
Morris AP, 12
Morton J, 32
Mosekilde L, 171
Moskovic DJ, 259
Muhandiramlage TP, 15
Mulatero P, 218
Murat A, 209
Murthy VL, 5
Mutharasan P, 250

N

Naik H, 26
Nair VV, 285
Naya M, 5

O

Okuzumi A, 71
Olthof MR, 76
Opitz R, 127
Orav EJ, 162

P

Palermo L, 173, 191
Palmert MR, 286
Papanastasiou L, 221
Pappa T, 221
Park JW, 113, 116
Parker BA, 206
Pasini M, 274
Paulides M, 100
Pazianas M, 180
Perneger TV, 166
Perrier ND, 215
Pierre A, 232
Popovsky E, 280
Pradhan A, 23
Prasad A, 25
Premaor M, 187

Pritchett Y, 160
Promintzer-Schifferl M, 101
Purnell JQ, 96

Q

Qi Q, 91
Qin J, 13

R

Rakhshandehroo M, 79
Rantala AS, 248
Recker RR, 185
Reginster J-Y, 198
Rejnmark L, 158
Repping S, 236
Rey R, 232
Ridker PM, 23
Ringe JD, 175
Riwanto M, 67
Robin G, 235
Robinson BG, 120
Robinson-Cohen C, 152
Rohrer L, 67
Romualdi D, 254
Roschitzki B, 67
Roth EM, 52
Roth MY, 242
Rubin MR, 205

S

Sabin MA, 285
Sai A, 164
Salerno P, 119
Sällström J, 138
Sattar A, 49
Sauer PJJ, 277
Schafer AL, 191
Schipper HS, 79
Seidell JC, 76
Sellmeyer DE, 191
Shaywitz AJ, 39
Shimada Y, 71
Siafarikas A, 14
Siemensma EPC, 270
Slatkovska L, 196
Sonigo C, 231, 266

Spremovic-Radjenovic S,
    123
Stamatakis E, 84
Steffes J, 282
Stein EA, 54
Stein EM, 94
Stern R, 166
Stevens GA, 89
Sun L, 144

T

Takeuchi K, 22
Tamburrino A, 119
Taniguchi T, 240
Tauber P, 218
Tébar FJ, 257
Tecco S, 274
Teeuwisse WM, 100
Templin T II, 164
Tepper PG, 230
Thadhani R, 160
Thomas T, 175
Thumbigere-Math V, 178
Timmermans S, 122
Tsigani T, 264
Tsujihata Y, 22
Tu L, 178
Tummers-de Lind van
    Wijngaarden RFA,
    270
Tura A, 101
Tybjærg-Hansen A, 30

U

Ueno Y, 71
Unger RH, 19
Unkila-Kallio L, 248

V

van Buuren S, 277
van de Graaf SFJ, 79
van der Wal R, 213
van Gaal L, 7
Varbo A, 30
við Streym S, 171
Visser W, 122

Viswanathan P, 20
Volkmar M, 13

W

Walls GV, 265
Walsh JB, 189
Wang H, 98
Wang M-Y, 18
Warensjö Lemming E, 156
Wasserman SM, 39
Wehrlé R, 134
Weidner C, 25
Wells SA Jr, 120
Widya RL, 100
Wildman RP, 230
Willett WC, 162
Wu J, 26

X

Xekouki P, 212
Xiao L, 82

Y

Yamamoto S, 64
Yan C, 4
Yancey PG, 64
Yang Y-M, 4
Yank V, 82
Yashiro H, 22
Yeap BB, 142
Young P, 94

Z

Zacharin M, 285
Zennaro MC, 218
Zhang HM, 215
Zhang W, 98
Zhang X, 98
Zhao L, 116
Zhou H, 185
Zhu L, 27
Zhu X, 116

Printed and bound by CPI Group (UK) Ltd, Croydon, CR0 4YY

08/05/2025

01864755-0007